Histopathological Diagnosis of Leprosy

Authored by

Cleverson Teixeira Soares

Laboratory of Anatomic Pathology
Instituto Lauro de Souza Lima (ILSL) and
Institute of Pathology of Bauru (ANATOMED) Bauru
Brazil

Histopathological Diagnosis of Leprosy

Author: Cleverson Teixeira Soares

ISBN (Online): 978-1-68108-799-3

ISBN (Print): 978-1-68108-800-6

ISBN (Paperback): 978-1-68108-801-3

need for a court order if at any point you breach any terms of this License Agreement. In no event will any delay or failure by Bentham Science Publishers in enforcing your compliance with this License Agreement constitute a waiver of any of its rights.

3. You acknowledge that you have read this License Agreement, and agree to be bound by its terms and conditions. To the extent that any other terms and conditions presented on any website of Bentham Science Publishers conflict with, or are inconsistent with, the terms and conditions set out in this License Agreement, you acknowledge that the terms and conditions set out in this License Agreement shall prevail.

Bentham Science Publishers Ltd.
Executive Suite Y - 2
PO Box 7917, Saif Zone
Sharjah, U.A.E.
Email: subscriptions@benthamscience.net

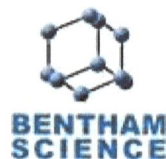

BENTHAM SCIENCE

CONTENTS

FOREWORD

I am pleased to present *Histopathological Diagnosis of Leprosy,* a book that focuses on medical pathology. It is a unique and special book that transcends the field and will certainly fill an important knowledge gap concerning the pathology of leprosy. This compendium of unique utility is written by Cleverson Teixeira Soares, a pathologist with extensive experience in subjects related to leprosy, who gained his educational expertise from the Hansenology School at the Lauro Souza Lima Institute (ILSL), Bauru, São Paulo, Brazil; a prestigious and prolific Brazilian Institute and the birthplace of brilliant hansenologists and pathologists, such as Professor Raul Negrão Fleury (*in memoriam*). This work continues his valuable legacy, as is much desired by surgical pathologists, dermatopathologists, medical students, and several professionals who clinically manage leprosy.

This book combines the author's extensive experience of the pathology of leprosy with an exhaustive effort to explain all the complex histopathological presentations of leprosy in a direct and simple manner. The book consists of eight chapters, with 214 figures in the form of panels containing 1,069 clinical and histopathological photographs. Additionally, it has an excellent microscopic record correlated with clinical and pathological findings and presented with all possible differential diagnoses for each leprosy type and its reaction phenomena; thereby, expanding the scope and utility of this subject.

I am convinced that this book will greatly help professionals who manage leprosy, a complex and clinically challenging disease.

Further, I am grateful on behalf of several individuals, especially pathologists and patients, who may benefit from the important knowledge mentioned and illustrated in this book.

José Fillus Neto
Dermatopathologist
Curitiba, Paraná
Brazil

PREFACE

Leprosy remains one of the biggest public health problems in many countries. It is a complex disease in several aspects, including clinical, histopathological, and molecular. This book is written to help different professionals (medical students, physicians, pathologists, researchers, and others) who handle this disease daily or are interested in it to understand the disease from the perspective of pathology. The histopathological characteristics of leprosy throughout its spectrum, reaction phenomena, and clinical presentation types are crucial for understanding the pathophysiology of the disease and guiding clinical conduct and research accordingly.

The book is organized into eight sequential chapters that allow the readers to gradually immerse themself in different histopathological aspects of leprosy. The clinical features discussed are accompanied by corresponding histopathological images presented as photo panels, along with key points that assist in understanding the described characteristics. Common histological sections stained by hematoxylin-eosin are complemented with those stained by Fite–Faraco to identify the different types of cells or tissues parasitized by *Mycobacterium leprae*. Immunohistochemical findings are used to clearly illustrate some characteristics observed in common histological sections. In some cases, more than one staining technique was used for the same histological section (for example, immunohistochemistry and Fite–Faraco), thereby contributing to a better understanding of the histopathological characteristics of the disease.

The interpretation of the histopathological characteristics of leprosy lesions is somewhat challenging. Each diagnosis depends on the close correlation between the findings of histopathology, bacilloscopy examination, and clinical data. In this context, histopathology is of great importance to confirm or dismiss a certain hypothesis and can guide teams to accurately interpret data and choose the best clinical and therapeutic conduct.

This book is intended to be a supplement to the leprosy literature found in journals and textbooks, offering the readers a background on leprosy-related histopathology that can improve their understanding of this disease.

Finally, I express deep gratitude toward the different support teams of the Lauro de Souza Lima Institute, especially that of the Laboratory of Anatomic Pathology, which contributed decisively to the conclusion of this book and to Dr. Cássio C. Ghidella for the numerous clinical photos that illustrate all chapters.

Cleverson Teixeira Soares
Laboratory of Anatomic Pathology
Instituto Lauro de Souza Lima (ILSL) and
Institute of Pathology of Bauru (ANATOMED) Bauru
Brazil

ACKNOWLEDGEMENTS

The whole endeavor of writing a book on the histopathology of leprosy was exhausting yet rewarding. Attempting to write all the chapters in a logical sequence of a disease complex and with different clinical-pathological presentations is challenging. Selecting the samples to be photographed and choosing those with greater representation on certain aspects of the disease were carried throughout a daily routine. For many years, writing, proofreading, and photographing were all executed after the daily routine of surgical pathology. All of these could not be done without the unconditional support and understanding of my family, Themis, Juliana, and Rafael. Numerous slides were made and added, especially for stains using different histochemical and immunohistochemical techniques. All of these are made possible by the exemplary dedication and excellent quality of the technical team of the Laboratory of Anatomic Pathology of the Instituto Lauro de Souza Lima (ILSL) and the Institute of Pathology of Bauru (ANATOMED). Several photographs with various clinical presentations of the different forms and reaction processes of leprosy were obtained from the archives of the ILSL library. The archives' collection contains precious materials such as photos, articles, books, and various notes that depict the rich history of leprosy even before the era of antibiotics began (pre-sulfonic era). These were made available so that I could use them in the preparation of the book, for which I extend my gratitude to the entire ILSL technical staff. I have no way of describing how thankful I am to countless people for their help in creating this book. Finally, I would also like to extend my gratitude to (1) Dr. Raul Negrão Fleury (*in memoriam*), a pathologist with a profound knowledge of leprosy and the founder of the Laboratory of Anatomic Pathology of the ILSL and (2) Dr. Cássio C. Ghidella for the gratifying anatomical and clinical discussions and the excellent clinical photographs observed throughout the book.

CONSENT FOR PUBLICATION

Not applicable.

CONFLICT OF INTEREST

The author declares no conflict of interest, financial or otherwise.

Cleverson Teixeira Soares
Laboratory of Anatomic Pathology
Instituto Lauro de Souza Lima (ILSL) and
Institute of Pathology of Bauru (ANATOMED) Bauru
Brazil

DEDICATION

Dedicated to
To Themis, Juliana, Rafael,
and
Raul Negrão Fleury (in memoriam)

CHAPTER 1

Classification and General Aspects of Leprosy

Abstract: Leprosy is a chronic infectious disease whose etiological agent is *Mycobacterium leprae*. Recently, *Mycobacterium lepromatosis* is also implicated as a causative agent and has been identified in different forms of the disease. Leprosy is a complex disease from a clinical, histopathological, and molecular point of view. The wide diversity of clinical presentation and histopathological characteristics observed throughout the disease spectrum and reactions render it a challenging disease in clinical and pathological practice. This chapter discusses the main aspects of the disease and its histopathological classification. An important approach to the bacilloscopic examination, which is fundamental for the histopathological classification of the disease, showing its quantitative and qualitative aspects, is discussed. The various photographic panels demonstrate the bacillus' ability to parasitize different types of tissues and cells of the skin and other organs of the human body. Multiple serial histological sections stained using different techniques allow the main points addressed in the text to be better understood through histopathological images. The entire content of this initial chapter (Chapter 1) will be the basis for understanding the other chapters. In the subsequent chapters, the clinical, histopathological, and bacilloscopic features of leprosy forms (Chapters 2, 3, and 4), the reactional phenomena (T1R - Chapter 5 and T2R - Chapter 6), the regressive changes observed in leprosy lesions during and after treatment or relapse (Chapter 7), and some variants with special clinical characteristics (Chapter 8) are discussed.

Keywords: Bacilloscopy, Hansen´s disease, Histopathology, Leprosy, *Mycobacterium leprae*, *Mycobacterium lepromatosis*, Ridley and Jopling.

INTRODUCTION

Leprosy is a chronic infectious disease whose etiological agent is *Mycobacterium leprae* [1]. Recently, *Mycobacterium lepromatosisis* is also implicated as a causative agent and has been identified in different forms of the disease [2, 3]. In fact, in some leprosy lesion samples from the skin, both bacilli were detected [3]. Leprosy affects millions of people globally, with hundreds of thousands of new cases diagnosed each year [4]. It is a major public health concern in Asian, African, and South American countries [4]. *Mycobacterium leprae* exhibits tropism in the peripheral nervous system (neural cutaneous branches and neural trunks in their more distal and superficial locations), and therefore, leprosy is initially a predominantly neural disease. As a strictly intracellular parasite, its elimination depends on cell-mediated immunity [1]. The ability of the host to produce an effective immunocellular reaction against *M. leprae* varies among individuals in a population. In endemic countries, it is estimated that 90% or more of the individuals infected with *M. leprae* develop a chronic granulomatous inflammatory reaction of a tuberculoid pattern, restricting the disease to one or a few cutaneous neural lesions that evolve spontaneously (tuberculoid pole) [1, 5]. However, some infected individuals fail to develop an effective immunocellular reaction, possibly due to the inadequate ability of their macrophages to destroy *M. leprae* and process the bacterial antigens [1, 5]. In this situation, phagocytosis of the bacilli by macrophages occurs, yet restriction of their proliferation and dissemination is ineffective. Thus, with the evolution of the disease, cutaneous neural lesions may be extensive and associated with compromised mucosae of the upper respiratory tract, lymph nodes, viscera (liver, spleen, kidneys, adrenals, *etc.*), eyeballs, testes, epididymides, synovial membranes, and bone marrow, among other tissues and organs (lepromatous pole) [1, 5].

The biological behavior of these polar forms of leprosy (tuberculoid and lepromatous) is antagonistic. They are stable manifestations of the disease, and there is likely no transformation from one form to another in its evolution, even after treatment [5]. Between these two stable poles, there is the dimorphous or borderline group, in which cutaneous neural lesions show intermediate characteristics between the two poles, suggesting partial immunity to *M. leprae*. The borderline group is unstable. That is, in the absence of treatment, these individuals tend to exhibit clinical, bacilloscopic, and histopathological characteristics shifted toward the lepromatous pole [5]. On the other hand, when treated, these patients may exhibit progression toward the tuberculoid pole of the disease spectrum [1, 5, 6] (Fig. **1**).

Aspects of the classification of leprosy will be discussed in this chapter. Furthermore, the important points of the bacilloscopic examination will be presented as these are crucial for the clinico-pathological classification of the disease. Likewise, its reaction phenomena will also be discussed in detail in the subsequent chapters.

CLASSIFICATION OF LEPROSY AND ITS REACTIONS

The South American classification for leprosy, officialized at the Congress of Madrid (1953), defines leprosy as a spectral disease, with polar forms, designated as tuberculoid (TT) and lepromatous (LL), and an intermediate or dimorphic group [7, 8]. Ridley and Jopling (R&J) subdivided the intermediate group into three subgroups—borderline-tuberculoid (BT), borderline-borderline (BB), and borderline-lepromatous (BL), establishing clinical, bacillary (0 to 6+), and histopathological variables for this classification [9]. In addition, they introduced the concepts of "downgrading," which is the evolutionary worsening toward the lepromatous pole, and "upgrading," in which there is an evolutionary improvement toward the tuberculoid pole [9] (Fig. **1**).

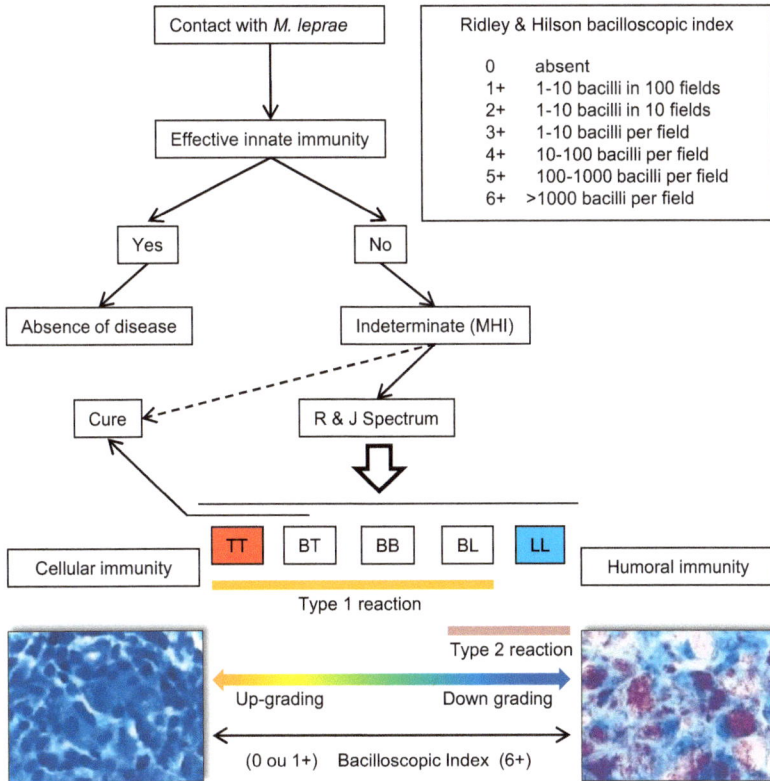

Fig. (1). Clinical spectrum and bacilloscopic index of leprosy forms and reactions. Patients who are exposed to *M. leprae* can eliminate the bacilli through the mechanisms of the primary immune response and do not develop the disease. If the primary immune defense cannot contain the proliferation of the bacilli, the patient develops indeterminate leprosy ("I"), the early stage of the disease preceding the polarized forms of the Ridley and Jopling (R&J) classification: tuberculoid (TT); borderline-tuberculoid (BT); borderline-borderline (BB); borderline-lepromatous (BL); and lepromatous or virchowian (LL). Late recognition of bacillary antigens by the individual may result in an intense and effective immune response (TT and BT pattern), which may lead to the destruction of the bacilli and spontaneous cure. TT individuals are those who have effective cellular immunity. If cellular immunity is not effective, the proliferation and dissemination of the bacilli persist, and the disease progresses toward the lepromatous pole. LL individuals are anergic and react to the bacilli through humoral immunity. Type 1 reactions (T1R) affect patients in the range from TT to BL. Type 2 reactions (T2R) affect patients on the lepromatous side (BL and LL). The bacilloscopic index ranges from 0 to 6+. The figure is partially adapted from Boggild *et al.* [21].

The low antigenicity of *M. leprae* may contribute to a delay in antigen recognition by the host immune system. Thus, in the first phase of the disease, while the amount of bacillary antigens in the tissues is not sufficient to trigger an immunocellular reaction, some parasitized cutaneous areas present discrete foci of non-granulomatous inflammatory infiltrate, predominantly composed of lymphocytes and macrophages selectively following or penetrating neural branches (neurocentric). At this early stage, leprosy is classified as indeterminate (I), as it precedes the clinicopathological conditions established in the R&J classification [1, 5] (Figs. **1** and **2**).

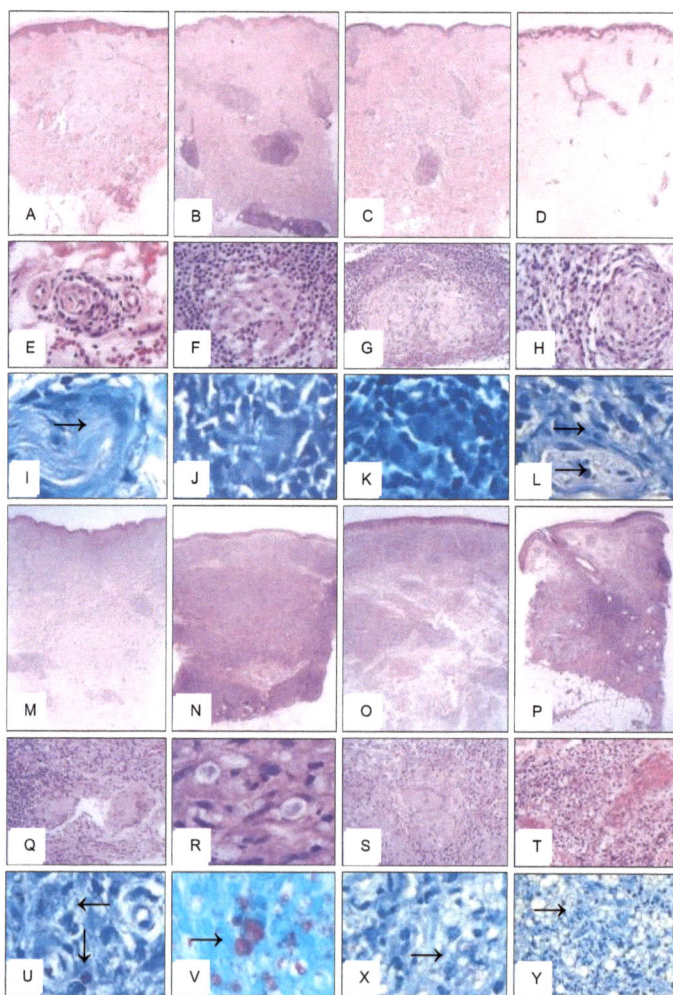

Fig. (2). Histopathological and bacilloscopic characteristics (→) common to clinical forms and leprosy reactions. "I" - (A, E, and I); "TT" - (B, F, and J); "BT" - (C, G, and K); "BB" - (D, H, and L); "BL" - (M, Q, and U); "LL" - (N, R, and V); "T1R" - (O, S, and X); and "T2R" - (P, T, and Y). HE (A-H, and M-T) and F-F (I-L, and U-Y) staining.

The progression of leprosy lesions occurs slowly, for years or decades, sometimes with few inflammatory signs in the lesions. Nerve involvement is also slow, with granulomas progressively accumulating, allowing endoneural structures to adhere to the immune response [6]. Functional changes are only noticed after a long duration of evolution. This behavior is likely due to the low antigenicity of *M. leprae*, stimulating a mild immune reaction without destructive alteration of the parasitized tissues. However, more intense and destructive inflammatory episodes, abrupt and occurring in cutaneous neural lesions or in any parasitized tissue, may arise during the course of the disease. These episodes are known as leprosy reactions [1, 5, 6]. There are two basic types of reactions in leprosy. One occurs in patients with varying degrees of preservation of the specific cellular immunity against *M. leprae*, known as the type 1 (T1R) reaction, and the other occurs in patients with poorly preserved or absent cellular immunity, known as type 2 (T2R) and corresponding to erythema nodosum leprosum (ENL) and its variants [1, 5, 6] (Figs. **1** and **2**).

BACILLOSCOPY

Identification of *M. leprae* in histological sections is generally performed using Fite-Faraco (F-F) or Wade-Fite stain [10 - 12]. F-F staining is a modification of the Ziehl-Neelsen (Z-N) method but yields superior results [10, 11]. The bacilli identified by F-F may not stain with Z-N, especially those that are fragmented, causing a decrease in the bacilloscopic index. Consequently, reduction in the bacilloscopic index and the non-identification of bacilli in the different types of parasitized tissues or cells may hinder or compromise both the bacilloscopic evaluation and lesion classification [10, 11] (Fig. **3**). The incomplete bacillus staining by the classical Z-N technique is probably due to the use of xylol, causing excessive removal of the fat from the bacillus cell wall, an important factor for its coloration. The re-fattening of the bacilli through the use of mineral oil or other oily substances allows the recovery of the staining properties of the bacilli [10, 11]. Like other mycobacteria, *M. leprae* is also stained by methenamine silver (Grocott) and, weakly, by Schiff's periodic acid (PAS) [13, 14] (Fig. **4**).

Bacilloscopic Index (BI)

The bacterial index commonly used for classification of leprosy lesions consists of a logarithmic scale proposed by Ridley and Hilson, ranging from 0 to 6+ [15]. The quantification is performed with an oil immersion objective (×100) as follows: (zero) absence of bacilli; (1+) 1–10 bacilli in 100 fields; (2+) 1–10 bacilli in 10 fields; (3+) 1–10 bacilli per field; (4+) 10–100 bacilli per field; (5+) 100–1,000 bacilli per field; and (6+) >1,000 bacilli per field (Fig. **1**).

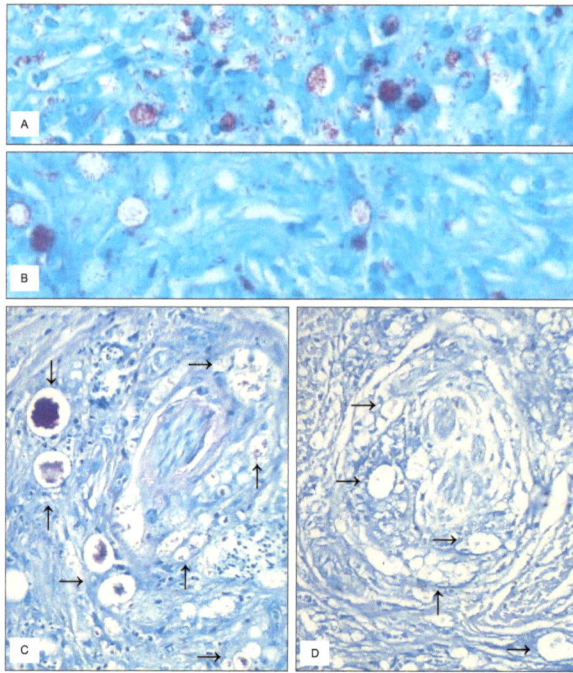

Fig. (3). Identification of *M. leprae* by Fite-Faraco (F-F) (A and C) and Ziehl-Neelsen (Z-N) (B and D) stains. Histological sections of **(A)** and **(B)** are from the same sample of active LL lesion. Those of **(C)** and **(D)** are of the same sample of LL lesion in regression after treatment. Note that in the active lesions, the staining of the bacilli (*M. leprae*) is strong with a large number of bacilli identified by F-F **(A)**, but there is a decrease in detection of bacilli when stained by Z-N **(B)**. In the regression lesions, where the bacilli are fragmented, the F-F technique identifies numerous faintly stained, fragmented bacilli (→) **(C)**, whereas the Z-N technique results in practically uncolored fragmented bacilli (→) **(D)**.

Qualitative Aspects of Bacilloscopy

In addition to quantification of the bacilli, the pathologist should assess the presence of the bacilli in granulomas and different tissues of the skin, nerve, or organ samples. *M. leprae* is an obligate intracellular parasite and can parasitize different types of cells and tissues. The presence of bacilli in macrophages, neural branches, endothelium of blood and lymphatic vessels, and smooth muscle cells of vessel walls and hair erector muscles is common in patients on the lepromatous side (BL and LL) (Figs. **5 – 9**). Less commonly, but not infrequently, *M. leprae* is observed within myoepithelial and epithelial cells of sweat glands, squamous epithelial cells of the epidermis and pilosebaceous follicle, nevus cells in the basal layer of the epidermis, mesenchymal cells of the dermis, and subcutaneous tissue (Figs. **10 – 16**). In lepromatous (LL) patients, there is intense parasitism of almost the entire skin in addition to the nasal and buccal mucosa (Fig. **17**). In autopsies of leprosy patients on the lepromatous side (BL and LL), bacilli were identified in many of the organs [6] (Fig. **18**). In our experience, we have also observed bacilli parasitizing neoplastic cells of neurofibroma, schwannoma, common melanocytic nevus, and even basal cell carcinoma (Figs. **19** and **20**). The presence of morphologically solid bacilli, or the persistence of fragmented bacilli in leprosy lesions and the different parasitized tissues is important for evaluating the effectiveness of treatment as well as disease relapse (Fig. **21**). These characteristics are discussed in detail in Chapter 8, which describes the clinical characteristics and histopathological changes observed before and after treatment initiation.

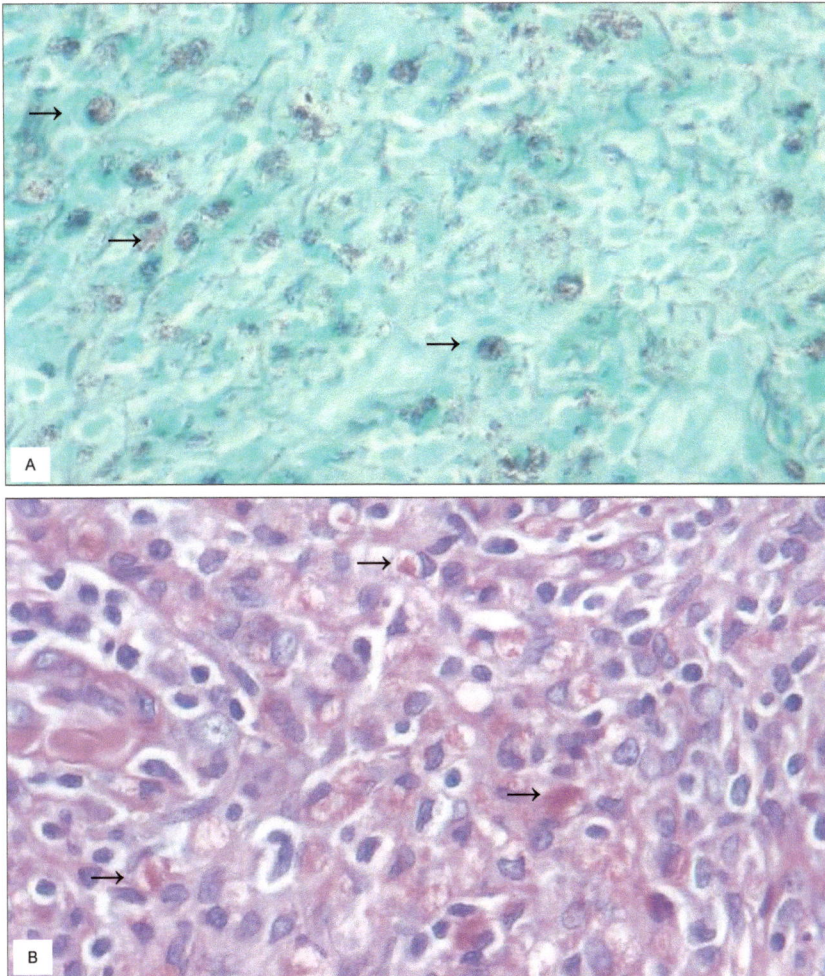

Fig. (4). *leprae* stained by the methenamine silver (Grocott) **(A)** and, weakly, by the periodic acid-Schiff (PAS) **(B)** techniques.

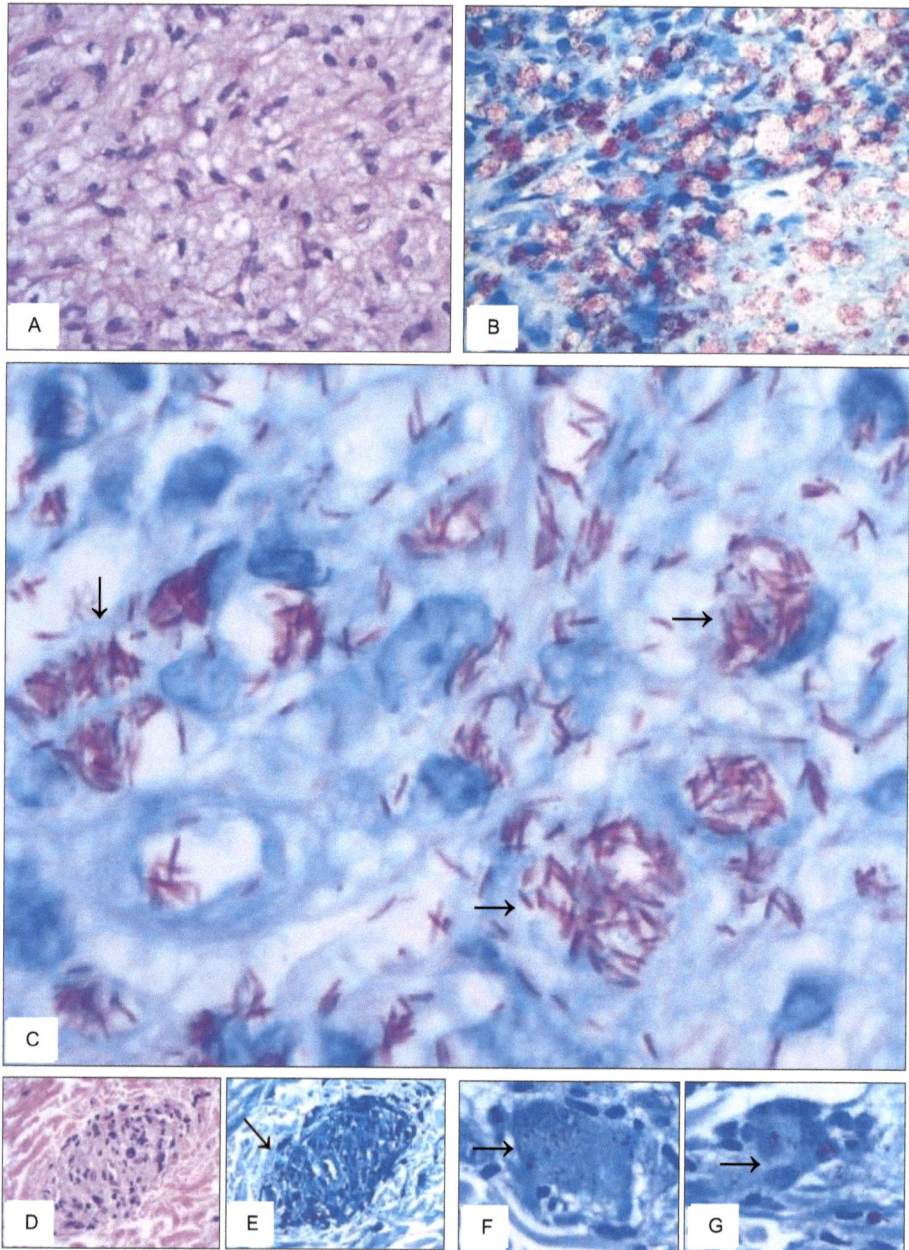

Fig. (5). *M. leprae* parasitizing macrophages (→). LL patient skin lesion with multivacuolated macrophages containing a large number of bacilli (A and B). In detail, the vacuoles filled by the bacilli **(C)**. Macrophage parasitism also occurs in epithelioid macrophages and in multinucleated giant cells. HE staining (A and D). F-F staining (B, C, E, F, and G).

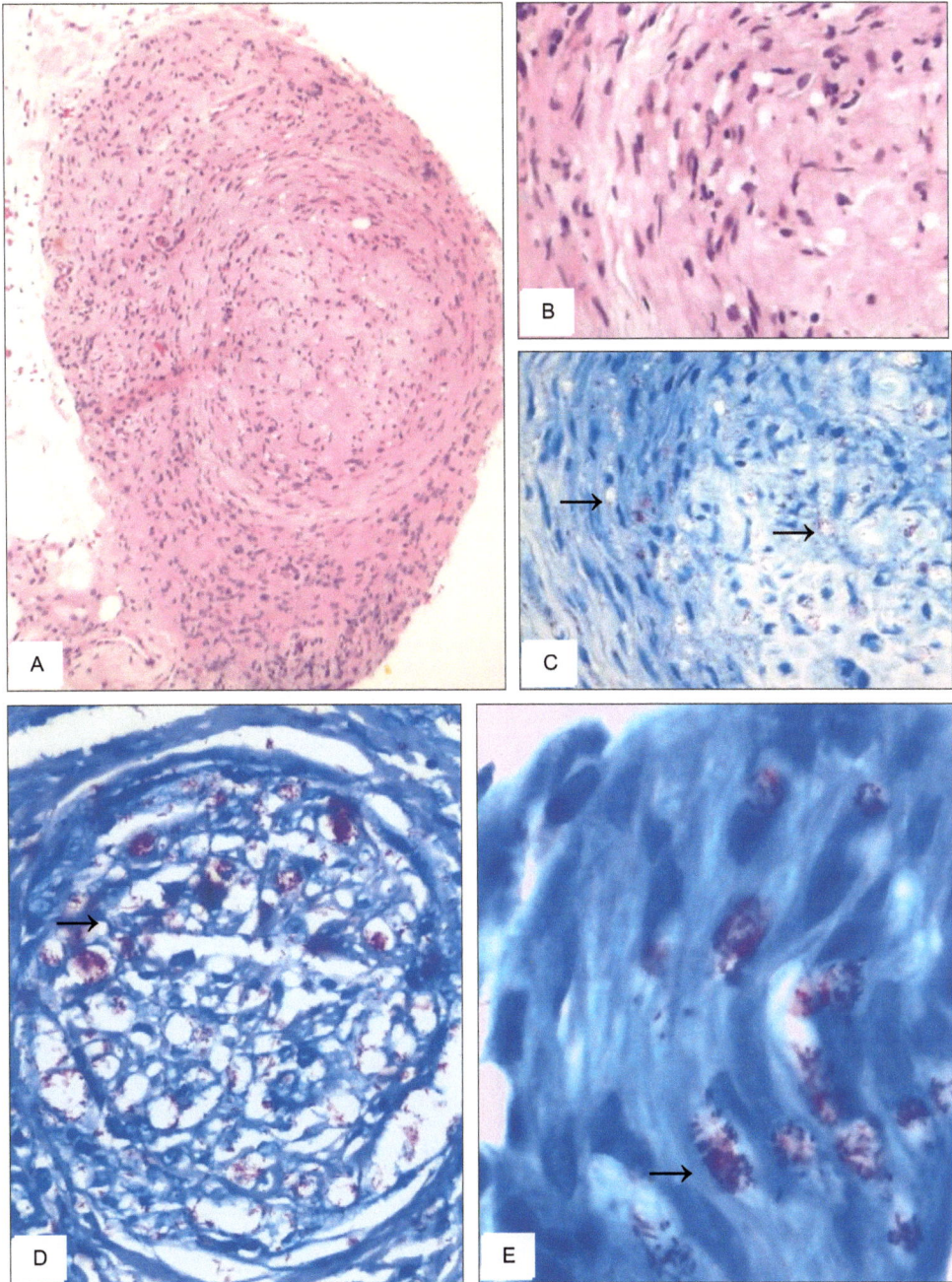

Fig. (6). *M. leprae* parasitizing neural branches (→). Nerve with peri- and intraneural inflammatory processes containing a large number of bacilli in all neural components (A, B, and C). Transverse **(D)** and longitudinal **(E)** sections of the neural branch with Schwann cells presenting intracytoplasmic vacuoles containing a large number of bacilli. HE staining (A and B). F-F staining (C, D, and E).

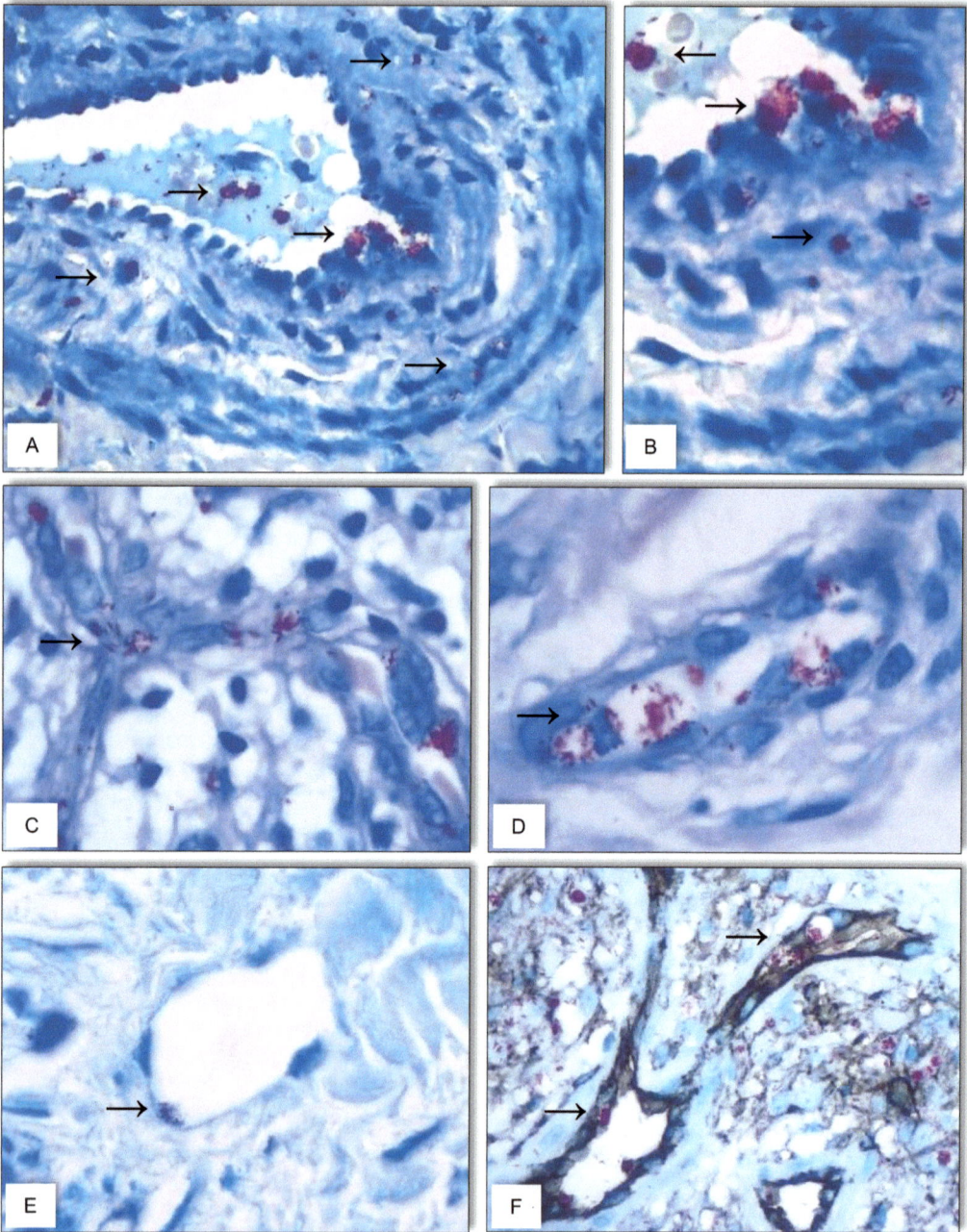

Fig. (7). *M. leprae* parasitizing vessels (→) (F-F). Presence of bacilli inside the blood vessel and parasitizing the endothelium and vessel wall (A and B). Capillary with intense parasitism of the endothelial cells throughout its path (C and D). Endothelial cells from lymphatic vessels parasitized by bacilli **(E)**. Double staining (F-F and anti-CD34) showing endothelial cells with vacuoles containing bacilli **(F)**.

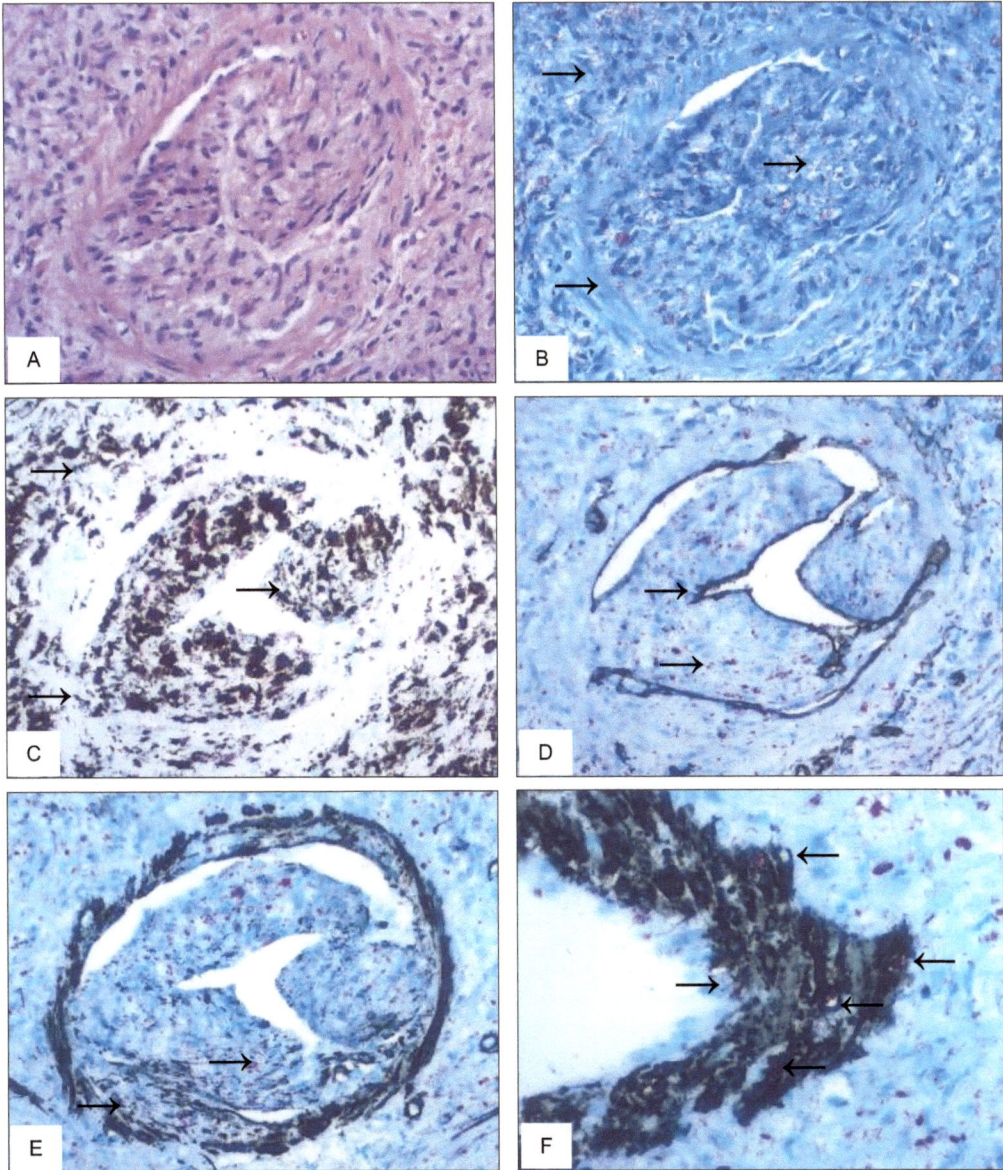

Fig. (8). *M. leprae* parasitizing vessels (→). HE staining vein presenting histiocytic infiltrate permeating the muscular wall and subintimal tissue **(A)**. F-F staining shows intense parasitism by *M. leprae* throughout the thickness of the vessel wall, the subintimal space, and the endothelium **(B)**. Double staining (anti-CD68 and F-F) demonstrates many bacilli-containing macrophages present in the perivascular, vessel wall, and subintimal tissues **(C)**. Double staining (anti-CD31 and F-F) showing endothelial proliferation and intense parasitism of subintimal cells and the vessel wall **(D)**. Double staining (anti-actin of smooth muscle-1A4 and F-F) showing intense parasitism of the vessel wall **(E)**. Double staining (anti-actin of smooth muscle-1A4 and F-F) showing smooth muscle cells parasitized by agglomerates of *M. leprae* bacilli in intracytoplasmic vacuoles **(F)**.

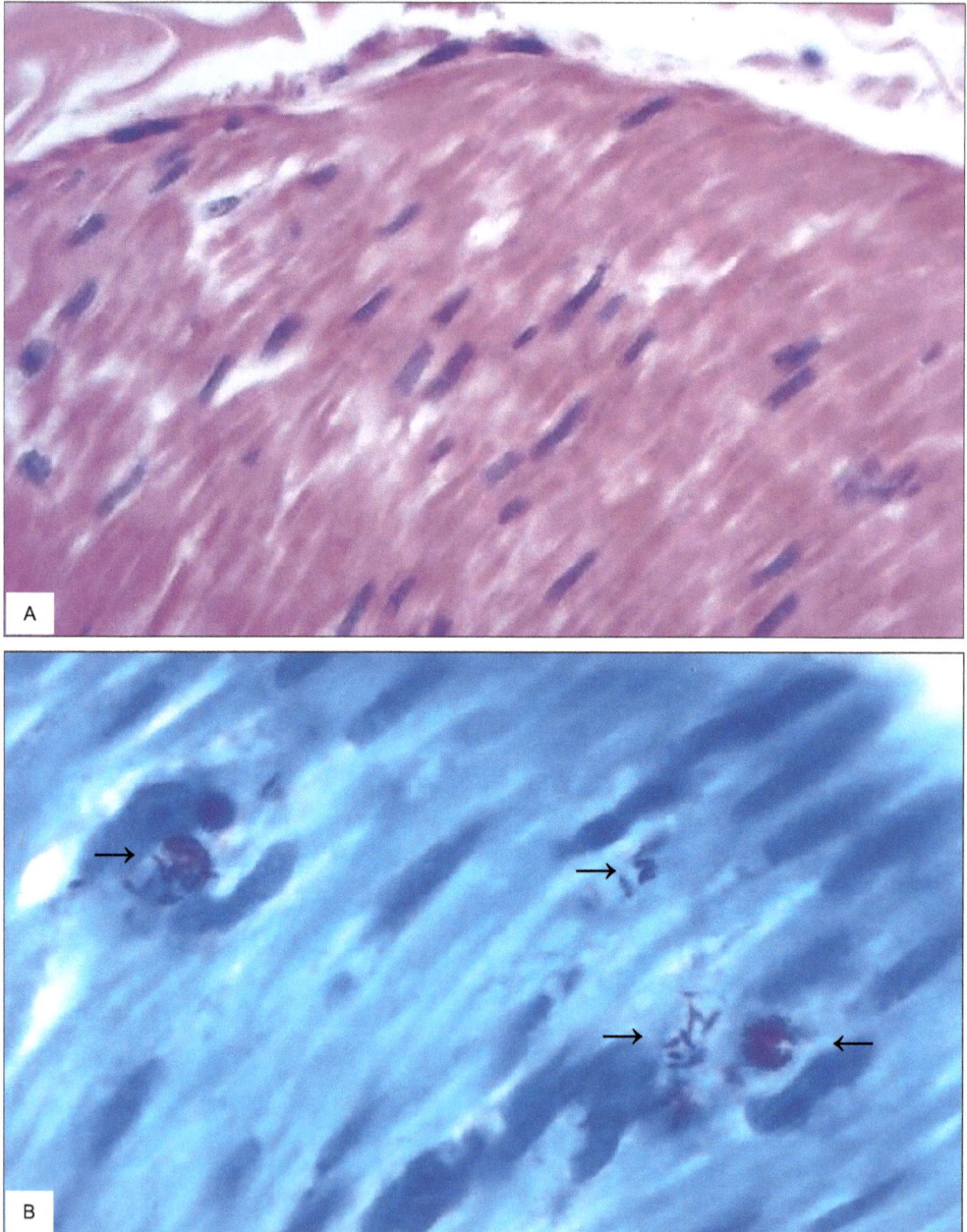

Fig. (9). *M. leprae* parasitizing the pili muscle (→). Smooth muscle cells of pili muscle without parasitism are observed in sections stained by HE **(A)**. In sequential sections stained with F-F, bacilli parasitizing the smooth muscle cells individually or intracytoplasmic vacuoles containing many bacilli are observed **(B)**.

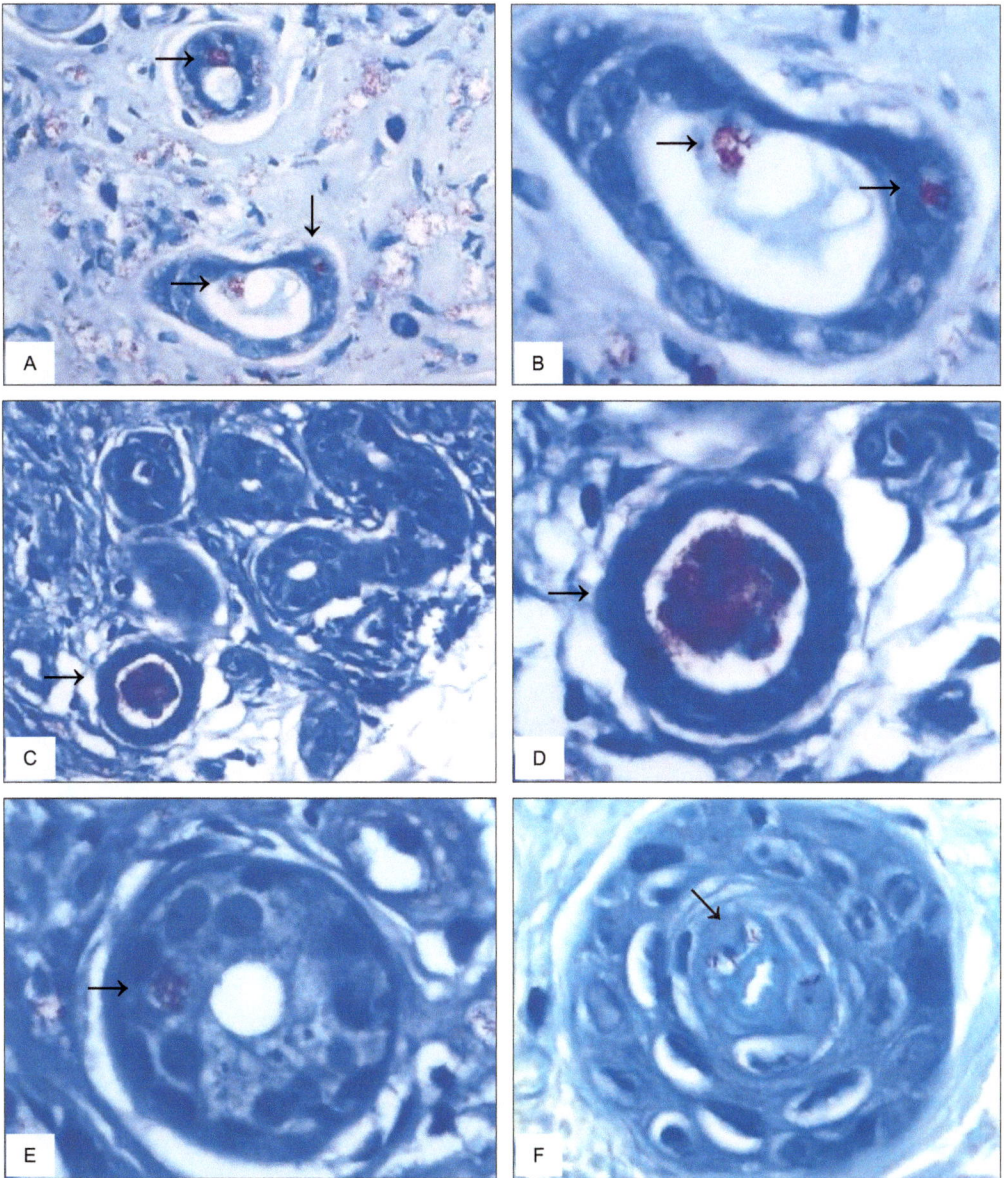

Fig. (10). *M. leprae* parasitizing eccrine glands (→). Parasitism of secretory epithelial cells and myoepithelial cells of the secretory portion of the sweat gland (A, B, C, D, and E). Intraluminal secretion with cells parasitized by *M. leprae* (B, C, and D). Parasitism of epithelial cells of the excretory component of the gland (**F**). F-F staining (A-F).

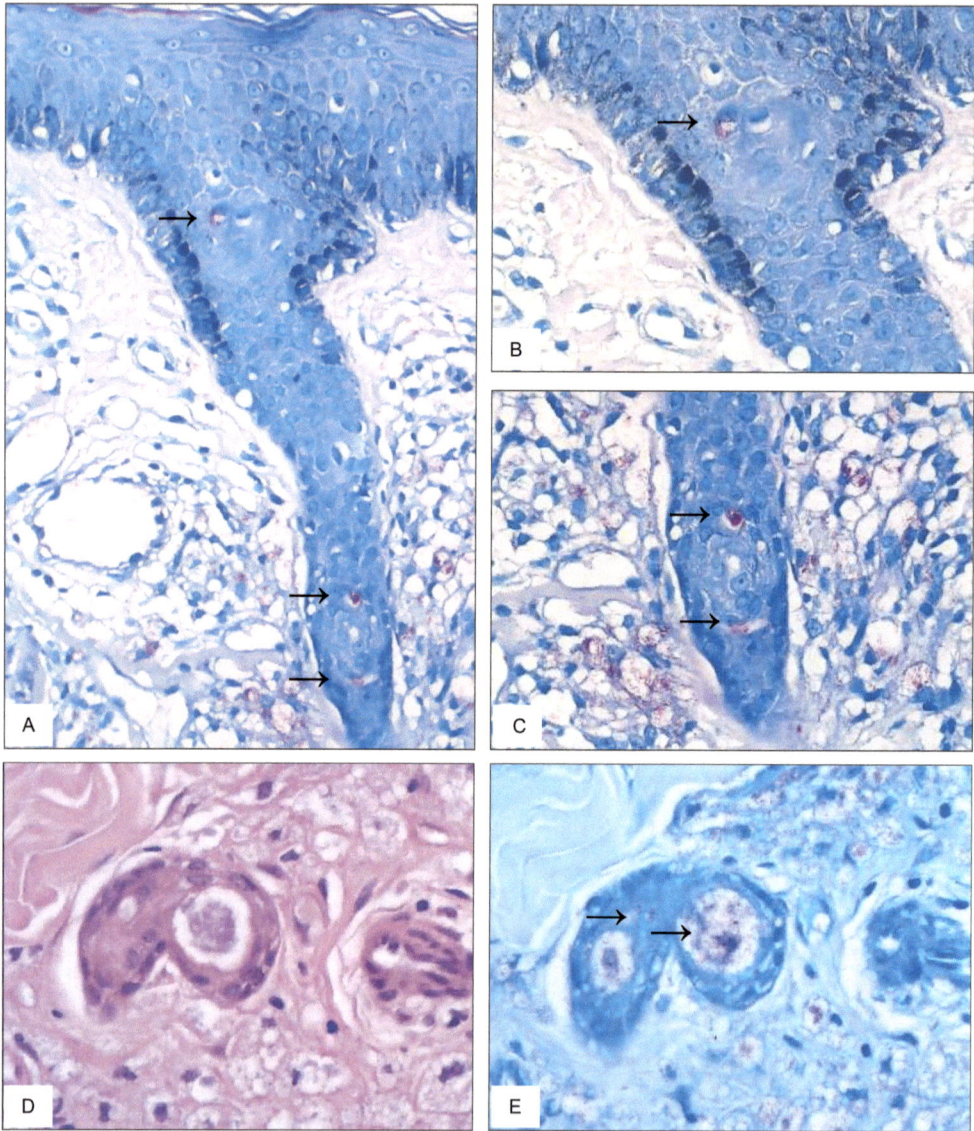

Fig. (11). *M. leprae* parasitizing eccrine glands (→). Parasitism of epithelial cells of the excretory component of eccrine glands (acrosyringium) (A, B, and C). Parasitism of epithelial cells of the secretory component of eccrine glands and intraluminal secretion containing a large amount of fragmented bacilli in a patient receiving treatment (D and E). F-F staining in **(A)**, **(B)**, **(C)**, and **(E)**. HE staining in **(D)**.

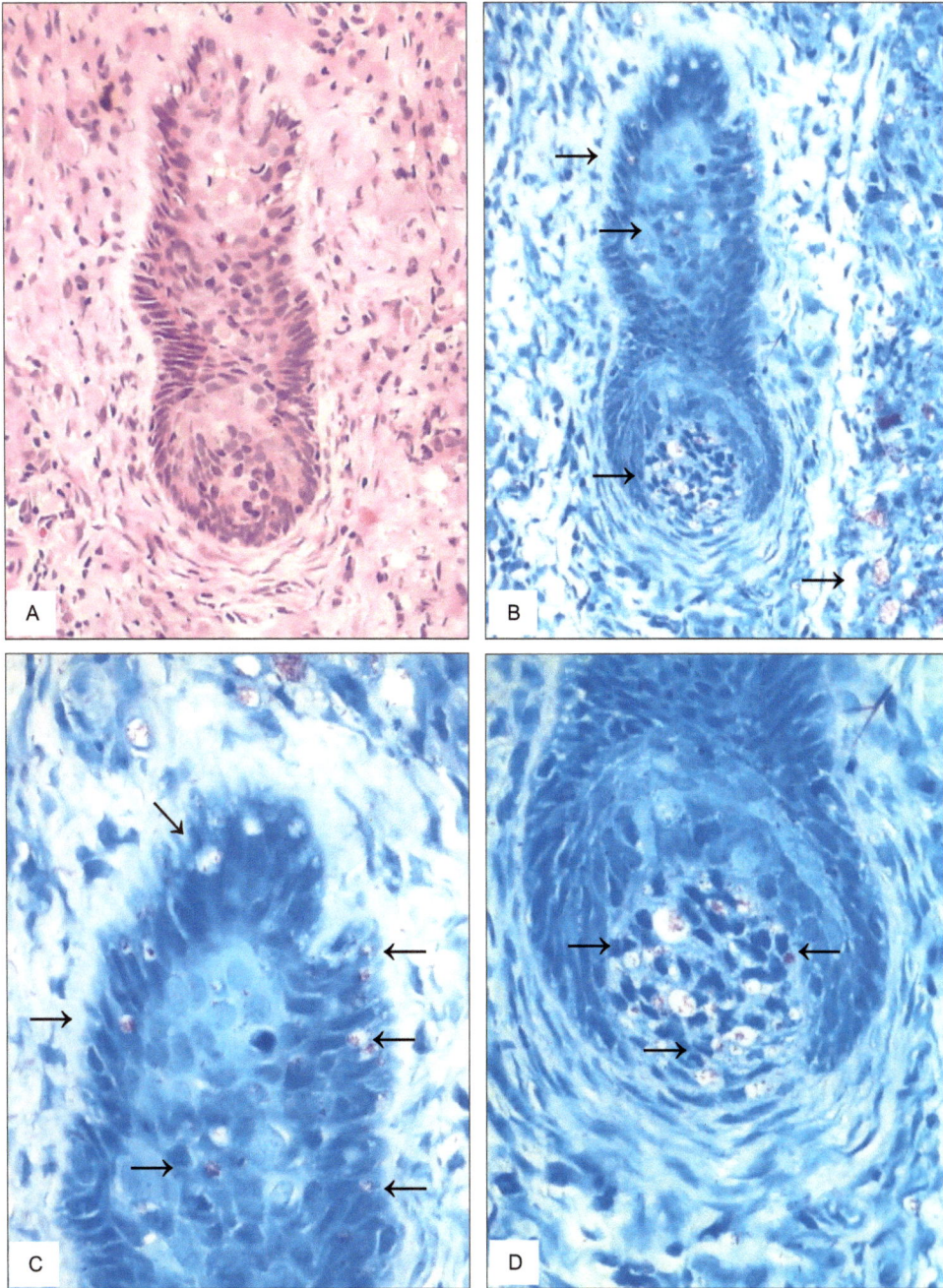

Fig. (12). *M. leprae* parasitizing a hair follicle (→). There is intense parasitism of squamous epithelial cells of the sheath and cells of the dermal papilla of the follicle (B and C). In tissues adjacent to the hair follicle, there is parasitism of macrophages and perifollicular tissues **(D)**. HE staining in **(A)**. F-F staining in **(B)**, **(C)**, and **(D)**.

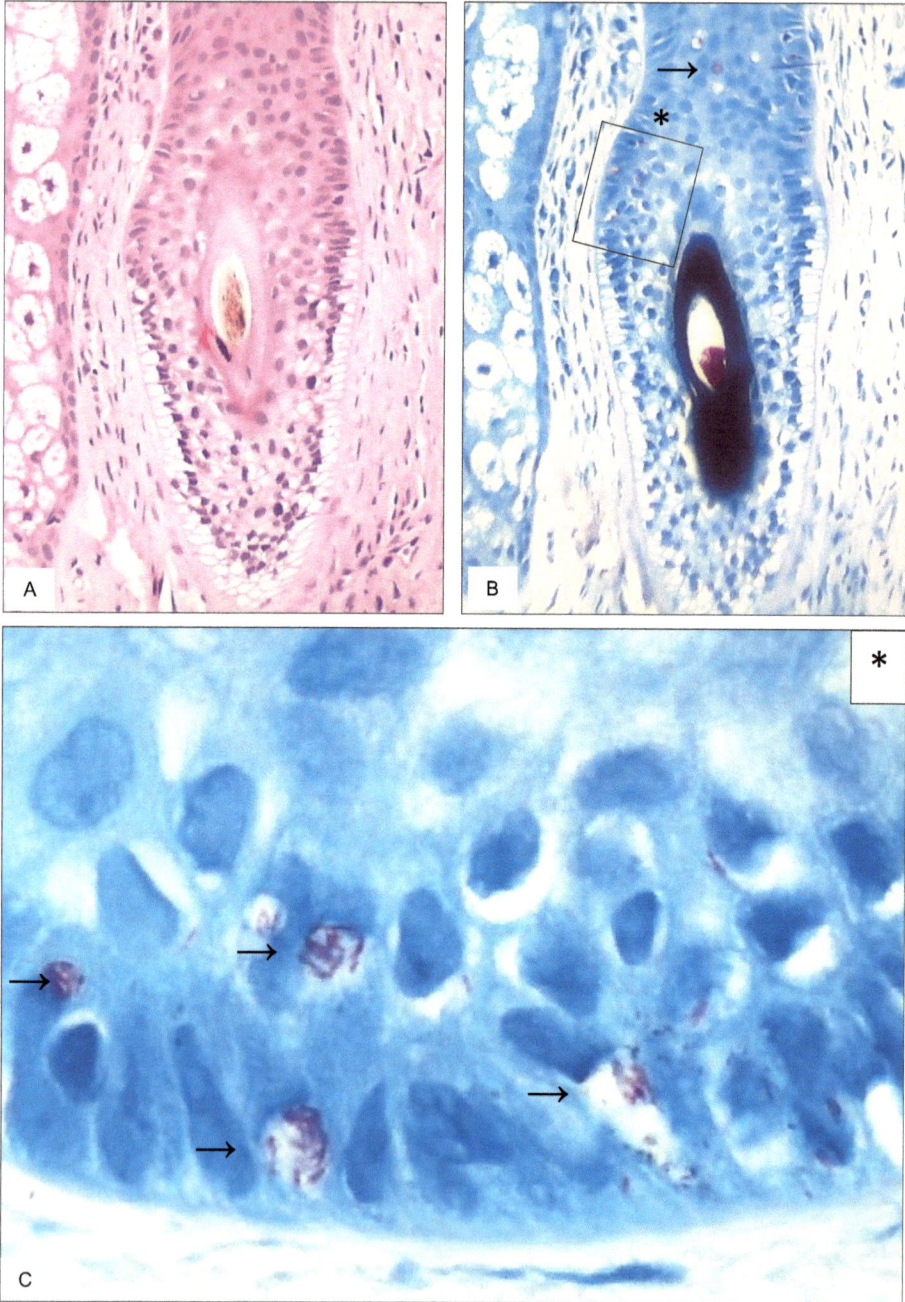

Fig. (13). *M. leprae* parasitizing a hair follicle (→). Pilosebaceous unit with intense parasitism of epithelial cells of the hair sheath **(B)** (*) and **(C)** (*). HE staining in **(A)**. F-F staining in **(B)** and **(C)**.

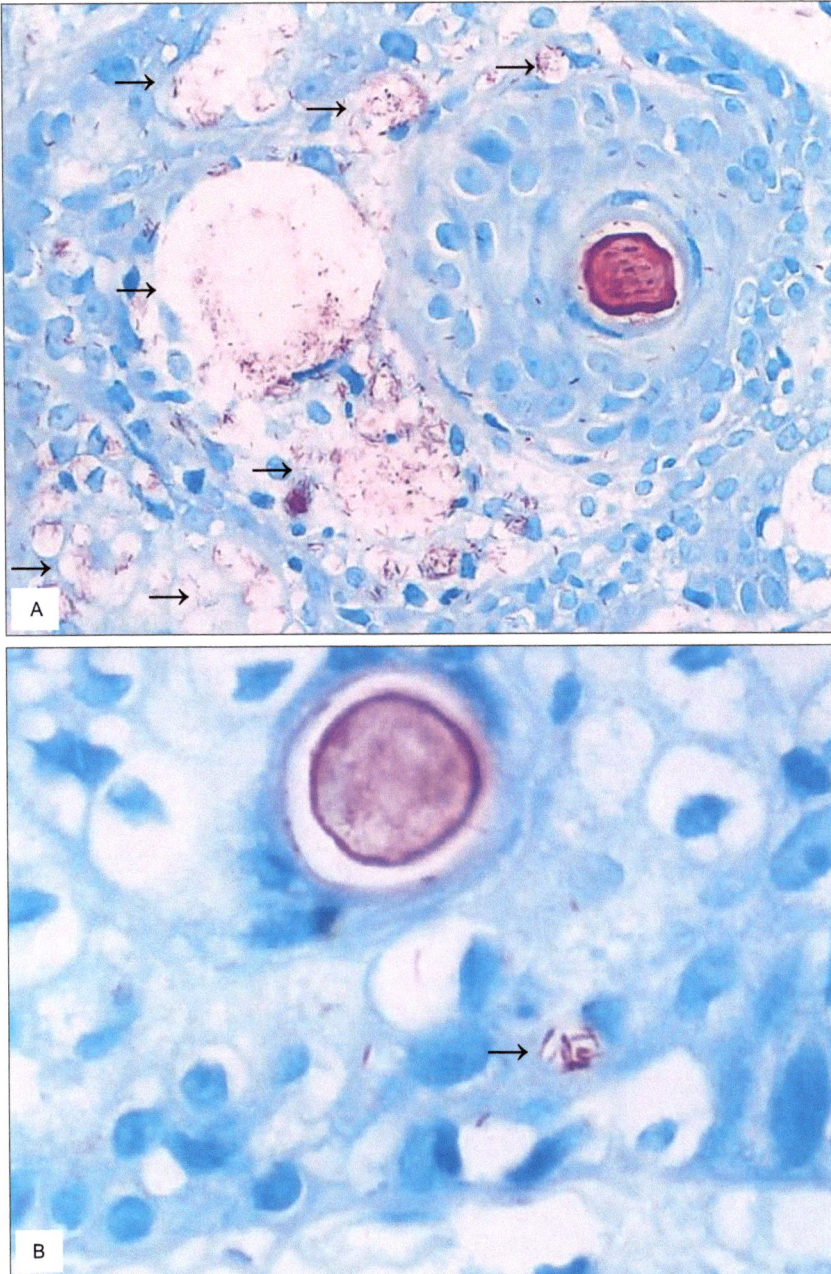

Fig. (14). *M. leprae* parasitizing a hair follicle (→). Pilosebaceous unit with intense parasitism of sebaceous cells and epithelial cells of the hair (A and B). F-F staining in both **(A)** and **(B)**.

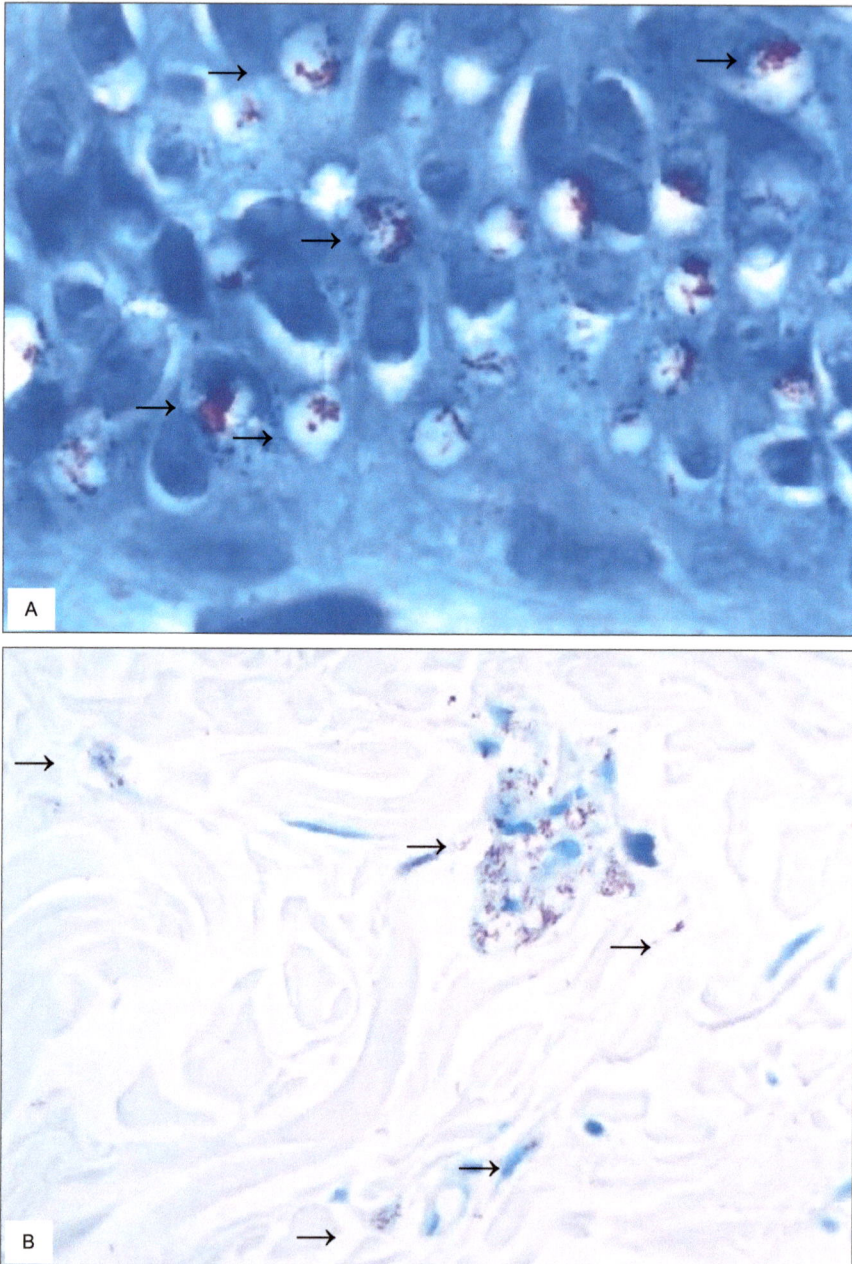

Fig. (15). *M. leprae* parasitizing the epidermis and dermis (→). In the epidermis, there is parasitism of epithelial cells at different levels of maturation **(A)**. In the dermis, different cell types (fibroblasts, macrophages, and vessels) are parasitized **(B)**. F-F staining in both **(A)** and **(B)**.

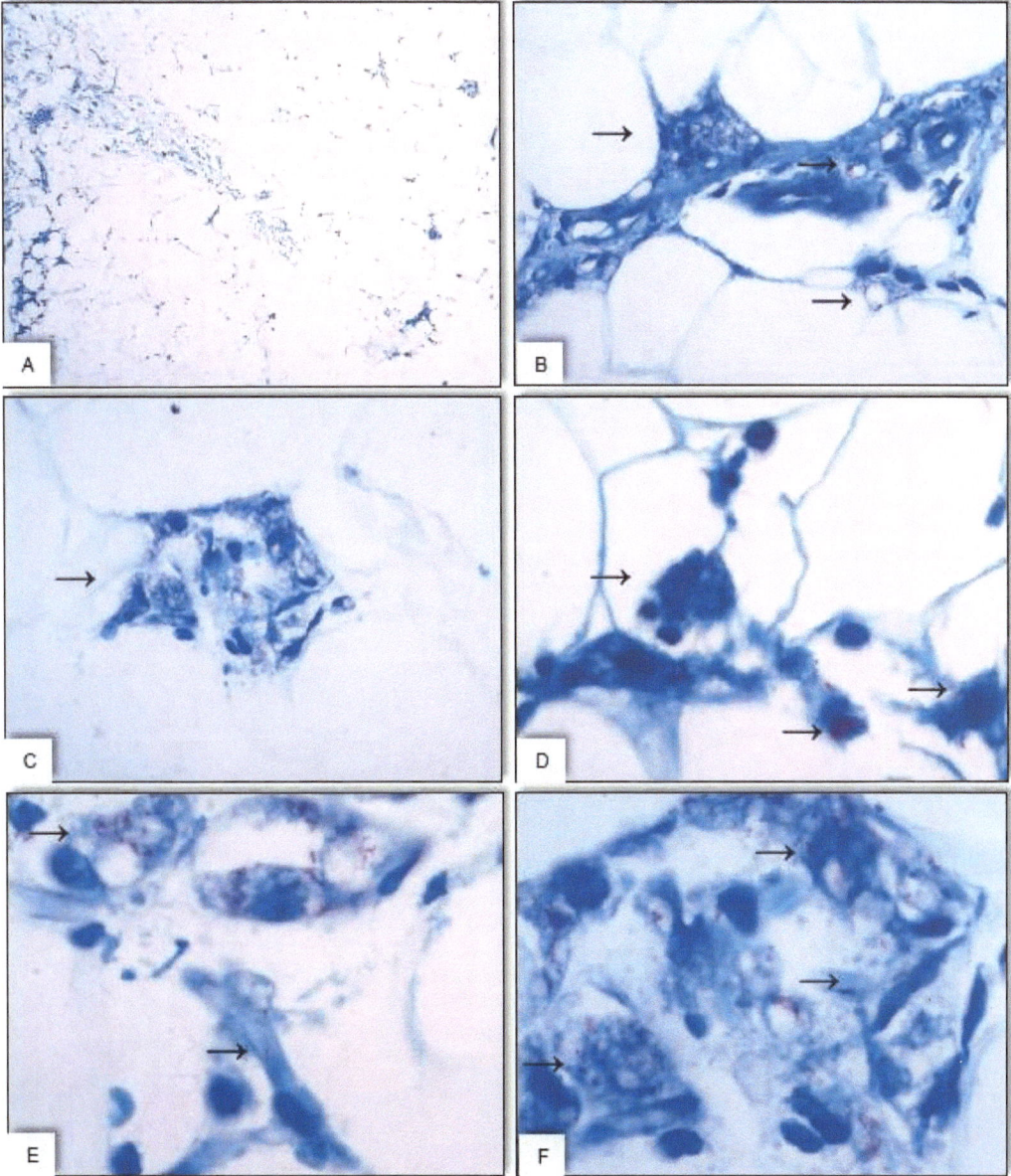

Fig. (16). *M. leprae* parasitizing the subcutaneous tissue (→). There are parasitized cells, mainly macrophages and vessels, involving adipose cells. F-F staining (A-F).

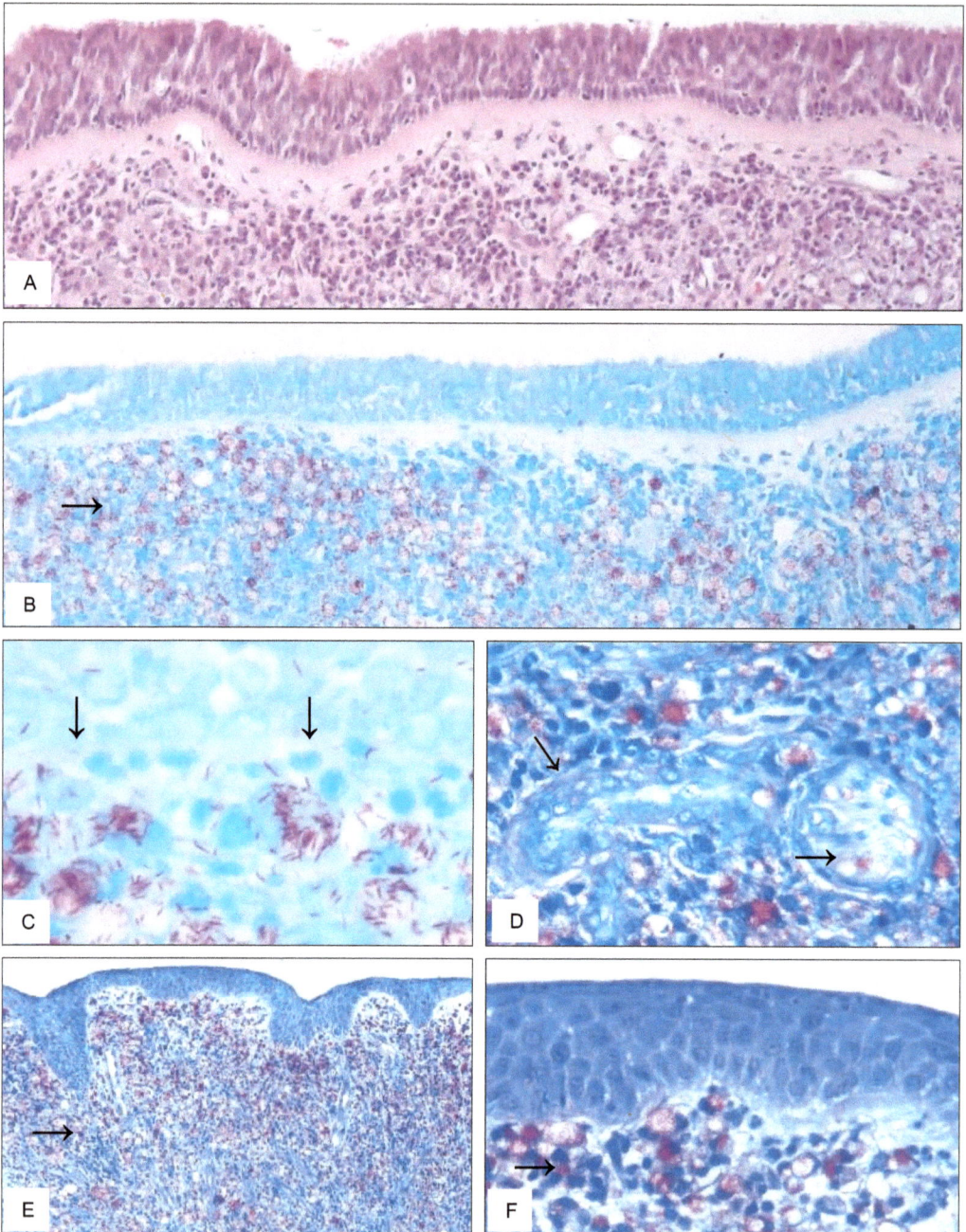

Fig. (17). *M. leprae* parasitizing the nasal and buccal mucosa (→). Nasal mucosa with macrophages, vessels, nerve, and other parasitized tissues (A, B, C, and D). Buccal mucosa with intense parasitism in different cells and tissues (E and F). HE staining in **(A)** and **(E)**. F-F staining in **(B)**, **(C)**, **(D)**, and **(F)**.

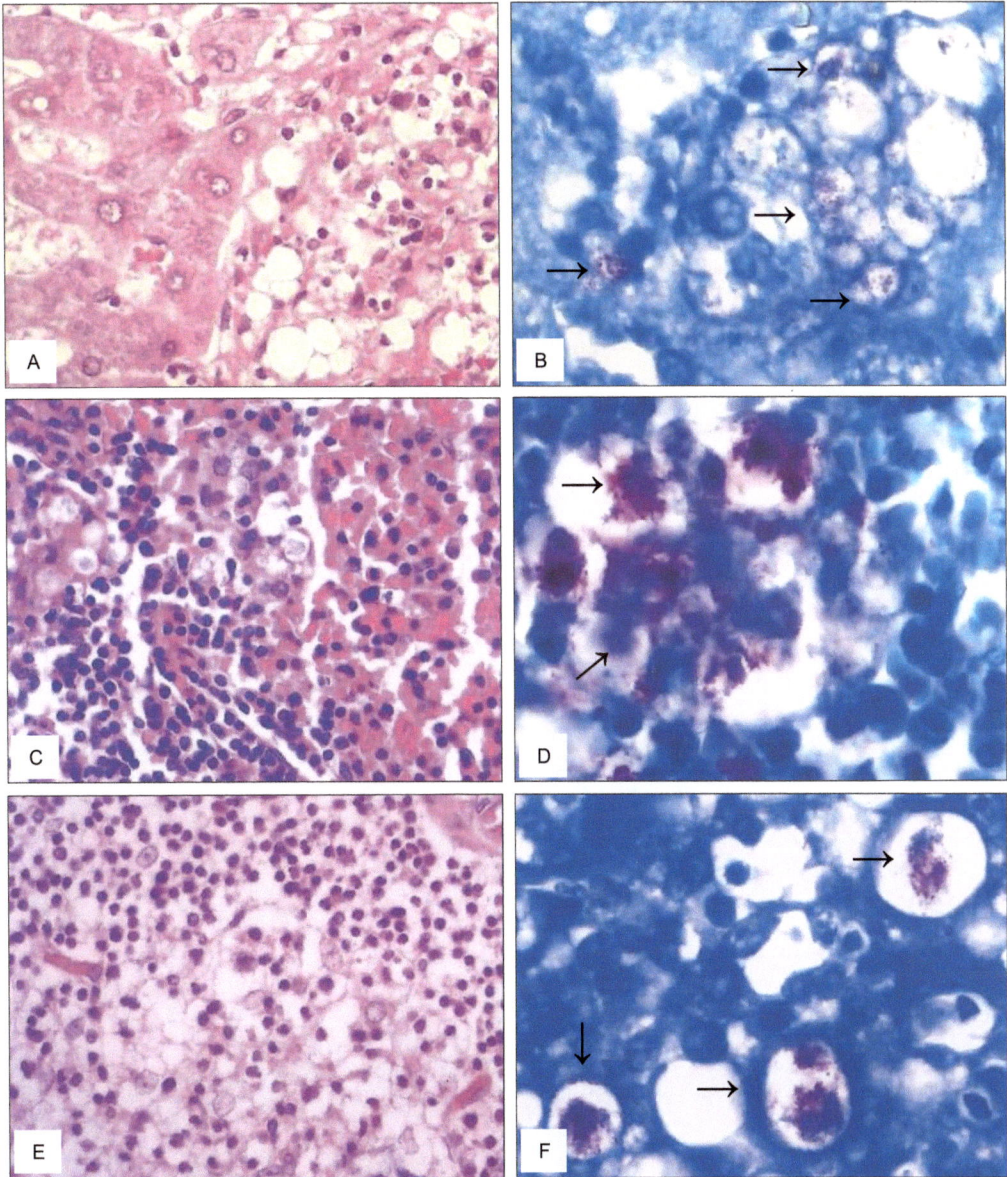

Fig. (18). *M. leprae* parasitizing the liver, spleen, and lymph node (→). Material obtained from autopsy of patients on the lepromatous side (BL and LL) who underwent polychemotherapy treatment for *M. leprae*. Fragmented bacilli in hepatic macrophages (A and B), splenic macrophages (C and D), and lymph node macrophages (E and F). HE staining in **(A)**, **(C)**, and **(E)**. F-F staining in **(B)**, **(D)**, and **(F)**.

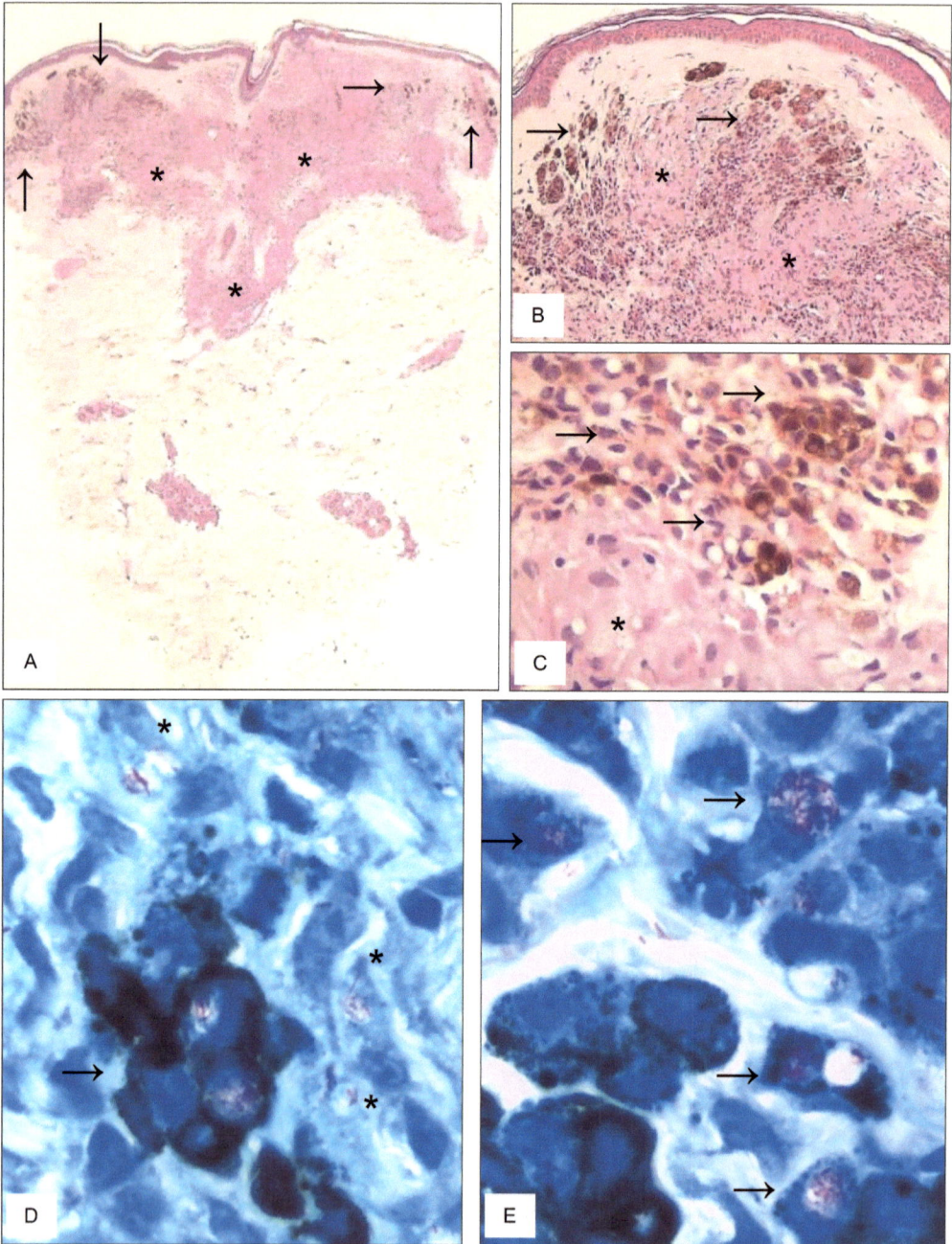

Fig. (19). *M. leprae* parasitizing melanocytic nevus (→). A lepromatous patient underwent excision of melanocytic nevus on the skin of the face. The histological sections show the dermal melanocytic nevi permeated by macrophages (*) of the leprosy lesion. Bacilli within intracytoplasmic vacuoles of nevus cells and within the cytoplasm of macrophages of the adjacent leprosy lesion are observed. HE staining in **(A)**, **(B)**, and **(C)**. F-F staining in **(D)** and **(E)**.

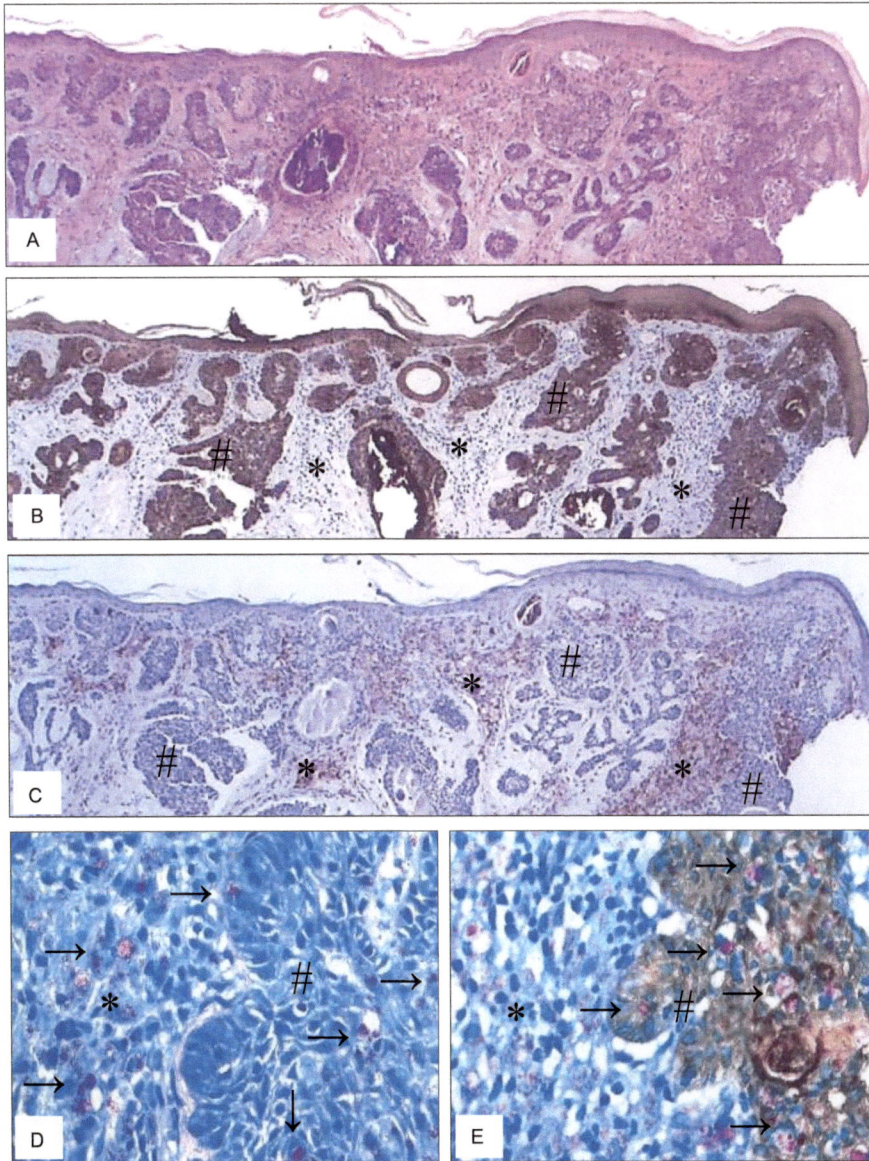

Fig. (20). *M. leprae* parasitizing basal cell carcinoma (→). A lepromatous patient underwent excision of basal cell carcinoma. **(A)** Histological sections show the carcinoma permeated by macrophages of the adjacent leprosy lesion. **(B)** Anti-cytokeratin/34BE12 staining demonstrates basal cell carcinoma (positive #) among macrophages (negative *) of the leprosy lesion. **(C)** Anti-CD68 staining demonstrates macrophages (positive *) of the leprosy lesion involving basal cell carcinoma (negative #). **(D)** F-F staining shows bacilli inside the macrophages and basal cell carcinoma cells. **(E)** Double staining (anti-cytokeratin/34BE12 and F-F) demonstrates basal cell carcinoma epithelial cells containing bacilli in intracytoplasmic vacuoles. Published in [22].

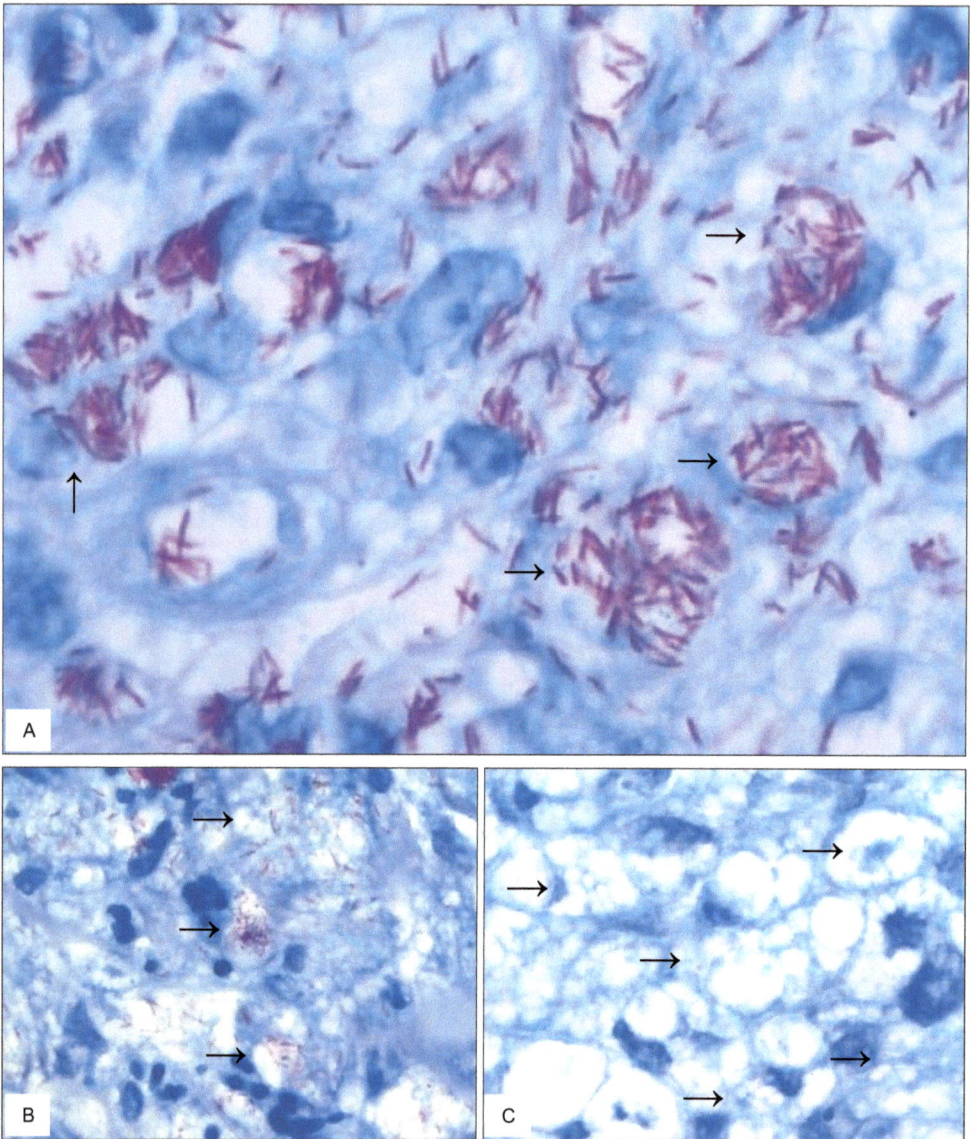

Fig. (21). Solid and fragmented *M. leprae* (→). Intact bacilli intensely stained in the cytoplasm of macrophages before the initiation of treatment. Fragmented bacilli strongly stained in the cytoplasm of macrophages after initiation of treatment. Multi-fragmented bacilli slightly stained or discolored in the cytoplasm of macrophages in the late phase of treatment. F-F staining (A-C).

GENERAL ASPECTS OF LEPROSY

Leprosy is a complex disease from a clinical, histopathological, and molecular point of view. The wide diversity of clinical presentation and the different histopathological characteristics observed throughout the disease spectrum and reactions render it a challenging disease in clinical and pathological practice. A large number of diseases, from inflammatory to neoplastic, are part of the differential diagnosis of leprosy. Late diagnosis of leprosy is not uncommon, occurring even months or years after the onset of signs and symptoms, leading to disease progression and increasing the probability of developing reactions. Because it is a spectral disease that can evolve over many years or decades, its clinical and pathological characteristics change slowly and steadily, often with overlap between the disease forms on the spectrum. There is also an overlap of histological patterns of reactions among forms and between reactions themselves. Therefore, it is unlikely that any classification could encompass and faithfully define the entire spectrum [16 - 19]. It is important to keep in mind the complexity of the disease and the difficulty of classifying it with any of the methods proposed to date. However, the classification proposed by R&J is considered the most representative. Therefore, the pathologist should strive to classify the disease, through assessment of clinical and histopathological characteristics, within the parameters proposed by R&J [8]. In addition, the pathologist must be able to recognize the histopathological characteristics of particular clinicopathological forms of the disease and identify the histopathological characteristics of the reactional phenomena (T1R and T2R) [6, 16 - 19]. It is critical to remember that the main histopathological characteristic of leprosy is the inflammatory infiltrate compromising neural branches since it is present in all clinical forms, including the indeterminate form. In histological sections of skin biopsies with inflammatory infiltrate involving neural branches, the pathologist should include leprosy among the diagnostic hypotheses. In endemic countries, if the inflammatory infiltrate is predominantly neural (neurocentric), the leprosy hypothesis is the most likely. In both situations, the pathologist must attempt to detect the bacillus by special staining or other techniques (F-F stain, immunohistochemistry, PCR, *etc.*). Other diseases may compromise the peripheral nerves with chronic inflammatory infiltrate, the most common of which are autoimmune diseases, syphilis, borreliosis, viral infections, and sarcoidosis [20].

In the subsequent chapters, the clinical, histopathological, and bacilloscopic features of leprosy forms (Chapters 2, 3, and 4), reactional phenomena (T1R - Chapter 5 and T2R - Chapter 6), the regressive changes observed in leprosy lesions during and after treatment or relapse (Chapter 7), and some variants with special clinical characteristics (Chapter 8) are discussed. The different histological characteristics of granulomas in the various forms of leprosy, in the reaction episodes, and in the regression will be discussed, respectively, in each chapter.

CONCLUSION

Leprosy is a long-term spectral disease that presents in several clinical forms with different histopathological aspects. Disease classification requires a careful correlation between its clinical and histopathologic or bacilloscopic characteristics.

REFERENCES

[1]　Hastings RC, Gillis TP, Krahenbuhl JL, Franzblau SG. Leprosy. Clin Microbiol Rev 1988; 1(3): 330-48.
　　　[http://dx.doi.org/10.1128/CMR.1.3.330] [PMID: 3058299]

[2]　Han XY, Seo YH, Sizer KC, *et al.* A new *Mycobacterium* species causing diffuse lepromatous leprosy. Am J Clin Pathol 2008; 130(6): 856-64.
　　　[http://dx.doi.org/10.1309/AJCPP72FJZZRRVMM] [PMID: 19019760]

[3]　Han XY, Aung FM, Choon SE, Werner B. Analysis of the leprosy agents *Mycobacterium leprae* and *Mycobacterium lepromatosis* in four countries. Am J Clin Pathol 2014; 142(4): 524-32.
　　　[http://dx.doi.org/10.1309/AJCP1GLCBE5CDZRM] [PMID: 25239420]

[4]　Global leprosy update, 2016: accelerating reduction of disease burden. Wkly Epidemiol Rec 2017; 92(35): 501-19.
　　　[PMID: 28861986]

[5]　Opromolla DVA. Manifestações clínicas e reações.Noções de Hansenologia. 2nd ed. Bauru, Brazil: Centro de Estudo Dr Reynaldo Quagliato, Instituto Lauro de Souza Lima 2000; pp. 51-8.

[6]　Fleury RN. Patologia e manifestações viscerais.Noções de Hansenologia. 2nd ed. Bauru, Brazil: Centro de Estudo Dr Reynaldo Quagliato, Instituto Lauro de Souza Lima 2000; pp. 63-71.

[7]　International Congress of Leprosy, Madrid. Report of the committee on classification. Int J Lepr 1953; 21: 504-16.

[8]　Rodrigues Júnior IA, Gresta LT, Noviello MdeL, Cartelle CT, Lyon S, Arantes RM. Leprosy classification methods: a comparative study in a referral center in Brazil. Int J Infect Dis 2016; 45: 118-22.
　　　[http://dx.doi.org/10.1016/j.ijid.2016.02.018] [PMID: 26928327]

[9]　Ridley DS, Jopling WH. Classification of leprosy according to immunity. A five-group system. Int J Lepr Other Mycobact Dis 1966; 34(3): 255-73.
　　　[PMID: 5950347]

[10]　Faraco J. Bacillos de Hansen e cortes de parafina: Methodo complementar para a pesquisa de bacilos de Hansen em cortes de material incluído em parafina. Rev Bras Leprol 1938; 6: 177-80.

[11]　Fite GL. The staining of acid-fast bacilli in paraffin sections. Am J Pathol 1938; 14(4): 491-507.
　　　[PMID: 19970405]

[12]　Wade HW. Demonstration of acid-fast bacilli in tissue sections. Am J Pathol 1952; 28(1): 157-70.
　　　[PMID: 14885412]

[13]　Xavier-Júnior JC, Ocanha JP, Marques ME, Marques SA. *Mycobacterium leprae* is usually positive to periodic acid-Schiff and Grocott stains. Am J Dermatopathol 2016; 38(4): 322-4.
　　　[http://dx.doi.org/10.1097/DAD.0000000000000360] [PMID: 26999344]

[14]　Wear DJ, Hadfield TL, Connor DH, *et al.* Periodic acid-Schiff reaction stains *Mycobacterium tuberculosis, Mycobacterium leprae, Mycobacterium ulcerans, Mycobacterium chelonei* (abscessus), and *Mycobacterium kansasii.* Arch Pathol Lab Med 1985; 109(8): 701-3.
　　　[PMID: 3925927]

[15]   Ridley DS, Hilson GR. A logarithmic index of bacilli in biopsies. I. Method. Int J Lepr Other Mycobact Dis 1967; 35(2): 184-6.
[PMID: 5338960]

[16]   Lastória JC, Abreu MA. Leprosy: review of the epidemiological, clinical, and etiopathogenic aspects - part 1. An Bras Dermatol 2014; 89(2): 205-18.
[http://dx.doi.org/10.1590/abd1806-4841.20142450] [PMID: 24770495]

[17]   Fleury RN. Difficulties in the use of the Ridley and Jopling classification--a morphological analysis. Hansenol Int 1989; 14(2): 101-6.
[PMID: 2562586]

[18]   Moorthy BN, Kumar P, Chatura KR, Chandrasekhar HR, Basavaraja PK. Histopathological correlation of skin biopsies in leprosy. Indian J Dermatol Venereol Leprol 2001; 67(6): 299-301.
[PMID: 17664782]

[19]   Scollard DM, Adams LB, Gillis TP, Krahenbuhl JL, Truman RW, Williams DL. The continuing challenges of leprosy. Clin Microbiol Rev 2006; 19(2): 338-81.
[http://dx.doi.org/10.1128/CMR.19.2.338-381.2006] [PMID: 16614253]

[20]   Katona I, Weis J. Diseases of the peripheral nerves. Handb Clin Neurol 2017; 145: 453-74.
[http://dx.doi.org/10.1016/B978-0-12-802395-2.00031-6] [PMID: 28987189]

[21]   Boggild AK, Keystone JS, Kain KC. Leprosy: a primer for Canadian physicians. CMAJ 2004; 170(1): 71-8.
[PMID: 14707226]

[22]   Teixeira CS, Montalvão PP, de Oliveira IT, Wachholz PA. Neoplastic cells parasitized by *Mycobacterium leprae*: report of two cases of melanocytic nevus and one of basal cell carcinoma. Surg Exp Pathol 2019; 2: 26.
[http://dx.doi.org/10.1186/s42047-019-0051-x]

CHAPTER 2

Indeterminate Leprosy

Abstract: Leprosy in its indeterminate form (I) is a clinical presentation of the disease preceding the forms described in the Ridley and Jopling (R & J) classification and any other special forms of leprosy or the reactions. In this chapter, the histopathological and bacilloscopic characteristics of the I form of leprosy are described, and the main differential diagnoses are discussed. The histopathological criteria that distinguish the I form from the other forms of leprosy and the reaction processes that may occur during the disease course are also discussed. The identification of the histopathological characteristics of I leprosy is of great importance with respect to the selection of the treatment. I leprosy should not be confused with other forms of leprosy, especially the multibacillary forms, which require more prolonged treatment and which can develop reaction phenomena, causing permanent sequelae.

Keywords: Bacilloscopy, Hansen's disease, Histopathology, Indeterminate leprosy, Leprosy, *Mycobacterium leprae*.

INTRODUCTION

Leprosy in its indeterminate form (I) is a clinical presentation of the disease preceding the forms described in the Ridley and Jopling (R & J) classification, as well as any other special forms of leprosy or its reactions [1, 2] (Fig. **1**). The recognition of the "I" form as a distinct form of leprosy is controversial in the literature [1]. Although some authors may doubt and not recognize the existence of the "I" form, it is recognized by many leprologists and has been described since the first proposal for the classification of leprosy [1]. There are several hypotheses that attempt to explain the onset and development of early lesions before the disease progresses into the R & J spectrum. One explanation is related to the low antigenicity and slow replication of the bacillus [3, 4]. *Mycobacterium leprae* is an obligate intracellular, gram-positive bacteria with a slow replication rate (approximately 12 days), a long incubation period, and only a small number of genes controlling its metabolism [3, 4]. These characteristics may hinder the passage of the bacillus through the individual's natural defenses, such as the integrity of the integuments, secretions, surface immunoglobulins, and the

Cleverson Teixeira Soares

mononuclear-phagocytic system. The main route of penetration of the bacilli is probably the upper airways, and from there, *via* the lymphohematogenous route, they continue to parasitize the Schwann cells and other cells [4, 5].

This chapter discusses the main histopathologic and bacilloscopic characteristics of leprosy and their significance in the identification of its initial presentation.

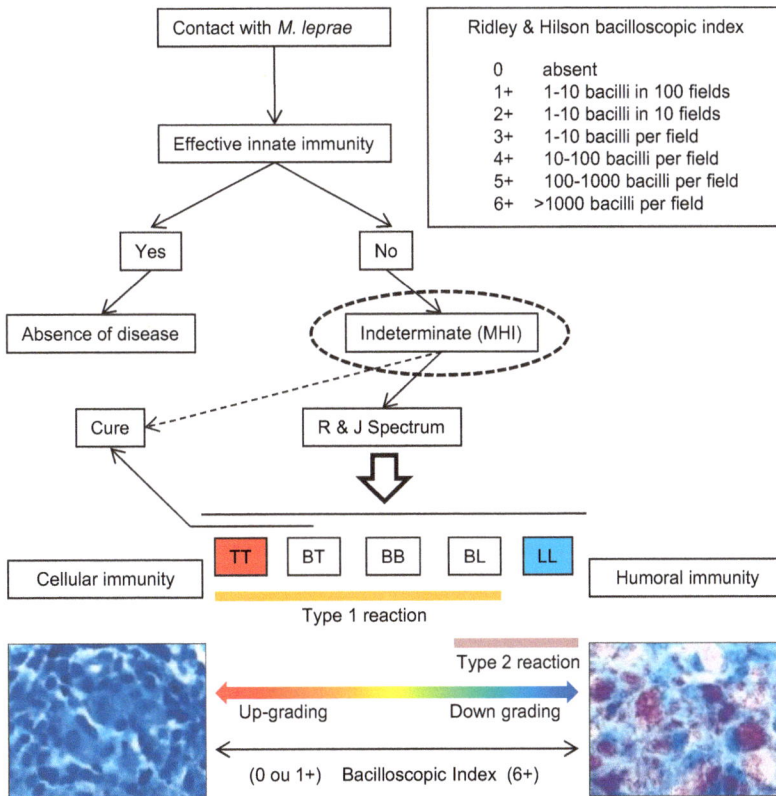

Fig. (1). Clinical spectrum and bacilloscopic index of leprosy forms and reactions. Patients who are exposed to *Mycobacterium leprae* can eliminate the bacilli through primary immune response mechanisms and do not develop the disease. If the primary immune defense cannot contain the proliferation of the bacilli, the patient develops indeterminate leprosy ("I"), the early stage of the disease preceding the polarized forms of the Ridley and Jopling (R&J) classification: tuberculoid (TT); borderline-tuberculoid (BT); borderline-borderline (BB); borderline-lepromatous (BL); and lepromatous or Virchowian (LL). Late recognition of bacillary antigens by the individual may result in an intense and effective immune response (TT and BT pattern), which may lead to the destruction of the bacilli and spontaneous cure. TT individuals are those who have an effective cellular immunity. If cellular immunity is not effective, the proliferation and dissemination of the bacilli persist, and the disease progresses toward the lepromatous pole. LL individuals are anergic and react to the bacilli through humoral immunity. Type 1 reactions (T1R) affect patients in the range from TT to BL. Type 2 reactions (T2R) affect patients on the lepromatous side (BL and LL). The bacilloscopic index ranges from 0 to 6+.

CLINICOPATHOLOGICAL ASPECTS OF INDETERMINATE LEPROSY

Some conditions seem to be important for an individual to develop leprosy. The person must be exposed to *M. leprae* for a long period of time, have a predisposition or significant deficiencies in the natural defenses specific to infection by the bacillus [4]. These conditions would be conducive for *M. leprae* to reach its place of preference, which is the peripheral nervous system, and parasitize the cutaneous sensory branches and superficial segments of the peripheral neural trunks [4]. Within the Schwann cells, the bacillus can survive and proliferate outside the reach of the defense mechanisms of the host immune system. It is estimated that this phase of parasitism restricted to the Schwann cells is long and can be between 5 to 10 years [4].

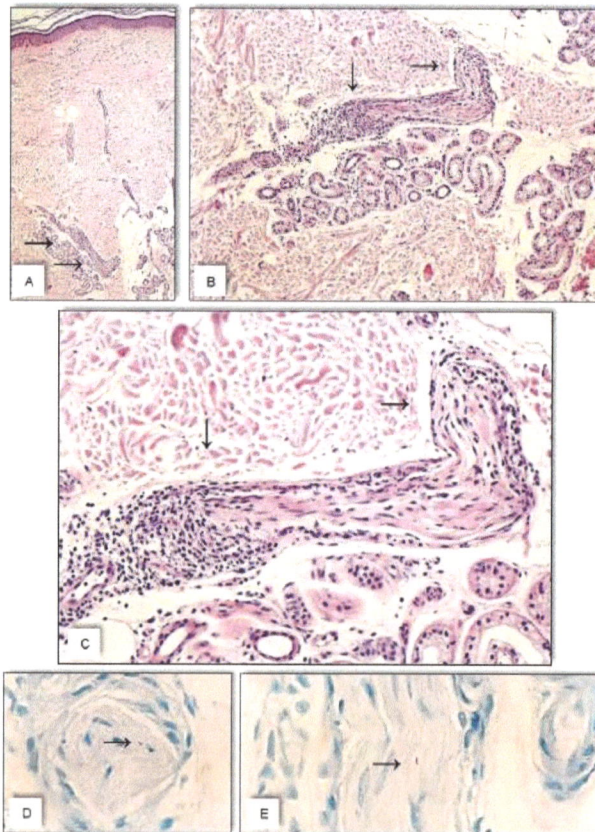

Fig. (2). Histopathological characteristics and bacilloscopic examination of indeterminate leprosy. (A and B) Discrete and focal inflammatory infiltrates appear lymphohistiocytic, non-tuberculoid, and selectively accompany or penetrate the neural branches (→), while other skin tissues show no histological changes (hematoxylin and eosin staining). (D and E) Bacilloscopic index of 1+ with bacillus within the neural branch (→) (Fite-Faraco staining). All images are obtained from the archives of the Lauro de Souza Lima Institute.

It is possible that the low antigenicity of *M. leprae* contributes to its poor recognition by the host immune system. Thus, in the first stage of the disease ("I" form), while the amount of bacillary antigens in the tissues is not enough to trigger an individual's own immunocellular reaction, the histological characteristics in the parasitized cutaneous areas indicate discrete lymphohistiocytic inflammation without tuberculoid granulomas, selectively involving the neural branches that accompany the vessels and cutaneous appendages [2, 4] (Figs. **2 - 4**). The detection of the bacillus within the neural branch allows the diagnosis of leprosy, though in most cases, the bacillus is not found (bacilloscopic index of 0 or 1+). It is important to note that even without the detection of the bacillus, the selectivity of the inflammatory infiltrates in the neural branches associated with the inflammatory delamination of the perineurium and the endoneurial infiltration by the inflammatory cells allows the diagnosis of "I" leprosy [1, 4]. These histopathological characteristics are clinically correlated with cutaneous areas presenting small changes in the thermal, pain, or tactile sensitivities. Minimal changes in sensitivities may or may not be associated with the concomitant dermatological lesions. In general, only hypochromic or erythematous-hypochromic macules are observed [1, 4 - 6], though in some other cases, circular normal-looking areas of the skin with discrete sensitivity disorders are detected (Fig. **5**).

In cases of clinical and pathological suspicion of leprosy, it is recommended that multiple and serial histological sections should be analyzed using both hematoxylin-eosin (HE) and Fite-Faraco (FF) staining. In our experience, this considerably increases the rate of detection of the bacilli, reaching up to 40% in lesions of the "I" form. The use of molecular techniques, such as the polymerase chain reaction, can further increase the detection rate of the bacilli [7, 8].

Clinicopathological Aspects that Differentiate the "I" Form from the other Forms and the Reactional Phenomena of Leprosy

The "I" form of leprosy is rare, and in general, biopsies of leprosy lesions that clinically suggest the "I" form actually present histological features of other forms of leprosy or its reactions. By concept, the "I" form of leprosy precedes the other forms of the R & J spectrum, and the inflammatory infiltrate involving the nerves is discrete and without formation of granulomas. Therefore, the diagnosis of the "I" form should be restricted to cases that are neurocentric, have minimal inflammatory infiltrate, and have a bacilloscopic index of 0 to 1+ in the histological sections. If the histological sections show granulomas of any size with a tuberculoid pattern, it indicates leprosy with a tuberculoid pattern (TT-TB) or type 1 reaction (Figs. **6** and **7**). Other important features that help differentiate the "I" form from other forms of leprosy are the bacilloscopic examination characteristics of the histological sections. The detection of bacilli in different types of cells or tissues as well as a bacilloscopic index greater than or equal to 2+ (multibacillary) should be an indication that it is not the "I" form. In such cases, the disease has probably progressed to some forms of the R & J classification and may be classified as either borderline leprosy with or without specifying the form or as multibacillary leprosy. In these cases, a close anatomical-clinical correlation may be crucial for the correct diagnosis.

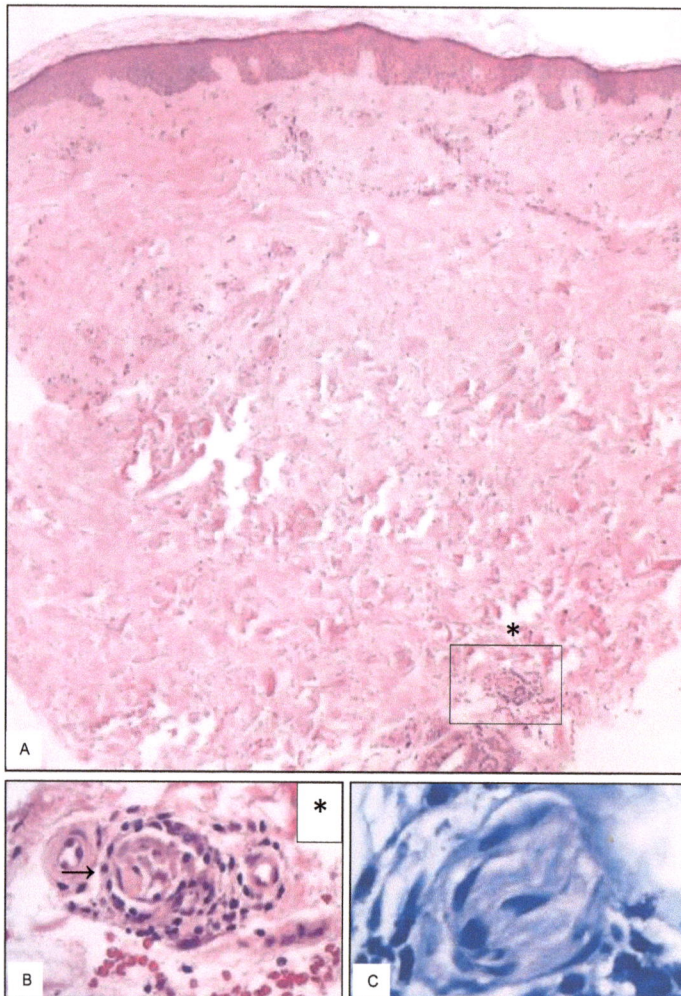

Fig. (3). Histopathological characteristics and bacilloscopic examination of indeterminate leprosy. Discrete and focal (*) inflammatory infiltrates appear lymphohistiocytic, non-tuberculoid, and selectively accompany or penetrate the neural branches (→), while other skin tissues show no histological changes. (A and B) Hematoxylin and eosin staining. Negative bacilloscopic index **(C)** by Fite-Faraco staining.

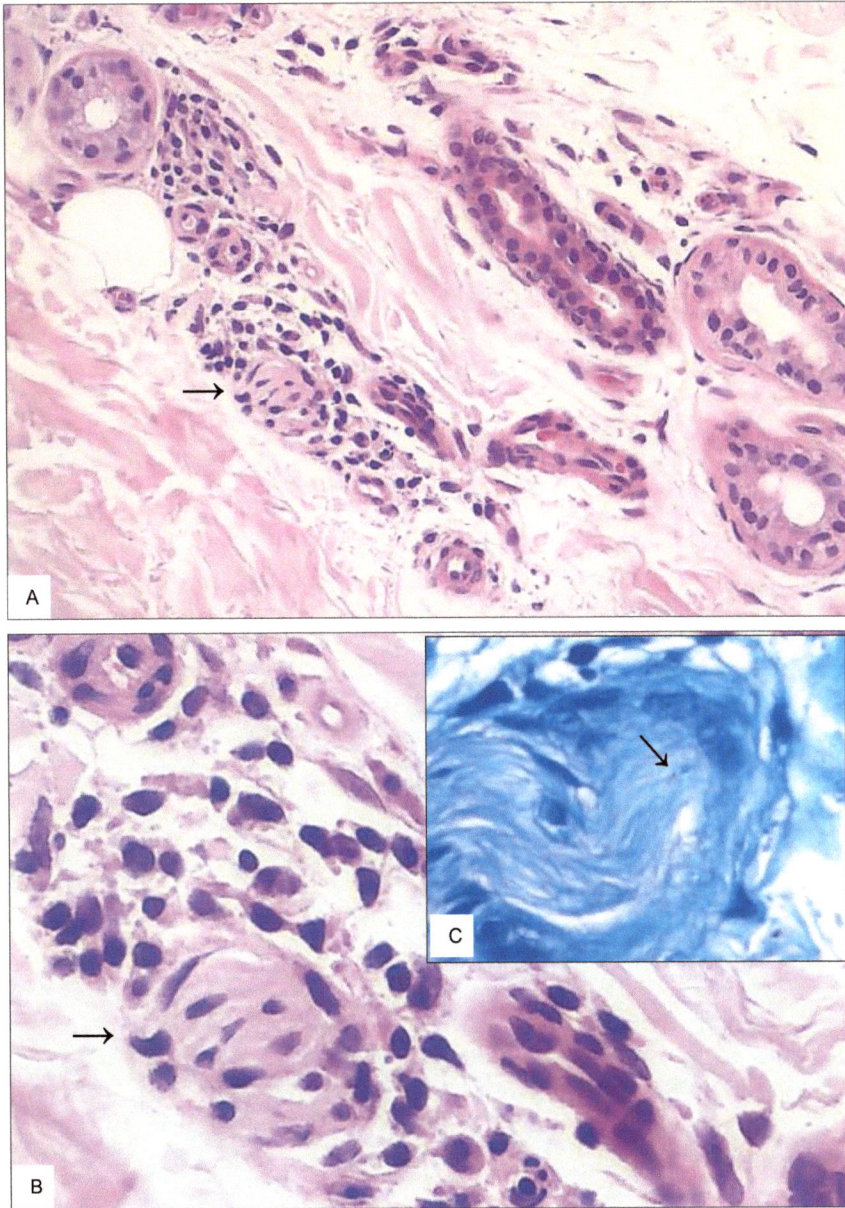

Fig. (4). Histopathological characteristics and bacilloscopic examination of indeterminate leprosy. Discrete and focal inflammatory infiltrates are lymphohistiocytic, non-tuberculoid, and selectively accompany or penetrate the neural branches (→), while other skin tissues show no histological changes. Bacilloscopic index of 1+ with bacillus within the neural branch (→) (Fite-Faraco (FF) staining). (A and B) Hematoxylin and eosin staining and **(C)** FF staining.

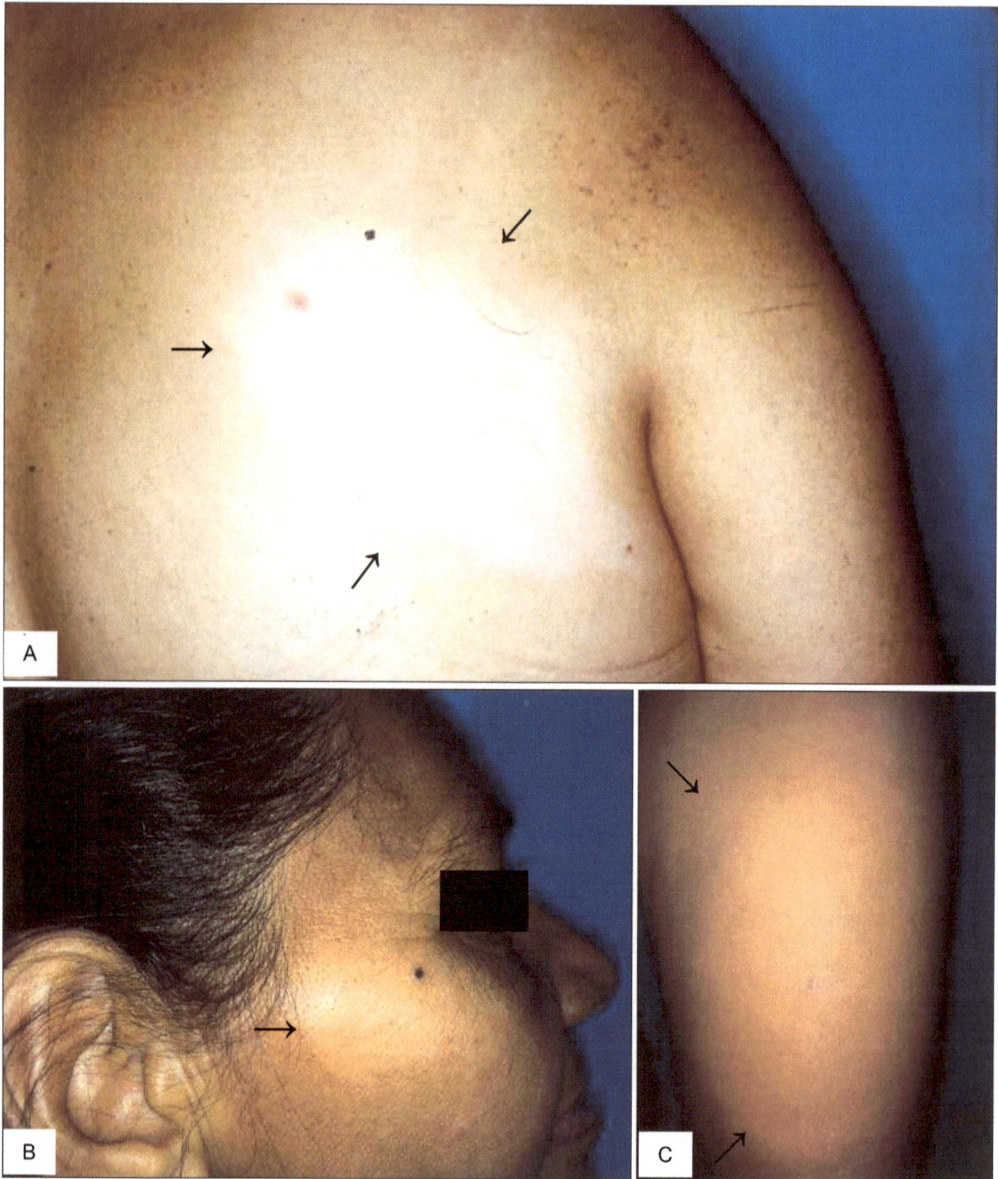

Fig. (5). Clinical characteristics of indeterminate leprosy lesions (→). **(A)** A hypochromic macula on the back with discrete sensitivity disorder (obtained from the archives of the Lauro de Souza Lima Institute). **(B)** A hypochromic macula on the face with slight marginal erythema and a slight decrease in sensitivity. **(C)** A hypochromic macula with sensitivity disorder affecting much of the anterior aspect of the left thigh ("B" and "C" courtesy of Dr. Cássio C. Ghidella).

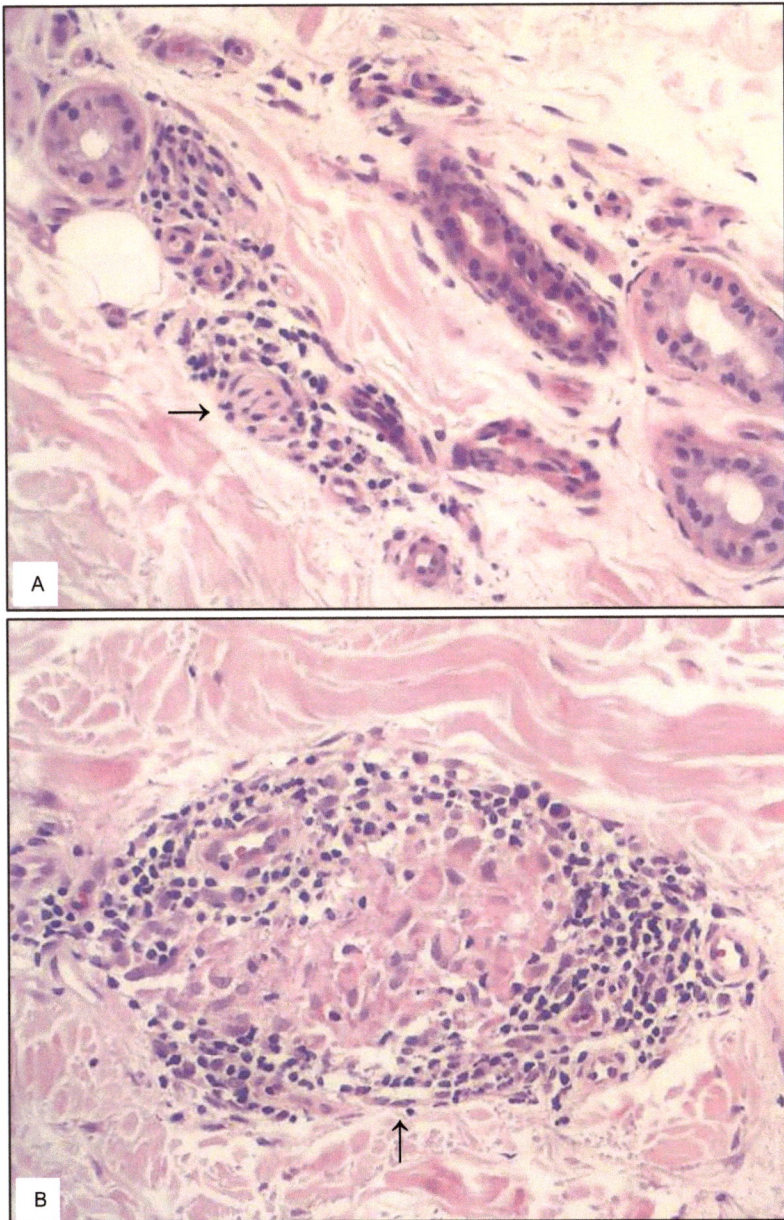

Fig. (6). Histological characteristics of the inflammatory infiltrate in the lesions of the indeterminate ("I") form of leprosy and in the tuberculoid granulomas. **(A)** Discrete inflammatory infiltrates appear lymphohistiocytic, non-tuberculoid, and selectively accompany or infiltrate the neural branches, which is characteristic of the "I" form (→). **(B)** A suspected case of the "I" form, but with a tuberculoid granuloma (→), suggestive of the tuberculoid forms (TT or BT) as per the R & J spectrum classification. A and B show hematoxylin and eosin staining.

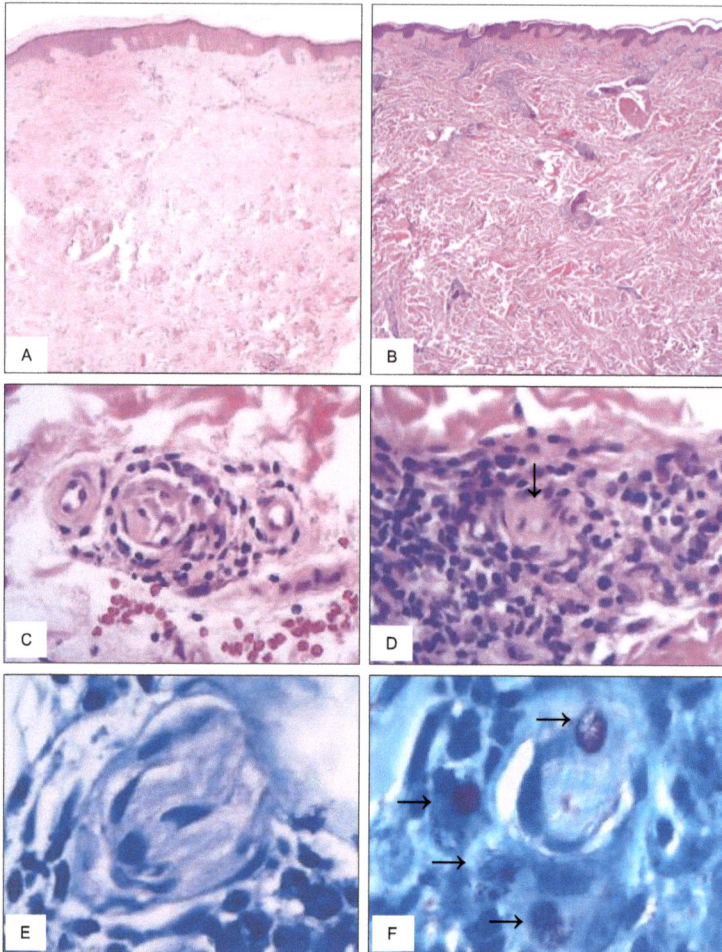

Fig. (7). Histological and bacilloscopic characteristics of indeterminate ("I") and borderline-borderline (BB) leprosy. (A, C and E) The "I" form shows the presence of discrete lymphohistiocytic inflammatory infiltrate selectively accompanying neural branches and with a bacilloscopic index of 0 or 1+. (B, D, and F) The BB form shows the presence of inflammatory lymphohistiocytic and plasmacytic infiltration, accompanying neural branches, vessels, and interstitium, with a bacilloscopic index greater than or equal to 3+. Bacilli (→) are present in the neural branches and macrophages in adjacent tissues (**F**). A, B, C, and D show hematoxylin and eosin staining, while E and F show Fite-Faraco staining.

Among the forms of leprosy of the R & J classification, the borderline-borderline form (BB) is the one that resembles "I" leprosy the closest (Chapter 4) (Fig. **8**). There are also cases of borderline-virchowian (BL) lesions, in which inflammatory infiltrates do not occupy large areas of the skin and can mimic the "I" form (Fig. **9**). In both these situations, the lymphohistiocytic infiltrates may be discrete and predominantly neurocentric. However, unlike the "I" lesions, these forms have a high bacilloscopic index (usually greater than or equal to 4+), with bacilli in different cell types or skin tissues. Additionally, the inflammatory infiltrates in these forms are always more extensive than those in the "I" form, with macrophages, lymphocytes and plasma cells involving vessels, periadnexial spaces, interstitium and subcutaneous adipose tissue (Figs. **8** and **9**).

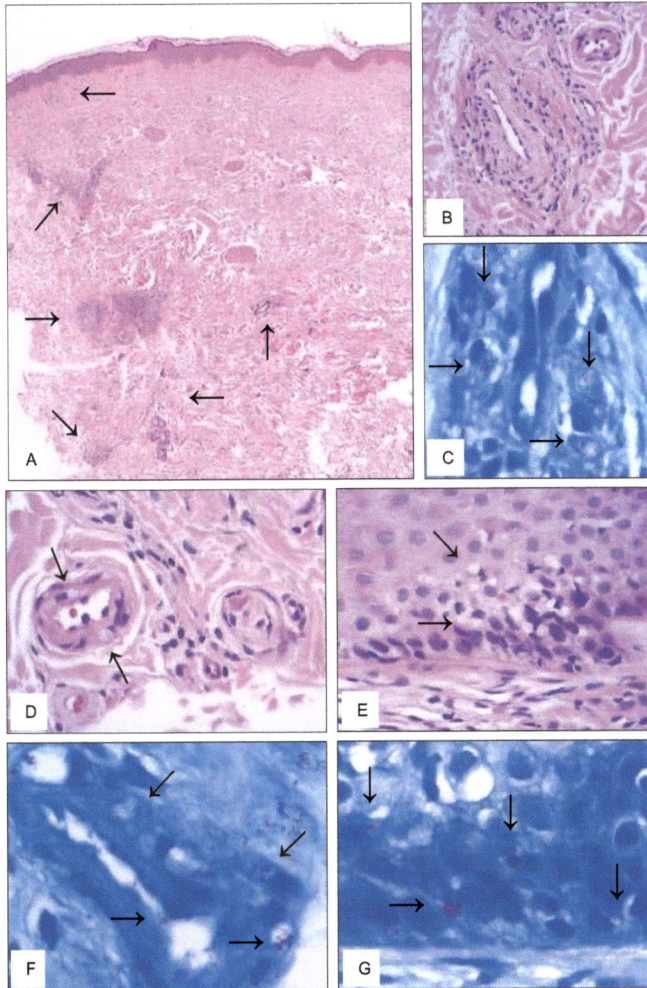

Fig. (8). Leprosy of the lepromatous side (BL-LL) clinically simulating the indeterminate form. (A, and B) Shown is the histology of discrete inflammatory lymphohistiocytic, plasma cells, and non-tuberculoid infiltrate, accompanying neural branches, vessels, and interstitium in a 22-year-old man, in the left upper limb and left foot. The presence of vacuoles on the vessel wall (→) **(D)** and squamous cells (→) **(E)** of the pilosebaceous follicle were observed. Bacilloscopy shows a large number of bacilli in the macrophages around the vessels (→) **(C)**, the vessel wall **(F)**, endothelium **(F)**, and the squamous cells of the pilosebaceous follicle **(G)**. While A, B, D, and E show hematoxylin and eosin staining, C, F, and G show Fite-Faraco staining.

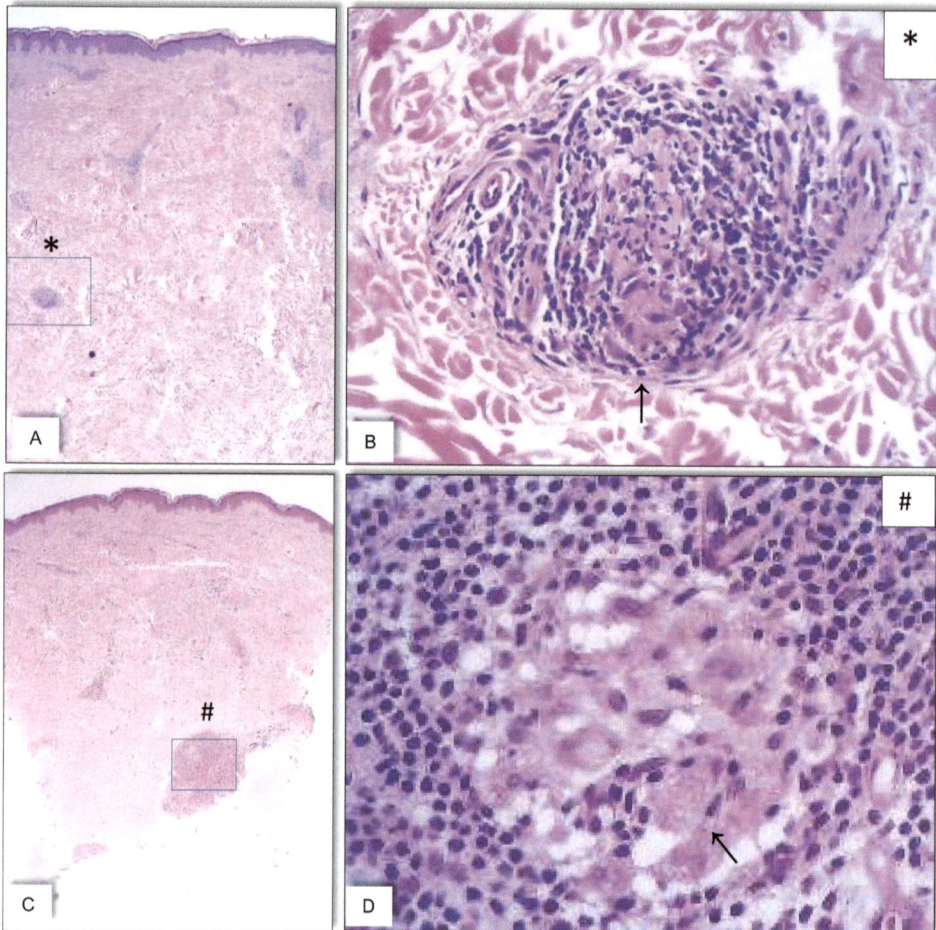

Fig. (9). Leprosy of the tuberculoid side (TT-BT) clinically simulating the indeterminate form. (A-B and C-D) Hematoxylin and eosin staining showing focal inflammatory infiltrates, with tuberculoid granuloma formation characterized by epithelioid macrophage clusters in the center and lymphocytes distributed in the periphery (→).

Lesions in other forms of leprosy associated with type 1 reaction (T1R) can also clinically mimic an "I" lesion (Chapter 5). Type 1 reaction occurs in Tuberculoid (TT) and borderline forms (BT, BB, and BL) and can be initiated by a single lesion with discrete clinical signs. After days or weeks, the reaction process may or may not extend to different parts of the body. At an early stage, with few lesions, T1R can clinically mimic the "I" form. However, the histological characteristics of the skin biopsies of these lesions include lymphohistiocytic infiltrates compromised of different skin components (nerve, vessels, perianexial and interstitial tissues), formation of granulomas simulating the tuberculoid pattern, and a bacilloscopic index ranging from 0+ to 5+, depending on the form of leprosy (TT, BT, BB or BL). These characteristics are typically observed in cases with type 1 reaction and help exclude the clinical diagnosis of "I" leprosy (Chapter 5) (Fig. **10**).

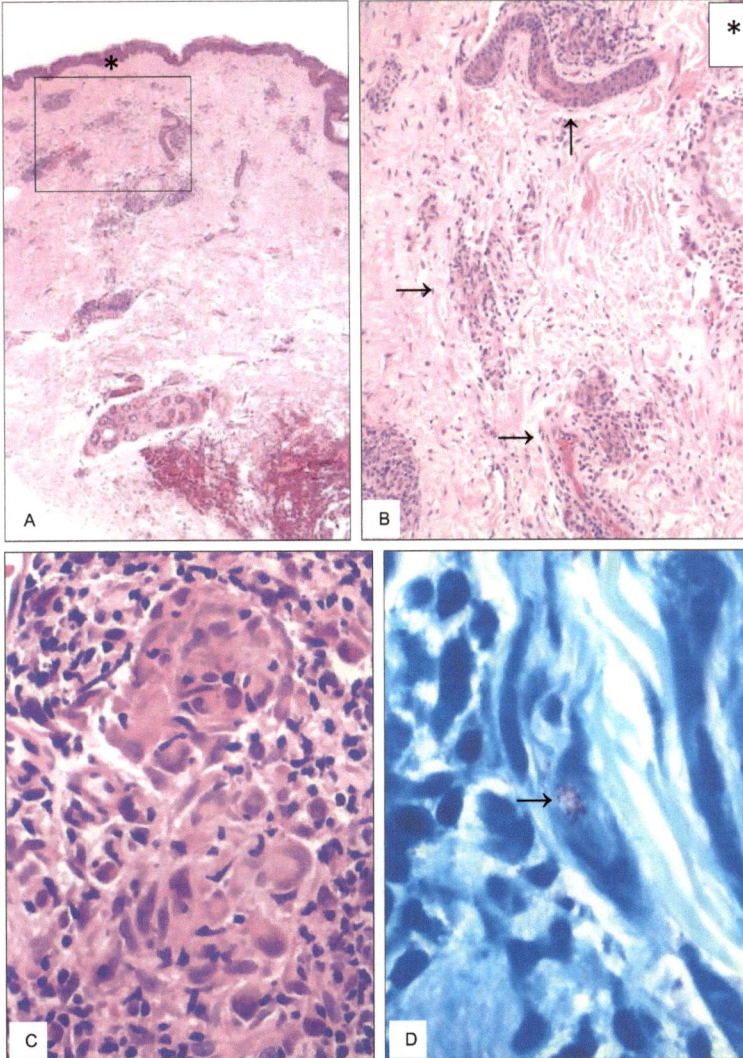

Fig. (10). Borderline leprosy (probably BB), associated with type 1 reaction (Borderline + T1R), clinically simulating indeterminate leprosy. (**A** and **B**) Hematoxylin and eosin (HE) staining shows perineural, perianexial and interstitial inflammatory infiltrates (→). (**C**) Granulomas with epithelioid macrophages, edema and lymphocytic infiltrate permeating the macrophages compatible with type 1 reaction (HE staining). (**D**) Fite-Faraco staining shows a bacilloscopic index of 4+ (→), with a predominance of fragmented bacilli.

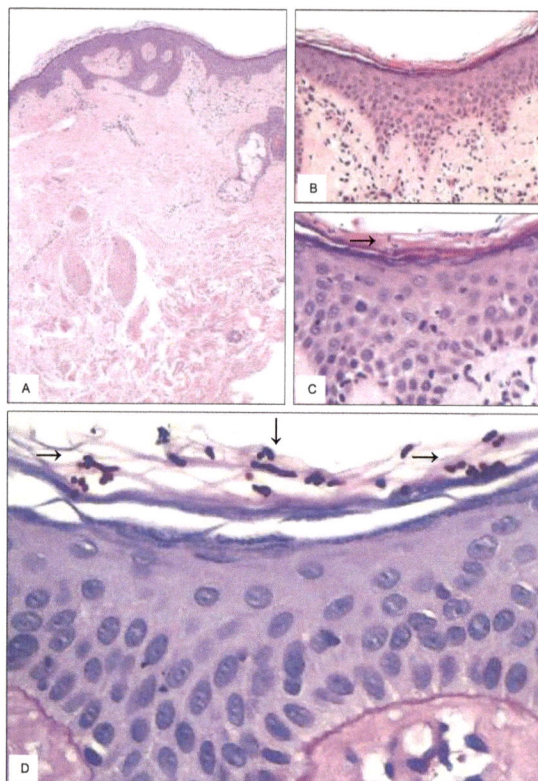

Fig. (11). Tinea versicolor (pityriasis versicolor) hypochromic clinically simulating indeterminate leprosy. **(A-C)** Hematoxylin and eosin staining shows discrete superficial inflammatory infiltrate in the superficial dermis associated with mild hypopigmentation of the basal layer, acanthosis, and hyperkeratosis. **(D)** Presence of short and septate hyphae (→) in the stratum corneum can be easily visualized by periodic acid-Schiff (PAS) staining.

Differential Diagnoses

Lesions of "I" leprosy may be undetectable based on just sensory changes. Clinically similar lesions (hypochromic or erythematous-hypochromic macules) (Figs. **11 - 13**) may be seen in a large number of diseases affecting the skin such as pityriasis alba, the hypochromic variant of pityriasis versicolor, solar hypochromiant dermatoses, achromic nevus, nevus anemicus, vitiligo, post-inflammatory hypopigmentation, fixed drug eruption, early-stage morphea, Lyme disease, cutaneous mycosis, and hypochromic mycosis fungoides among others [6, 9, 10]. However, due to the different histopathological characteristics of these diseases, they can be differentiated relatively easily from leprosy. In general, they do not present with an inflammatory infiltrate composed of neural branches (neurocentric), a characteristic that is present in all forms of leprosy. It is important to distinguish the neurocentric inflammatory infiltrate in "I" leprosy from the diffuse, perianexial or perivascular infiltrates that eventually involve the neural branches in the other diseases. In these diseases, the neural involvement is secondary to the inflammatory infiltrate present in the skin and the subcutaneous tissues. Moreover, there is no direct effect on the nerve, with the presence of endoneural lymphocytes or macrophages, as observed in "I" leprosy. Some cutaneous lesions of syphilis may also present with an inflammatory infiltrate involving neural branches. However, the difference is the presence of perivascular lymphoplasmacytic infiltrate, occasionally at the interface with the epidermis, and perineural plasma cells, which are rare or non-existent in the inflammatory infiltrates of the "I" form. Additionally, while the syphilis lesions are negative for FF staining, they are generally positive for *Treponema pallidum* by immunohistochemistry (Fig. **12**). In hypochromic mycosis fungoides, the lymphocytic infiltrate is superficial and practically restricted to the papillary derma. Additionally, it is associated with epidermotropism and is composed predominantly of $CD3^+$ and $CD8^+$ T lymphocytes [11] (Fig. **13**).

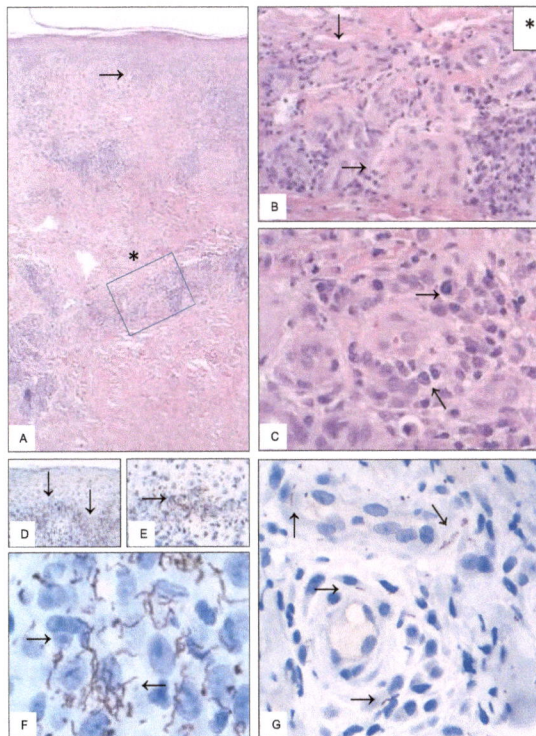

Fig. (12). Secondary syphilis (syphilids) clinically mimicking indeterminate leprosy. Hematoxylin and eosin staining shows discrete inflammatory infiltrate with plasma cells in the (**A**) papillary dermis (→), perivascular and perineural spaces (→) (**B** and **C**). Immunohistochemistry using anti-*Treponema pallidum* antibodies reveals numerous spirochetes (→) at the dermo-epidemic junction (**D-F**) and vessels (**G**).

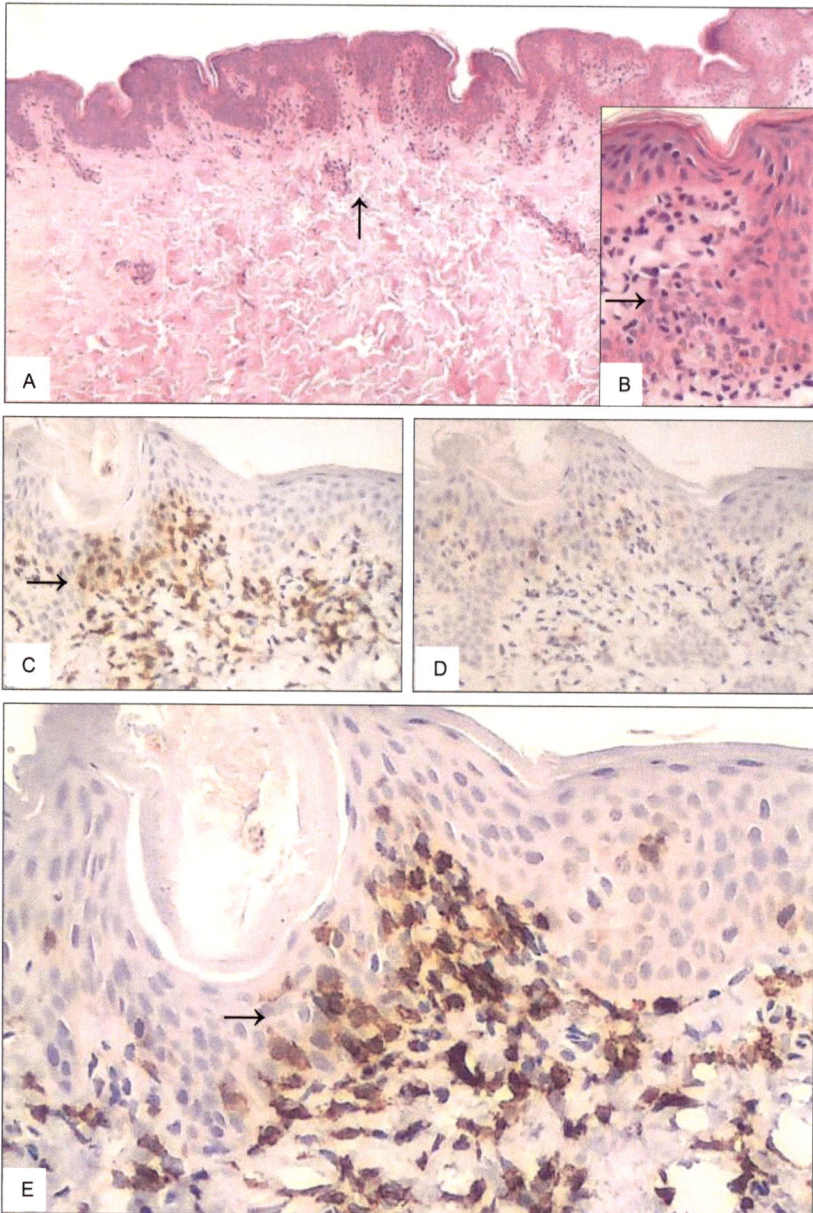

Fig. (13). Mycosis fungoides-associated hypopigmentation simulating clinically indeterminate leprosy. (A and B) Hematoxylin and eosin staining shows the presence of discrete lymphocytic infiltrate in the papillary dermis associated with epidermotropism and absence of neural impairment (→) (predominantly CD3$^+$ / CD8$^+$ "T" cells). Immunohistochemistry shows positivity for **(C)** CD3, **(D)** CD4, and **(E)** CD8.

CONCLUSION

Indeterminate leprosy is a presentation of the disease that precedes any of its other forms or reaction phenomena. A close correlation between its clinical and histopathologic characteristics is crucial for its diagnosis. However, it may also be excluded if tuberculoid granulomas, characteristics of the reaction phenomena, or a bacilloscopic index of ≥ 2+ are observed.

REFERENCES

[1]   Browne SG. Indeterminate leprosy. Int J Dermatol 1985; 24(9): 555-9.
        [http://dx.doi.org/10.1111/j.1365-4362.1985.tb05848.x] [PMID: 3905636]

[2]   Hastings RC, Gillis TP, Krahenbuhl JL, Franzblau SG. Leprosy. Clin Microbiol Rev 1988; 1(3): 330-48.
        [http://dx.doi.org/10.1128/CMR.1.3.330] [PMID: 3058299]

[3]   Cole ST, Eiglmeier K, Parkhill J, *et al.* Massive gene decay in the leprosy bacillus. Nature 2001; 409(6823): 1007-11.
        [http://dx.doi.org/10.1038/35059006] [PMID: 11234002]

[4]   Fleury RN. Patologia e manifestações viscerais.Noções de Hansenologia. 2nd ed. Bauru: Centro de Estudo Dr Reynaldo Quagliato, Instituto Lauro de Souza Lima 2000; pp. 63-71.

[5]   Opromolla DVA. Manifestações clínicas e reações.Noções de Hansenologia. 2nd ed. Bauru: Centro de Estudo Dr Reynaldo Quagliato, Instituto Lauro de Souza Lima 2000; pp. 51-8.

[6]   Giridhar M, Arora G, Lajpal K, Singh Chahal K. Clinicohistopathological concordance in leprosy - a clinical, histopathological and bacteriological study of 100 cases. Indian J Lepr 2012; 84(3): 217-25.
        [PMID: 23484336]

[7]   Natrajan M, Katoch K, Katoch VM, Bharadwaj VP. Enhancement in the histological diagnosis of indeterminate leprosy by demonstration of mycobacterial antigens. Acta Leprol 1995; 9(4): 201-7.
        [PMID: 8711981]

[8]   Banerjee S, Biswas N, Kanti Das N, *et al.* Diagnosing leprosy: revisiting the role of the slit-skin smear with critical analysis of the applicability of polymerase chain reaction in diagnosis. Int J Dermatol 2011; 50(12): 1522-7.
        [http://dx.doi.org/10.1111/j.1365-4632.2011.04994.x] [PMID: 22097999]

[9]   Talhari C, Talhari S, Penna GO. Clinical aspects of leprosy. Clin Dermatol 2015; 33(1): 26-37.
        [http://dx.doi.org/10.1016/j.clindermatol.2014.07.002] [PMID: 25432808]

[10]   Patel AB, Kubba R, Kubba A. Clinicopathological correlation of acquired hypopigmentary disorders. Indian J Dermatol Venereol Leprol 2013; 79(3): 376-82.
        [http://dx.doi.org/10.4103/0378-6323.110800] [PMID: 23619442]

[11]   Misra RS, Ramesh V. Hypopigmented macules in mycosis fungoides. Indian J Dermatol Venereol Leprol 1987; 53(3): 189-90.
        [PMID: 28145339]

CHAPTER 3

Polar Forms (TT and LL)

Abstract: Leprosy is a spectral disease. Its two polar forms, tuberculoid (TT) and lepromatous (LL), are distinct presentations of the disease, both from a clinical and histopathological/bacilloscopic point of view. In this chapter, the histopathological characteristics that define the two polar forms (TT and LL) are presented, and their main differential diagnoses are discussed. These two forms also have significant differences in their treatment protocol. Histopathological recognition of both forms of the disease is important for choosing the correct treatment. Also, there are a large number of diseases that can have a clinical presentation similar to the TT and LL forms of leprosy. In this context, histopathological examination is essential for defining the diagnosis of leprosy.

Keywords: Hansen's disease, Lepromatous leprosy (LL), Leprosy, *Mycobacterium leprae*, Tuberculoid leprosy (TT).

INTRODUCTION

Although the vast majority of individuals are resistant to *Mycobacterium leprae* [1, 2], the population of an endemic region exhibits different degrees of cellular immune responses to antigens of *M. leprae* (Mitsuda reaction) [1]. The degree of variation ranges from maximum resistance (tuberculoid pole – TT) to minimal or anergic resistance (virchowian or lepromatous pole – LL). When exposed to *M. leprae,* individuals develop effective cellular immune responses capable of preventing the proliferation and spread of the bacteria, followed by elimination of the bacterial antigens. Because *M. leprae* is an intracellular parasite, resistance to it depends on cell-mediated immunity characterized by phagocytosis of the bacilli by macrophages, followed by intracytoplasmic antigenic processing and presentation of antigenic determinants to lymphocytes and other cells of the immune system. In this microenvironment, the stimulated immune cells differentiate, proliferate, and secrete lymphokines and chemokines that stimulate the influx and fixation of macrophages and other cell types in the tissue areas with bacillary proliferation, thereby potentiating the immune response and the destructive action of macrophages on phagocytosed bacilli and parasitized tissues [2].

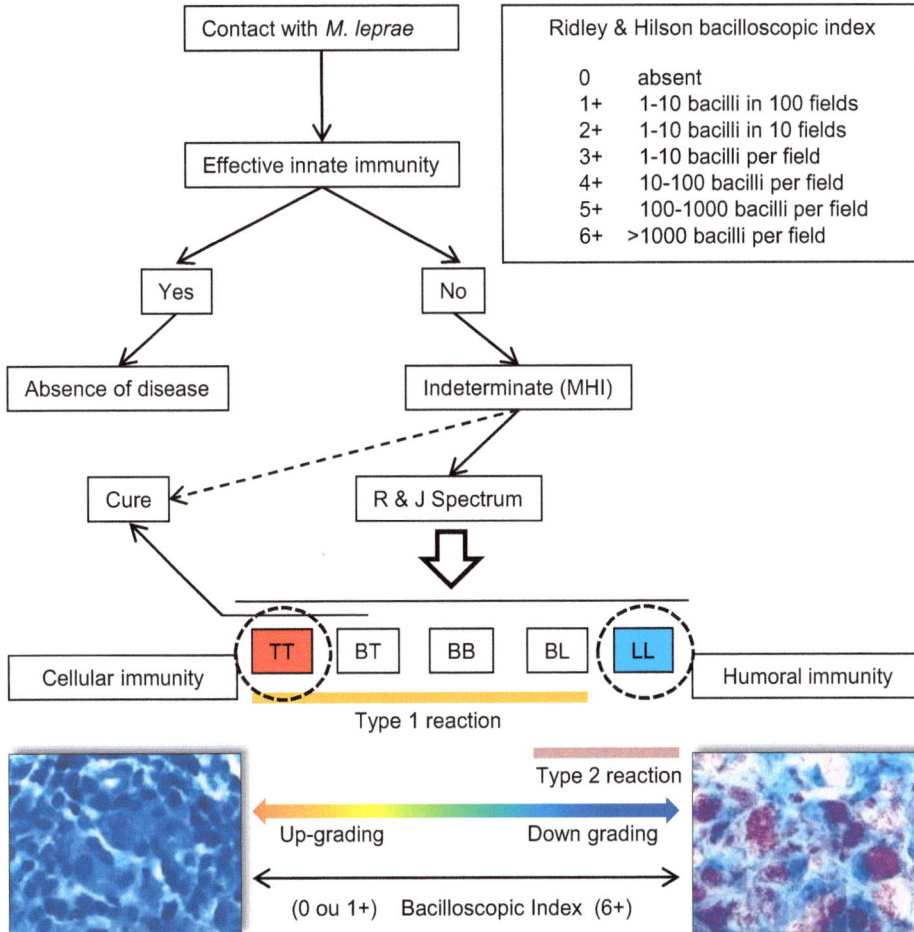

Fig. (1). Clinical spectrum and bacilloscopic index of leprosy forms and reactions. Patients who are exposed to *M. leprae* can eliminate the bacilli through the mechanisms of the primary immune response and do not develop the disease. If the primary immune defense cannot contain the proliferation of the bacilli, the patient develops indeterminate leprosy (I), the early stage of the disease preceding the polarized forms of the Ridley and Jopling (R&J) classification: tuberculoid (TT); borderline-tuberculoid (BT); borderline-borderline (BB); borderline-lepromatous (BL); and lepromatous or virchowian (LL). Late recognition of bacillary antigens by the individual may result in an intense and effective immune response (TT and BT pattern), which may lead to the destruction of the bacilli and spontaneous cure. TT individuals are those who have an effective cellular immunity. If cellular immunity is not effective, proliferation and dissemination of the bacilli persist, and the disease progresses toward the lepromatous pole. LL individuals are anergic and react to the bacilli through humoral immunity. Type 1 reactions (T1R) affect patients in the range from TT to BL. Type 2 reactions (T2R) affect patients on the lepromatous side (BL and LL). The bacilloscopic index ranges from 0-6+.

The biological behavior of the polar forms of leprosy (TT and LL) is antagonistic. They are stable manifestations of the disease, with no change or progression from one type to another during the course of the disease, even after the beginning or end of treatment (Fig. **1**) [3]. The histopathological characteristics of these two forms are also different (Fig. **2**). In all likelihood, both polar forms are rare. The majority of cases diagnosed as TT are borderline tuberculoid (BT), with or without a type 1 reaction. Moreover, most cases diagnosed as LL are actually borderline-borderline (BB) or borderline-lepromatous (BL), in which the disease has progressed for years or decades towards the lepromatous pole ("downgrading"), displaying clinical and histopathological features of the LL form [3]. These borderline patients in whom the disease has progressed for a long time and who may present clinically and histologically with characteristics similar to LL are called subpolar lepromatous patients (LLsp) [3].

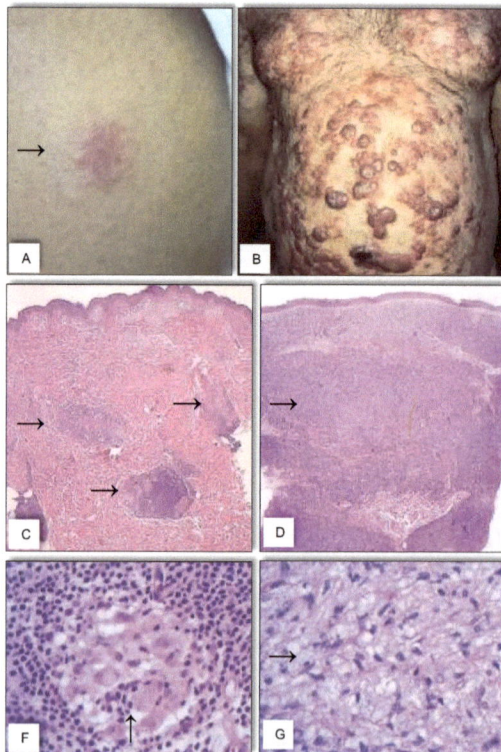

Fig. (2). Common clinical and histopathological features of the polar forms of leprosy show two completely different forms. In tuberculoid leprosy (TT), **(A)** the lesions are well delimited with raised borders, and (B and C) tuberculoid granulomas accompanying the neural branches consist of epithelioid macrophages at the center and lymphocytes at the periphery (→). In lepromatous leprosy (LL), **(D)** lesions are disseminated with the formation of papules or nodules formed by (E and F) diffuse granulomas with multivacuolated macrophages permeated by rare lymphocytes (→). (B, C, E, and F) Hematoxylin and eosin staining. (A and B) Courtesy of Dr. Cássio C. Ghidella.

TUBERCULOID LEPROSY (TT)

The tuberculoid granulomatous reaction of TT is intense and destructive in parasitized tissues. Consequently, healing is accompanied by sensory, motor, and trophic deficits in cutaneous lesions and limbs. The immunocellular response of TT patients is effective even against small amounts of the bacillary antigen. This results in a greatly reduced number of TT lesions. In general, there is one or several dermatological lesions with precise borders and limited and asymmetric impairment of neural trunks [2 - 4]. Predominant well-delimited macules are surrounded by well-defined papules or plaques with significant alteration of sensitivity, occasionally even anesthesia (Fig. **3**). Histopathologically, TT is characterized by granulomas composed of epithelioid macrophages grouped in the center of the granuloma, surrounded by a mantle of lymphocytes and other cells (Fig. **4**). In the skin, tuberculoid granulomas accompany the neural branches, resulting in an ascending arboriform structure (Fig. **4**). The deepest granulomas are larger and more organized than superficial granulomas located in the papillary dermis. In addition to granulomas in the neural branches, granulomas are occasionally observed involving the pili muscle and penetrating the basal layer of the epidermis (Fig. **4**). Some lymphocytes can be observed permeating the basal layer of the epidermis and are associated with mild epithelial hyperplasia, hyperkeratosis, and parakeratosis (Fig. **5**). Excluding the areas compromised by tuberculoid granulomas (neural branches, erector muscles of the hair, and neural filaments around cutaneous appendages and the dermal papilla), all skin components are commonly preserved (Fig. **5**). In the initial lesions and also in granulomas of the papillary derma, the number of lymphocytes around epithelioid macrophages is small. In these situations, the well-defined lymphocytic halo around the macrophages may not be observed (Fig. **6**). Granulomas in the deep dermis and subcutaneous layer present a thick lymphocytic halo around the macrophages (Fig. **6**). The epithelioid macrophages at the center of the tuberculoid granulomas are of the M1 (CD68+ and CD163-) profile (Fig. **7**) [5]. Capillary vessels are present around the periphery and are rare in the center of the granulomas (Fig. **7**). The lymphocytic infiltrate of granulomas is polyclonal with a predominance of B-lymphocytes compared to T-lymphocytes (Fig. **8**). Among T-lymphocytes, CD4+ predominates over CD8+ (CD4 > CD8, 2:1) [5]. Few plasma cells and other cells permeate B- and T-lymphocytes at the periphery of tuberculoid granulomas [5]. Rarely, lymphocytes permeate the macrophages in the center of granulomas (Fig. **8**). Neural branches within tuberculoid granulomas are dissociated, fragmented, or destroyed. In general, it is difficult to identify them in histological sections stained using hematoxylin and eosin (Fig. **9**) [6]. In this context, the use of immunohistochemical markers (S-100 and CD56 proteins) can be of great help in identifying neural fragments (Schwann cells) among macrophages (Fig. **9**) [6]. The intense neural involvement and the destruction of the neural branches lead to a significant decrease in sensitivity or anesthesia of the cutaneous lesions. The bacilloscopic examination (Fite-Faraco staining) is also of importance. In general, the bacilloscopic index of TT lesions is 0 or 1+. In approximately 40% of cases, rare bacilli (1+) can be identified mainly if multiple serial histological sections are stained using the Fite-Faraco method. Bacilli are more easily identified in partially compromised neural branches, in macrophages in the more peripheral portions of granulomas, and in mononuclear cells in the papillary dermis (Fig. 10). Bacilli are rarely found in epithelioid macrophages at the center of tuberculoid granulomas. Polymerase chain reaction (PCR) may be useful for the identification of bacillary antigens in lesions in which the BI is negative (0+) [7]. Bacilli are not observed in the interstitium, vessel wall, endothelium, glandular epithelial cells, or epidermis.

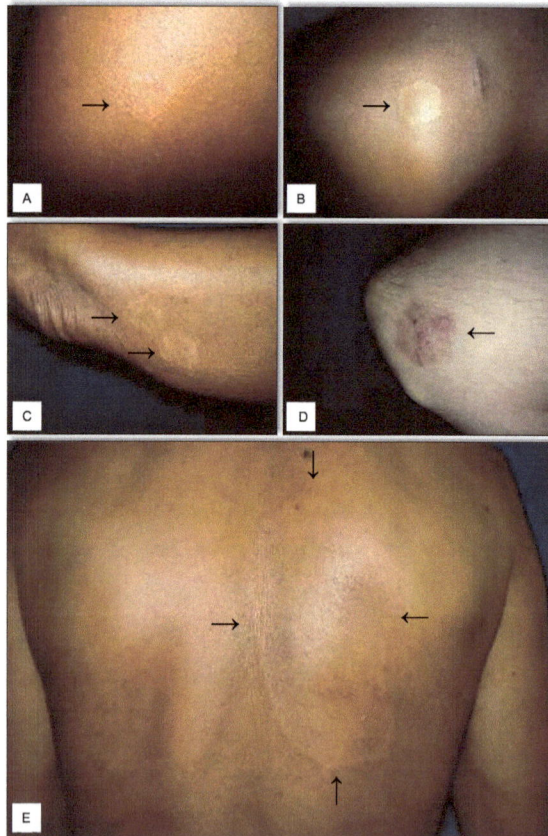

Fig. (3). Different clinical presentations of the tuberculoid (TT) form (→). **(A)** A brownish plaque with a slightly raised surface and infiltrated edges with minute papules. **(B)** A plaque lesion with a homogeneous infiltrative appearance. **(C)** An infiltrated lesion with slight atrophy. **(D)** An atrophic and purpuric lesion. **(E)** Large lesion involving part of the back. Courtesy of Dr. Cássio C. Ghidella.

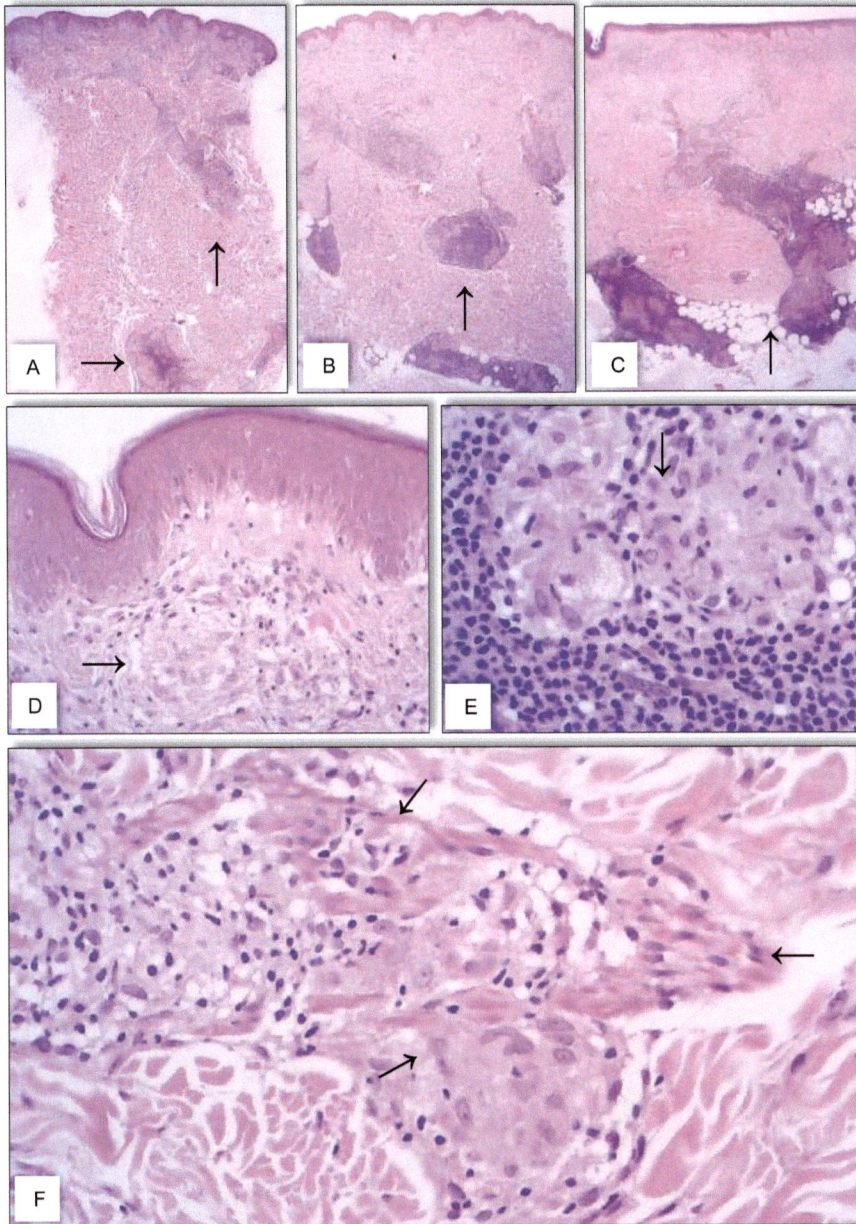

Fig. (4). Histopathological characteristics of tuberculoid leprosy (TT) lesions. (A, B, and C) The granulomas follow the ascending path of the neural branches, from the subcutaneous to the superficial portions of the dermis (→). **(D)** Superficial granulomas in the papillary dermis have few lymphocytes involving macrophages and can focally permeate the epidermis (→). **(E)** Deep granulomas are well organized with epithelioid macrophages at the center and a thick mantle of lymphocytes at the periphery (→). **(F)** Granulomas commonly involve the pili muscle (→). (A-F) Hematoxylin and eosin staining.

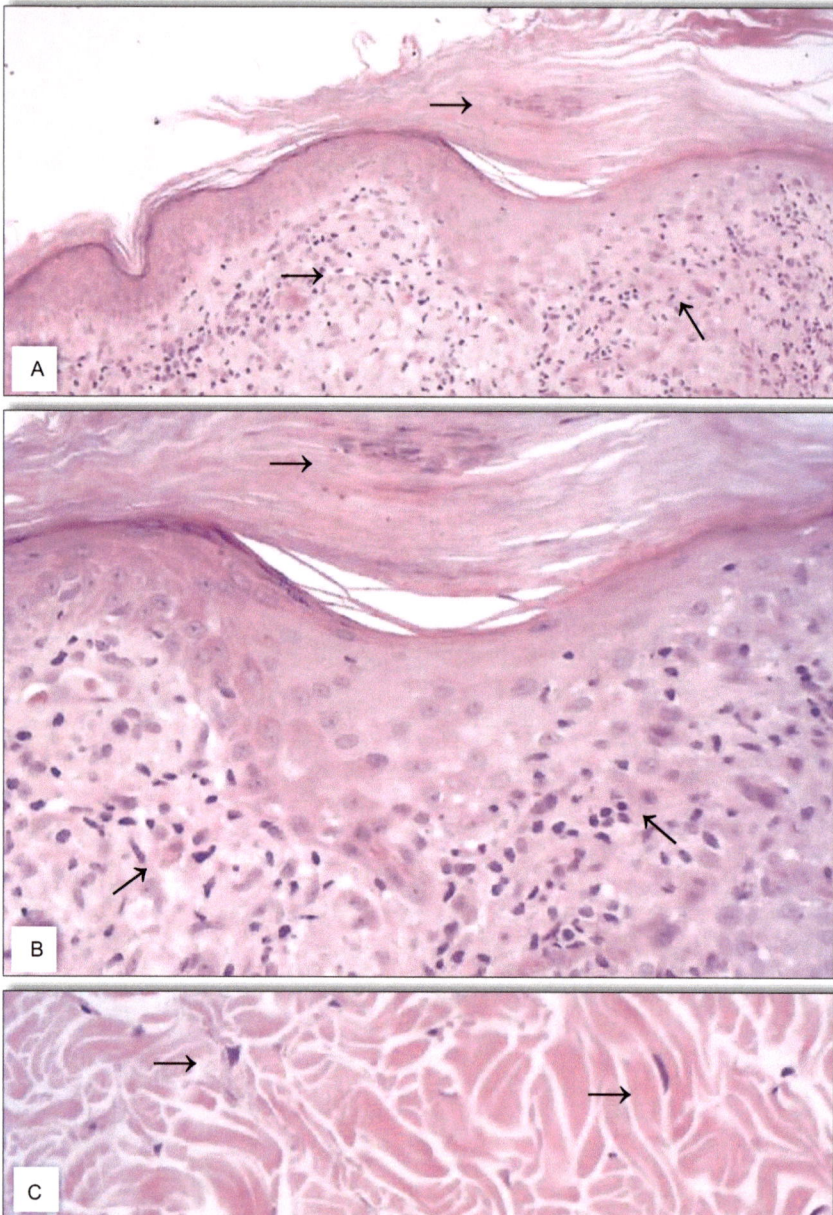

Fig. (5). Histopathological characteristics of tuberculoid leprosy (TT) lesions. (A and B) A small number of lymphocytes can be observed permeating the basal layer of the epidermis and are associated with discrete epithelial hyperplasia, hyperkeratosis, and parakeratosis (→). **(C)** Interstitial fibroblasts are not parasitized (→). (A, B, and C) Hematoxylin and eosin staining.

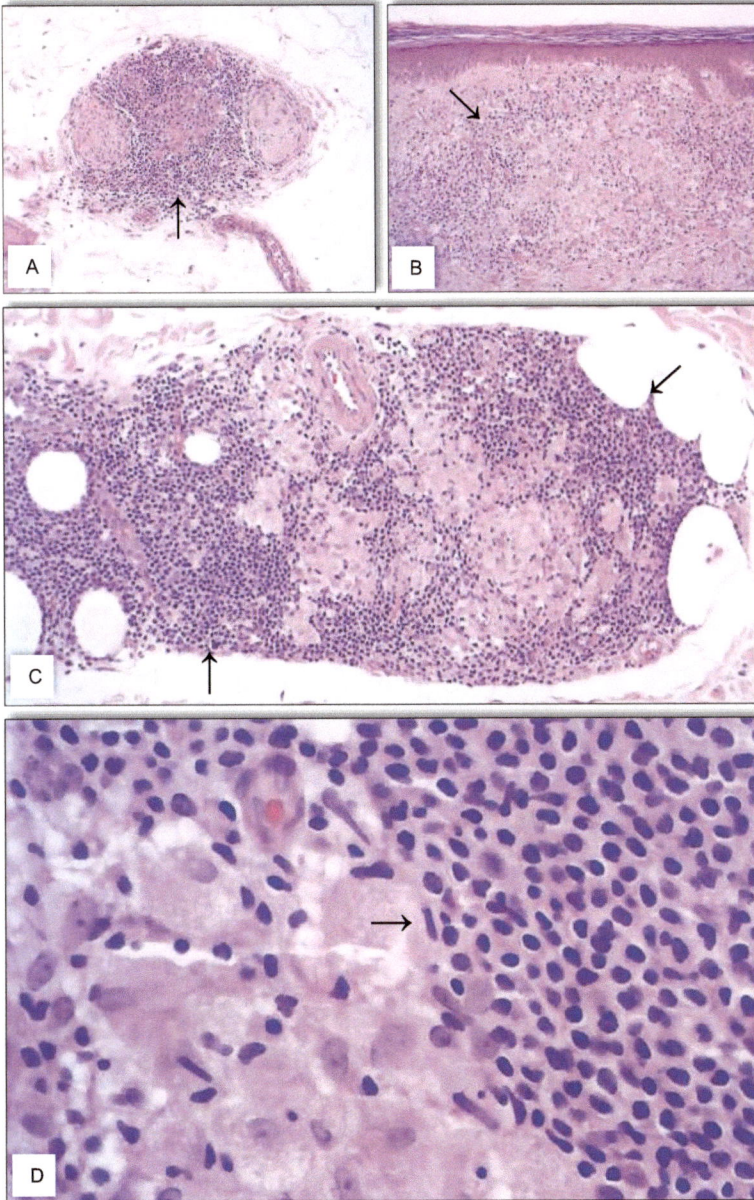

Fig. (6). Histopathological characteristics of tuberculoid leprosy (TT) lesions. **(A)** In the initial lesions when tuberculoid granulomas are forming and in granulomas in the papillary dermis **(B)**, the number of lymphocytes around the epithelioid macrophages is small and there may be no well-defined lymphocytic halo. (C and D) Granulomas in the deep and subcutaneous dermis present a thick lymphocytic halo around the epithelioid macrophages. (A-D) Hematoxylin and eosin staining.

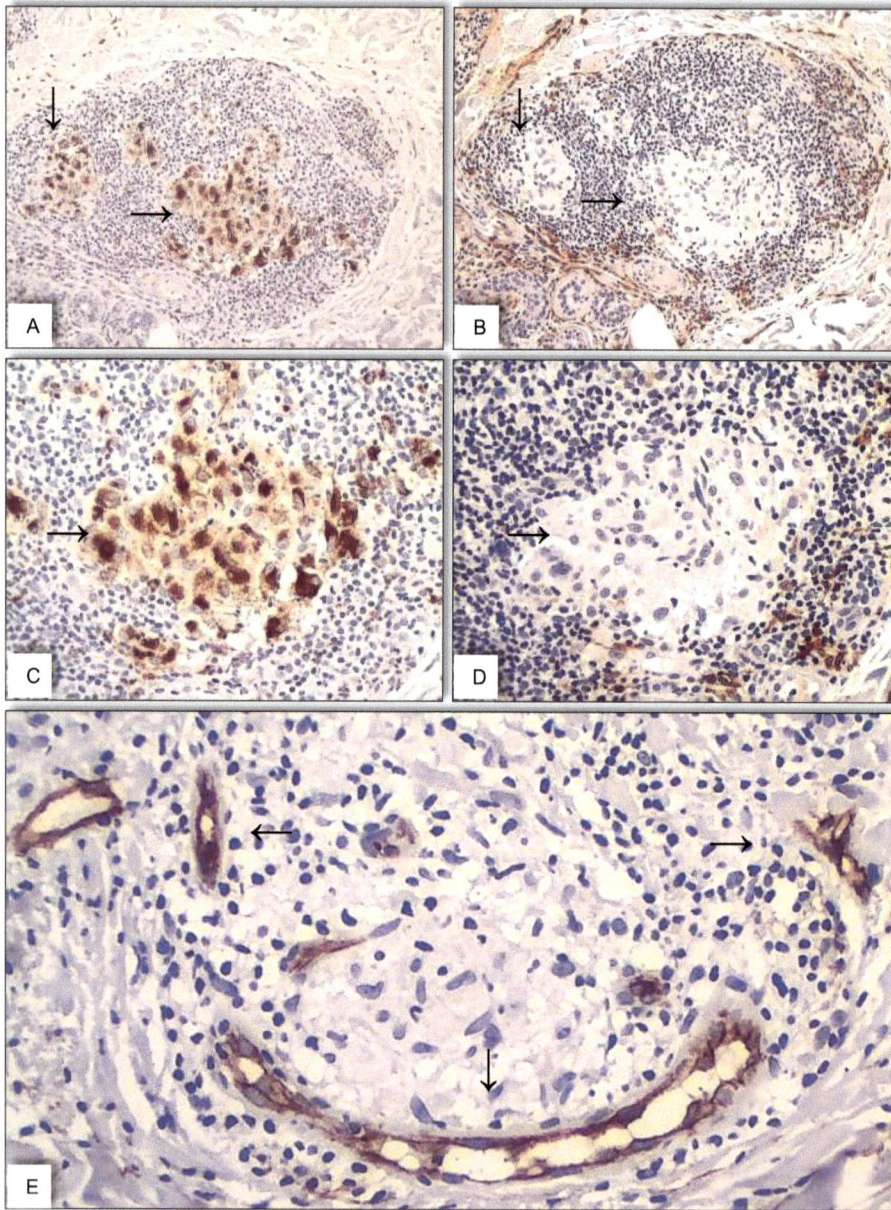

Fig. (7). Histopathological characteristics and immunohistochemical profile of tuberculoid leprosy (TT) lesions. (A and B) The epithelioid macrophages at the center of the TT granulomas are of the M1 profile (CD68+ and CD163-). (A and C) Expression of CD68 in macrophages (→). (B and D) Absence of CD163 expression in epithelioid macrophages (→). **(E)** Capillary vessels predominate on the periphery of granulomas (→) (CD31). (A-E) Immunohistochemistry.

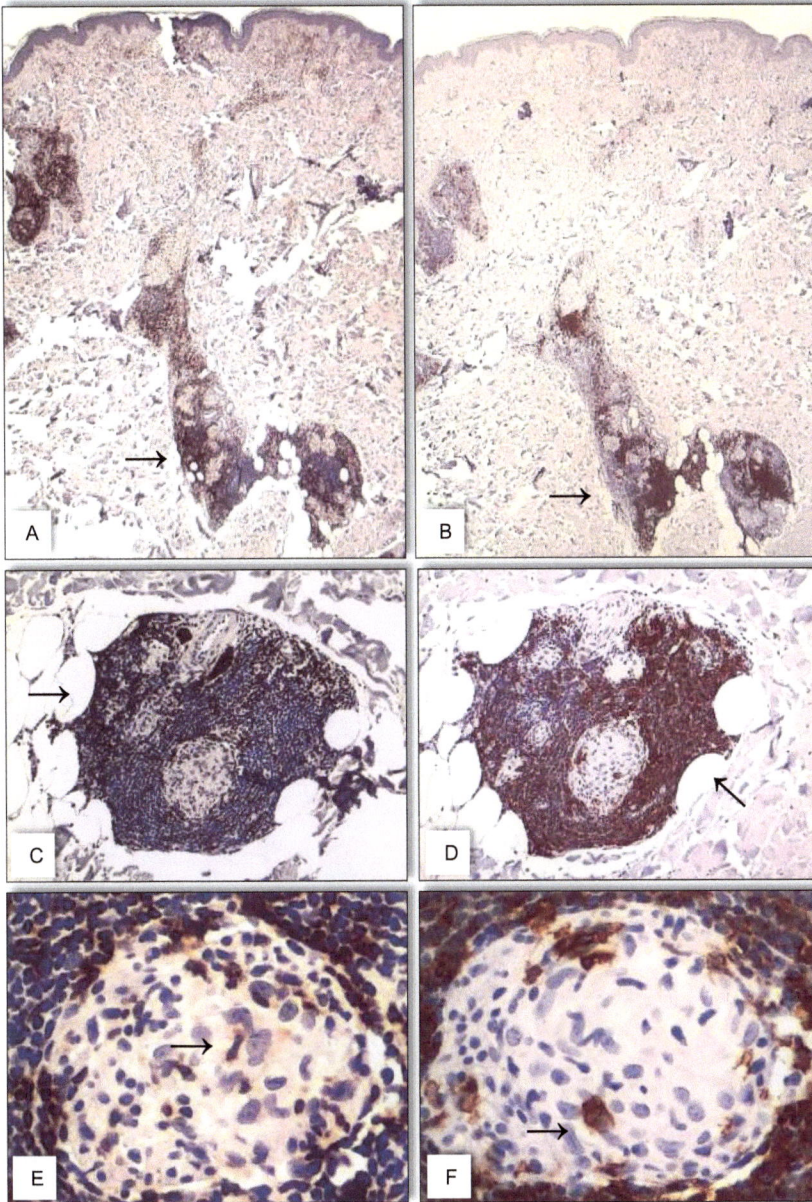

Fig. (8). Immunohistochemical profile of lymphocytes present in the granulomas of tuberculoid leprosy (TT) lesions. Sequential sections for CD3 and CD20 (→) immunostaining. (A, C, and E) Expression of CD3 in T-lymphocytes at the periphery of granulomas are rare, permeating the epithelioid macrophages to the center. (B, D, and F) Expression of CD20 on B-lymphocytes in the same granulomas. Note that in deep granulomas there is a predominance of "B" lymphocytes (CD20+) in relation to "T" lymphocytes (CD3+). (A-F) Immunohistochemistry.

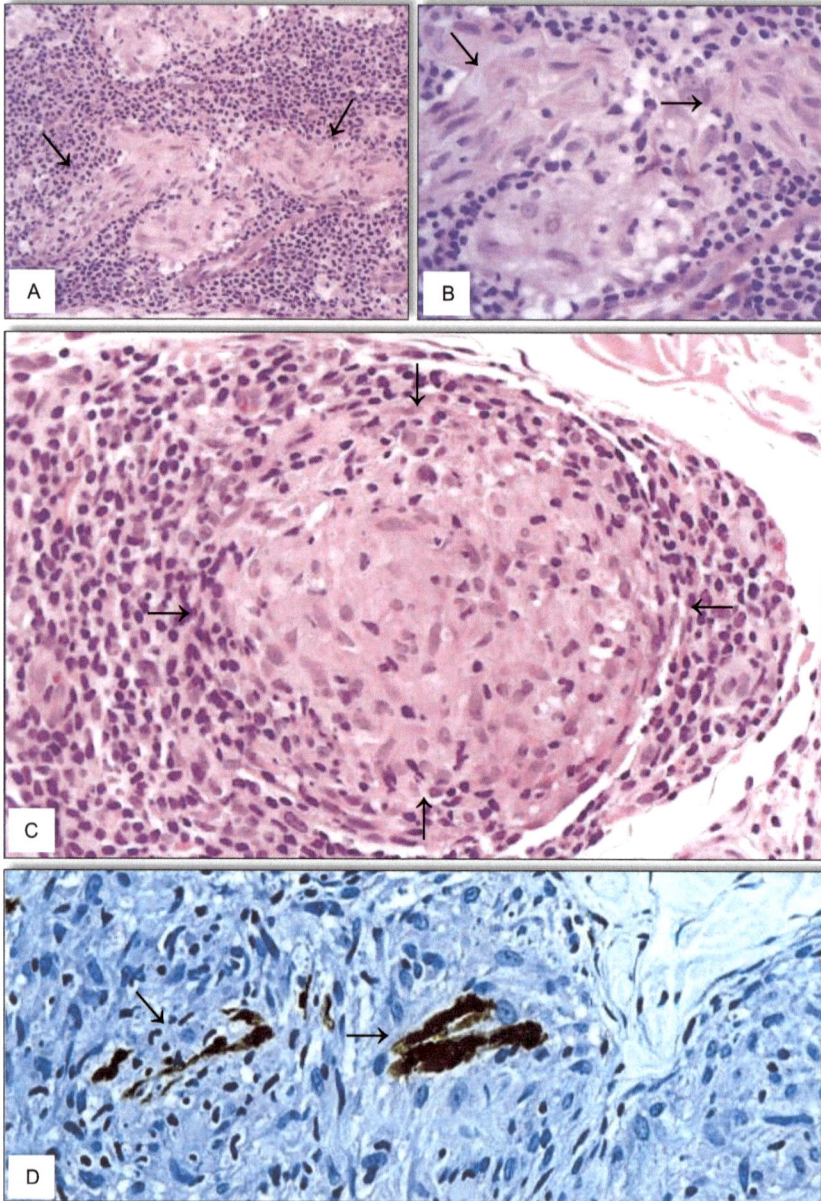

Fig. (9). Histopathological characteristics of the granulomas of tuberculoid leprosy (TT) lesions. (A and B) Tuberculoid granuloma involving fragmenting neural branches (→). **(C)** Tuberculoid granuloma compromising the entire nerve associated with the expansion of neural boundaries by epithelioid macrophages (→). **(D)** Presence of Schwann cells (S-100+ protein) within the tuberculoid granuloma with extensive neural involvement, evidencing nerve remnants (→). (A-C) Hematoxylin and eosin staining. **(D)** Immunohistochemistry.

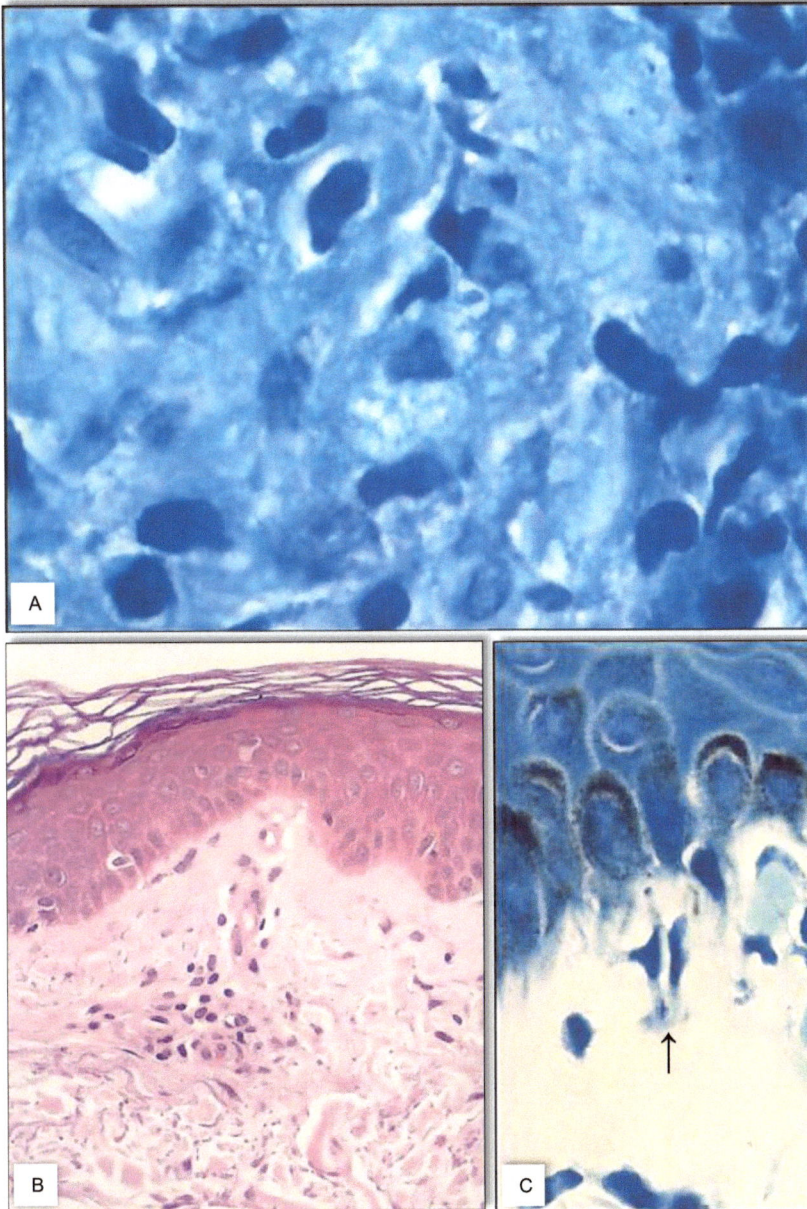

Fig. (10). Characteristics of the bacilloscopic examination of tuberculoid leprosy (TT) lesions. **(A)** Absence of bacilli within the tuberculoid granulomas (BI 0+). (B and C) Bacilli present, probably in small neural branches, in the papillary dermis (→). (A and C) Fite-Faraco staining. **(B)** Hematoxylin and eosin staining.

The main differential diagnoses are other infectious and non-infectious cutaneous granulomatous diseases, such as paracoccidioidomycosis, late secondary syphilis, annular granuloma, and diseases with histological characteristics of necrobiosis, tuberculosis, and sarcoidosis [8, 9]. In these diseases, the granulomas are not characteristically neurocentric, and there is no destruction of the neural branches. Moreover, the presence of eosinophilic infiltrate is common in fungal infections but rare in all forms of leprosy including reactive leprosy (T1R and T2R) (Figs. **11** and **12**). Another important point is the differentiation between tuberculoid granulomas (TT) and type 1 reaction (T1R) granulomas by pathologists. Although they have similarities, certain histological features can be used to distinguish them; these features are discussed in detail in Chapter 5.

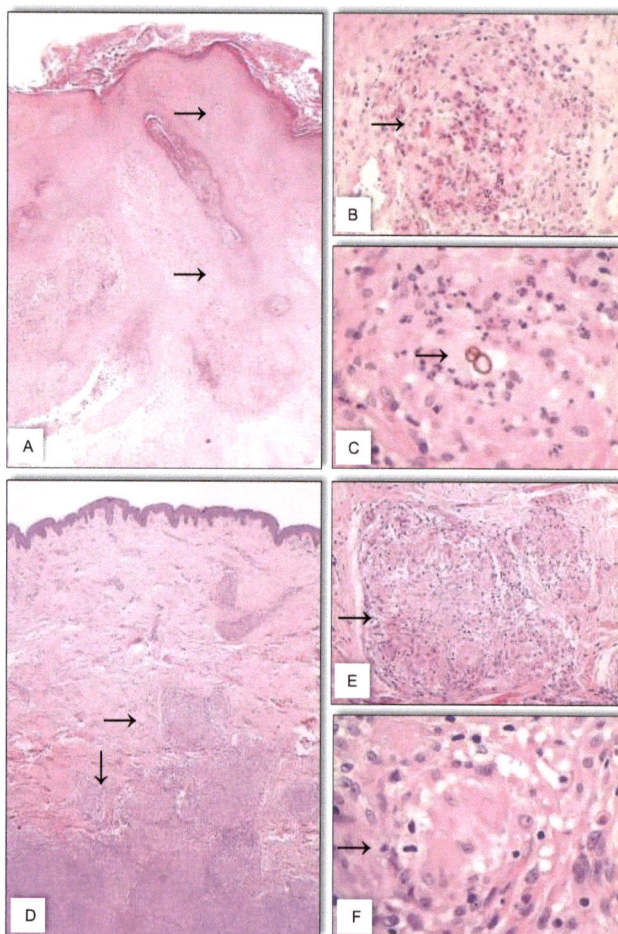

Fig. (11). Histopathological differential diagnoses of tuberculoid leprosy. (A, B, and C) Skin lesion with a clinical hypothesis of TT and histopathological diagnosis of chromoblastomycosis. Note the intense epithelial hyperplasia **(A)**, granulomas containing eosinophils, and the presence of the pigmented fungus involving neutrophils inside the granuloma **(C)** (→). (D, E, and F) Histopathological characteristics of sarcoidosis, showing granulomas that do not follow the path of the neural branches and do not present the thick lymphocytic mantle of TT granulomas (→). (A-F) Hematoxylin and eosin staining.

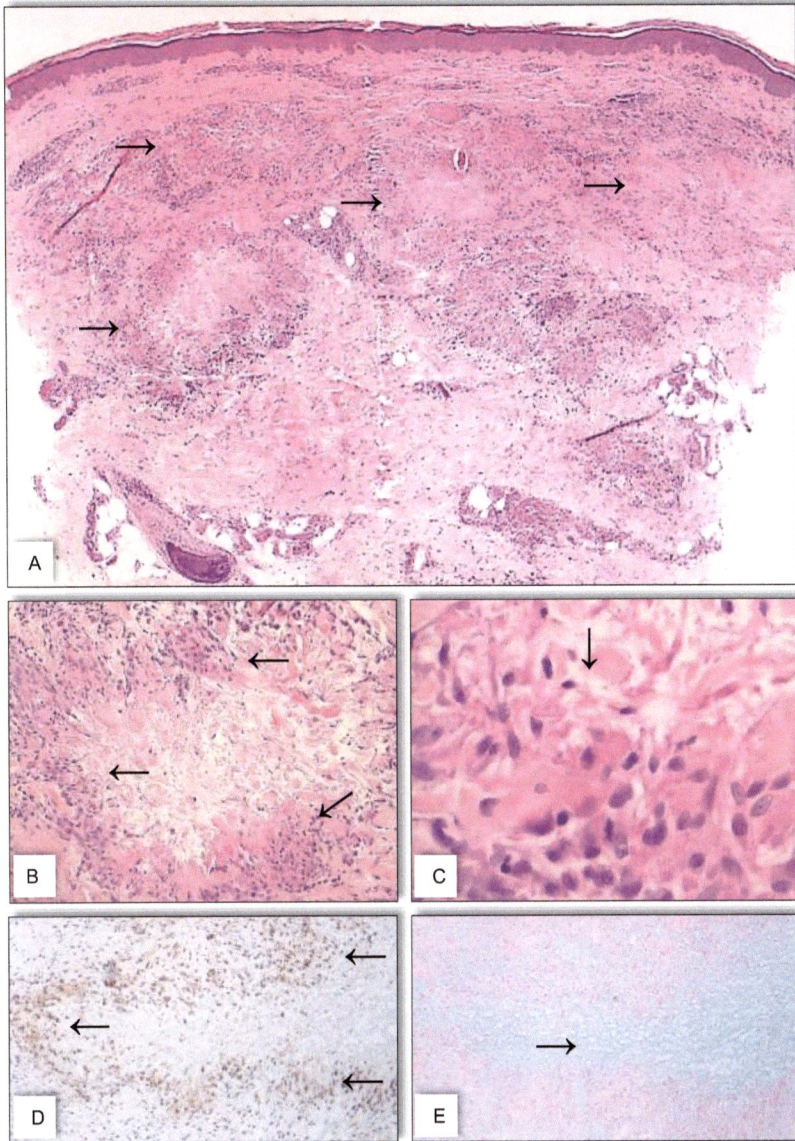

Fig. (12). Histopathological differential diagnosis of tuberculoid leprosy (TT). Clinically suspected lesion of TT leprosy and histopathological diagnosis of annular granuloma. (A, B, and C) Granulomas without ascending involvement of the neural branches and with a central area of necrobiosis surrounded by macrophages (→). **(D)** Positivity to CD68 (→) showing macrophages in the periphery and **(E)** alcian blue staining showing mucin deposition in the center of the granuloma (→). (A-C) Hematoxylin and eosin staining. **(D)** Immunohistochemistry. **(E)** Alcian blue staining.

Therefore, the main clinical-pathological features for the diagnosis of TT are: (1) tuberculoid granulomas accompanying the neural pathway from the deep layer to the surface (ascending neurocentric granulomas); (2) well-organized deep granulomas with epithelioid macrophages at the center and a thick lymphocytic mantle; (3) negative or positive smear microscopy (BI 0-1+), identification of bacilli in granulomas, neural branches, or mononuclear cells in the papillary dermis, and (4) sensitivity changes present in almost all lesions, sometimes with anesthesia.

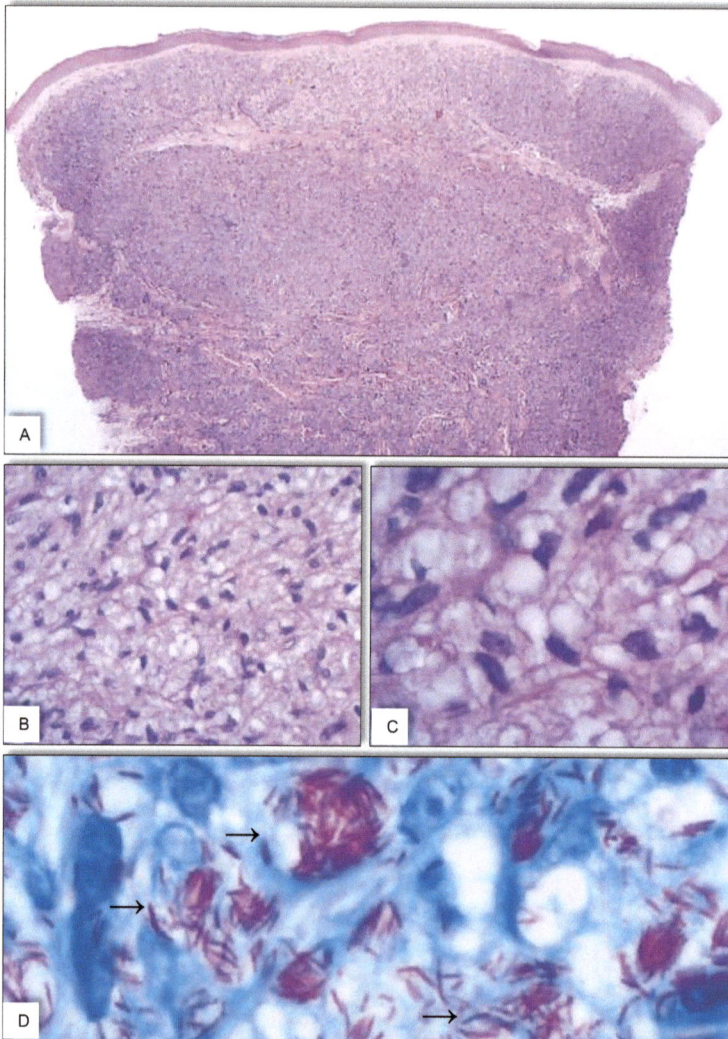

Fig. (13). Histopathological characteristics and bacilloscopic examination of lepromatous leprosy (LL) lesions. **(A)** Granulomas are extensive and compromise most of the dermis and subcutaneous tissue. (B and C) Macrophages are multivacuolated with rare adjacent lymphocytes. **(D)** Intracytoplasmic vacuoles contain a large number of bacilli (→). (A, B, and C) Hematoxylin and eosin staining. **(D)** Fite-Faraco staining.

VIRCHOWIAN OR LEPROMATOUS LEPROSY (LL)

In contrast to the vast majority of the population that have different degrees of immunocellular reaction against *M. leprae*, a small portion presents very low resistance or is anergic to the bacillus [1]. Individuals in this latter group, when infected with *M. leprae*, will develop the lepromatous polar (LL) form of leprosy. Upon the proliferation of *M. leprae* in the tissues, they will present a reaction almost exclusively composed of macrophagic granulomas where the macrophages are multivacuolated containing a large number of bacilli (Fig. **13**). There is no restriction on the proliferation and spread of the bacilli. Cutaneous lesions are generalized and consist of diffuse infiltrations, papules, or nodules (Figs. **14** and **15**) [2 - 4]. In all likelihood, macrophages phagocytose the bacilli but are unable to destroy them to present antigenic determinants that can stimulate the immune system. In addition to the skin and neural branches, there is involvement of the mucous membranes of the airways, lymph nodes, spleen, liver, adrenal glands, bone marrow, synovium, epididymis, testes, and eyeballs, among others [2].

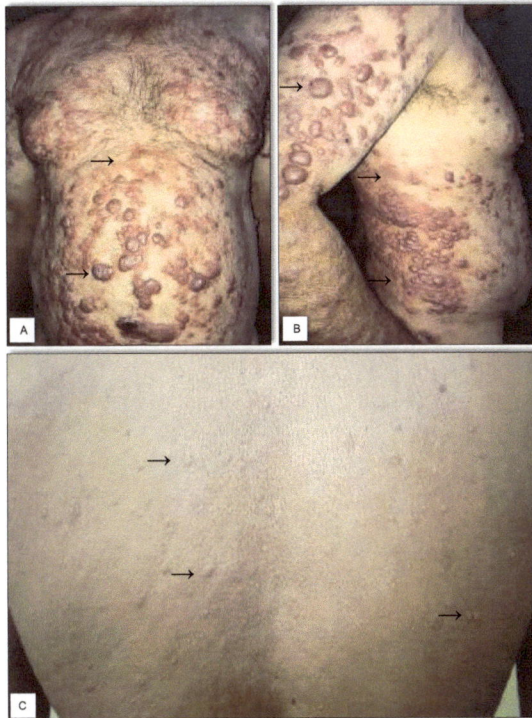

Fig. (14). Different clinical presentations of lepromatous leprosy (LL) (→). (A and B) Exuberant clinical presentation of plaques, nodules, and tubers. The entire integument is compromised by specific infiltration. (**C**) Another example less exuberant but with diffuse infiltration of the entire integument. Courtesy of Dr. Cássio C. Ghidella.

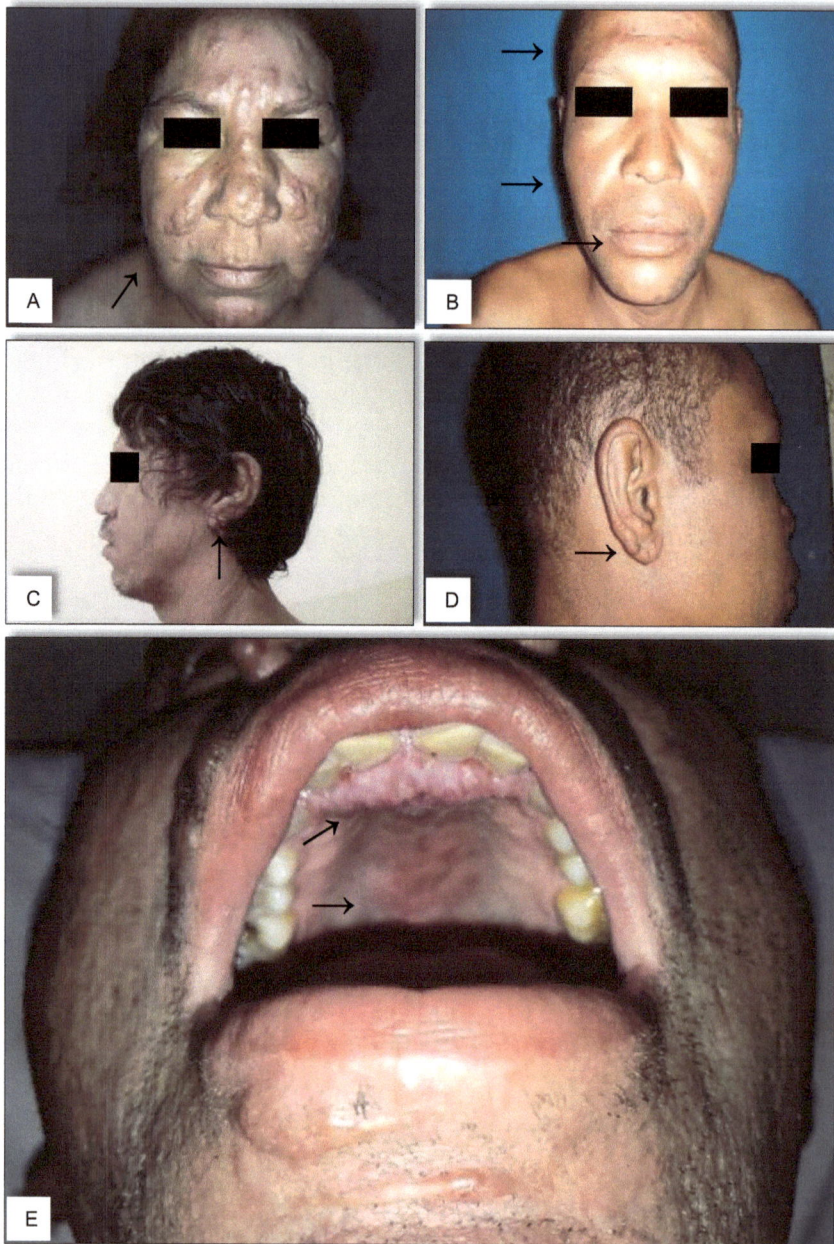

Fig. (15). Different clinical presentations of lepromatous leprosy (LL) (→). **(A)** Diffuse infiltration of the face with multiple nodules and a clinical history of disease progression for many years. **(B)** Diffuse infiltration of the skin and the formation of small nodules on the forehead. (C and D) Uniform infiltration of the skin of the face and the presence of nodules (lepromas) on the ear lobes. **(E)** Infiltration of the gingival mucosa and hard palate. Courtesy of Dr. Cássio C. Ghidella.

Inflammatory infiltrates of LL lesions are extensive and compromise a large part of the tissues of the dermis but do not destroy the affected tissues (Fig. **13**). All layers of the neural branches are permeated by multivacuolated macrophages containing large numbers of bacilli. The endoneural structures adapt to the macrophagic infiltrate. It is only after the long-term evolution of the disease that neurological "deficits" begin to be observed. Therefore, although the neural branches are intensely parasitized by the bacilli and infiltrated by macrophages, they remain relatively well preserved (Fig. **16**). The epidermis is commonly atrophic and linear. There is a collagenized and acellular band (the grenz zone) located in the papillary dermis, between the basal layer of the epidermis and the macrophagic infiltrate in the dermis, called the Unna band (Fig. **17**). Bacilli are rare or absent in the Unna band (Fig. **17**). Subcutaneous adipose tissue and a large part of the dermal interstitium are also impaired (Fig. **18**). Unlike tuberculoid granulomas, where macrophages are accompanied by a large number of lymphocytes, lepromatous granulomas are composed mostly of macrophages with multivacuolated cytoplasm and vesicular nuclei permeated by a small number of lymphocytes and rare plasma cells (Fig. **19**). These macrophages almost exclusively have the M2 profile (CD68+ and CD163+) (Fig. **19**). The vacuoles inside the macrophages are filled with fragmented and solid bacilli. Intense bacillary proliferation occurs within the intracytoplasmic vacuoles, with large numbers of bacilli arranged in overlapping, stacking structures called globi (Fig. **19**).

The bacilloscopic examination presents important characteristics of LL. The bacilloscopic index is 5 + or 6 +. In addition to the bacilli-parasitizing macrophages, neural branches, and erector muscles of the hair, it is common to observe bacilli in the vascular (blood and lymphatic) endothelium, in the smooth muscle cells of the vessel wall, and in mononuclear cells in the vessel lumen (bacillemia) (Fig. **20**). In some cases, it is possible to observe the parasitism of epithelial and myoepithelial cells of the sweat glands, squamous and sebaceous cells of the pilosebaceous follicles, squamous and melanocytic cells of the epidermis, and all the cells that make up the tissues of the nasal and oral mucosae (Figs. **21 - 24**). This indicates that patients with the LL form can eliminate *M. leprae* through the mucosa, the secretions of the sweat glands and the pilosebaceous follicles, and also through the transepidermal route. Generally, patients with intense and diffuse parasitism of the tissues by the bacilli are those with an extended period of evolution of the disease (many years or decades), resulting in the detection of the bacilli in virtually any segment of the skin, including the nail bed and scalp, as well as tissues of the internal organs. In our experience, we have observed *M. leprae* parasitism of neoplastic cells in neurofibroma, schwannoma, melanocytic dermal nevus, and basal cell carcinoma in leprosy patients with lepromatous forms of the disease (BL and LL). There are two special clinical presentations of LL: (1) Wade's histoid leprosy and (2) leprosy of Lucio-Latapi ("lepra bonita"). Both are described in detail in Chapter 8.

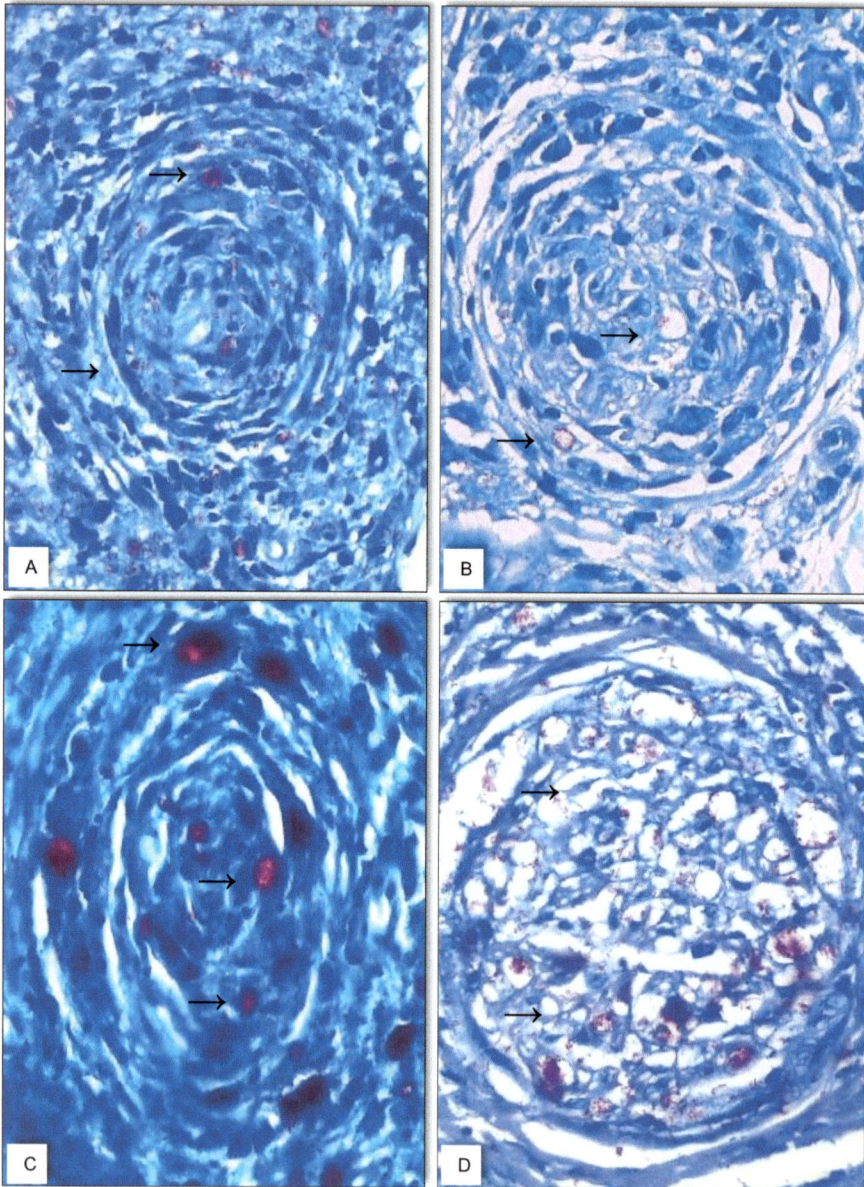

Fig. (16). Neural branches in lepromatous leprosy (LL) lesions are permeated in all its layers by multivacuolated macrophages containing large numbers of bacilli (→). (A-D) The infiltration pattern of the neural branches is concentric ("target" or "onion" type). (A-D) Fite-Faraco staining.

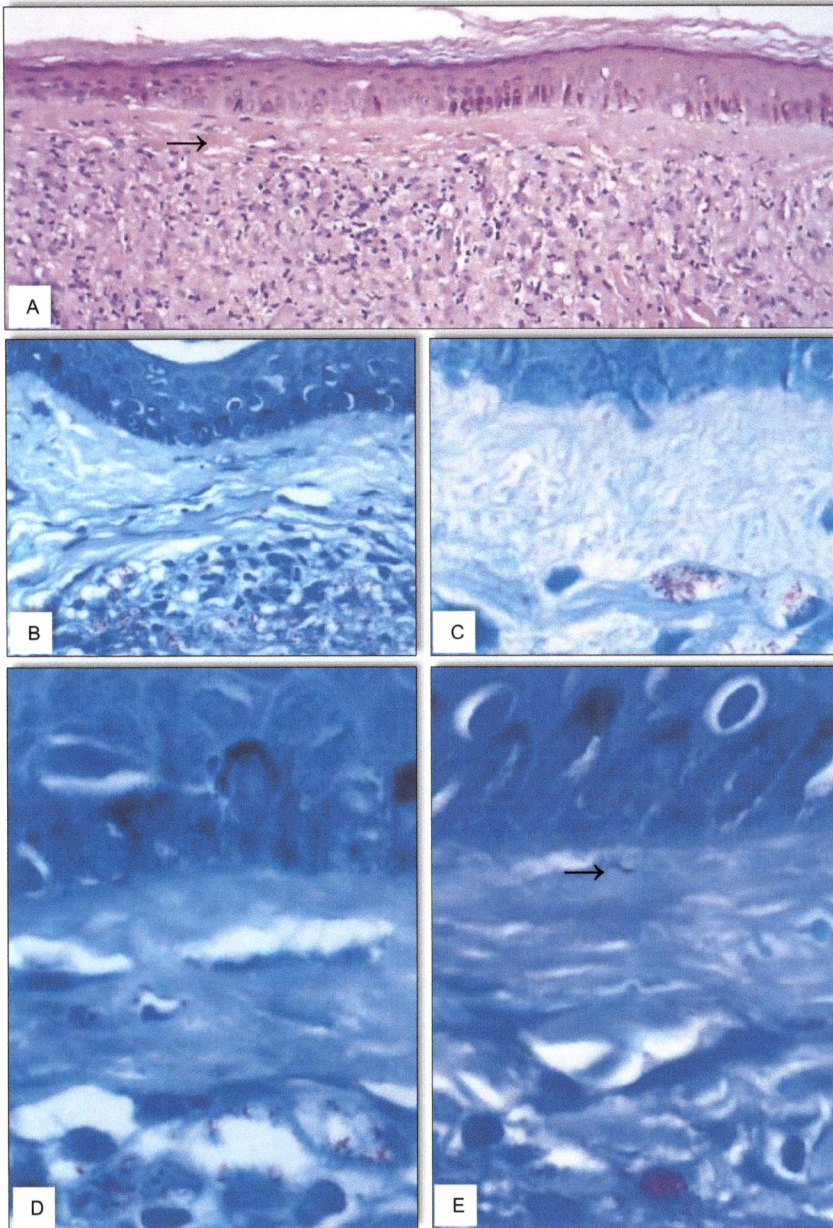

Fig. (17). (A) In lepromatous leprosy (LL) lesions, the epidermis is usually atrophic and rectified. There is a collagenized zone occupying the papillary dermis (the grenz zone) between the basal layer and the macrophage infiltrate just below, known as the Unna band (→). **(B-E)** Bacilli are rare or absent in the Unna band (→). **(A)** Hematoxylin and eosin staining. **(B-E)** Fite-Faraco staining.

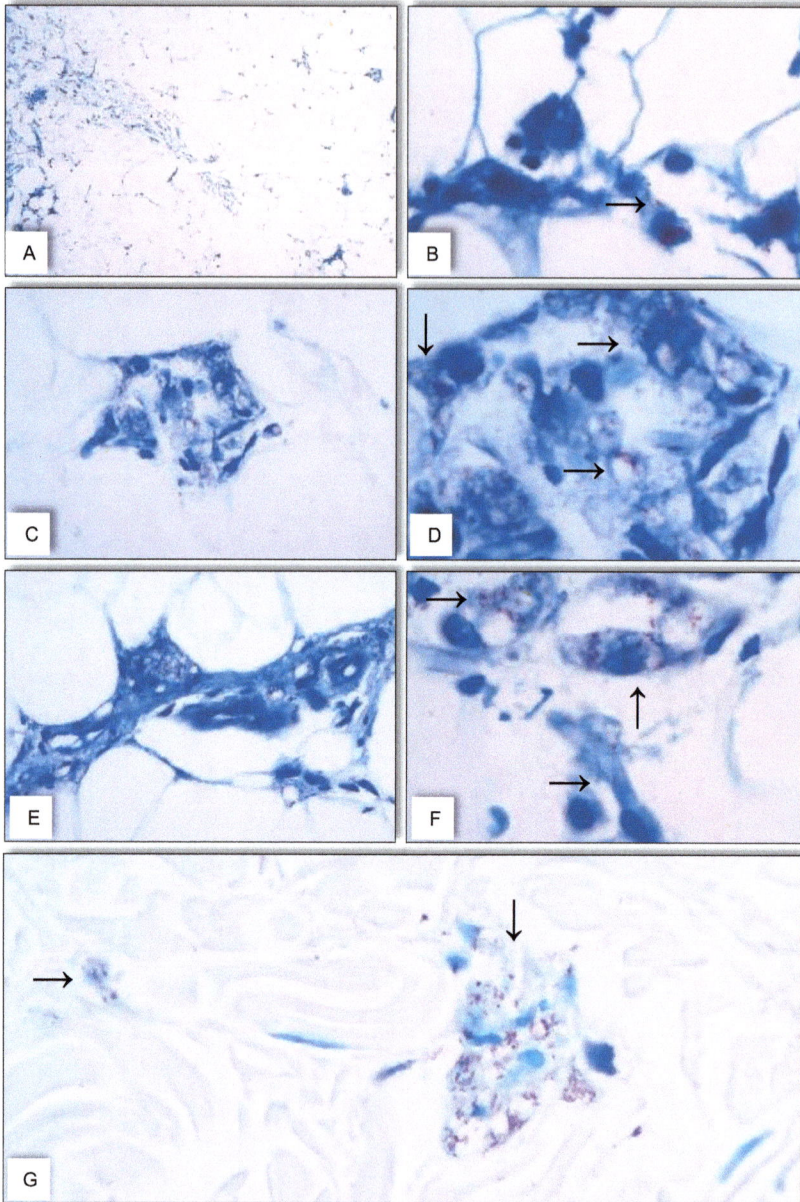

Fig. (18). (A-G) Lepromatous leprosy (LL) lesion with involvement of subcutaneous adipose tissue and a large part of the dermal interstitium. *M. leprae*, parasitizing macrophages, vessels, adipose cells, and fibroblasts (→). (A-G) Fite-Faraco staining.

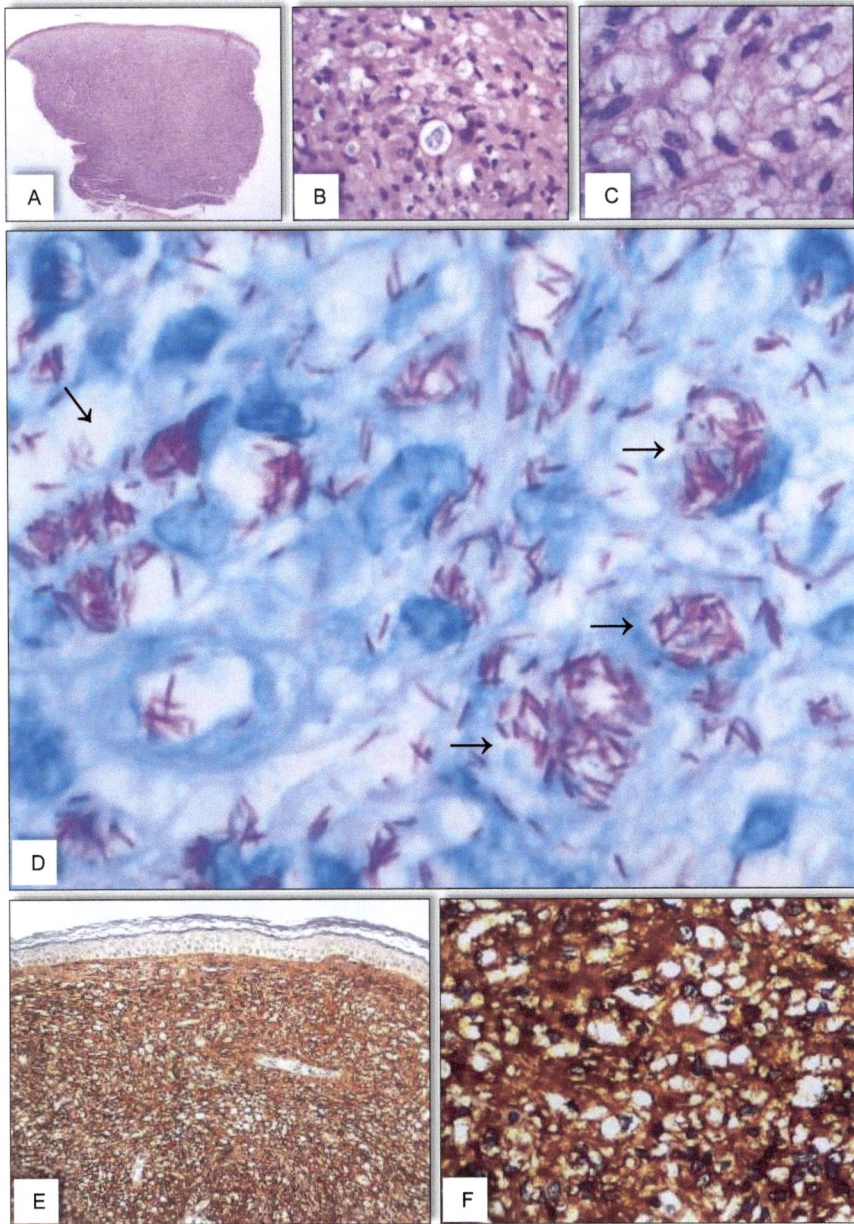

Fig. (19). (A-C) Lepromatous leprosy (LL) granulomas consist largely of macrophages with vacuolated cytoplasm and vesicular nuclei permeated by rare lymphocytes and plasma cells. **(D)** Vacuoles in the cytoplasm of macrophages are filled by bacilli. There is intense bacillary proliferation within the vacuoles, with many bacilli arranged in layers called globi (→). These macrophages are almost exclusively of the M2 profile (CD68+ and CD163+). (A-C) Hematoxylin and eosin staining. **(D)** Fite-Faraco staining. Immunohistochemistry **(E)** CD68+ and **(F)** CD163+.

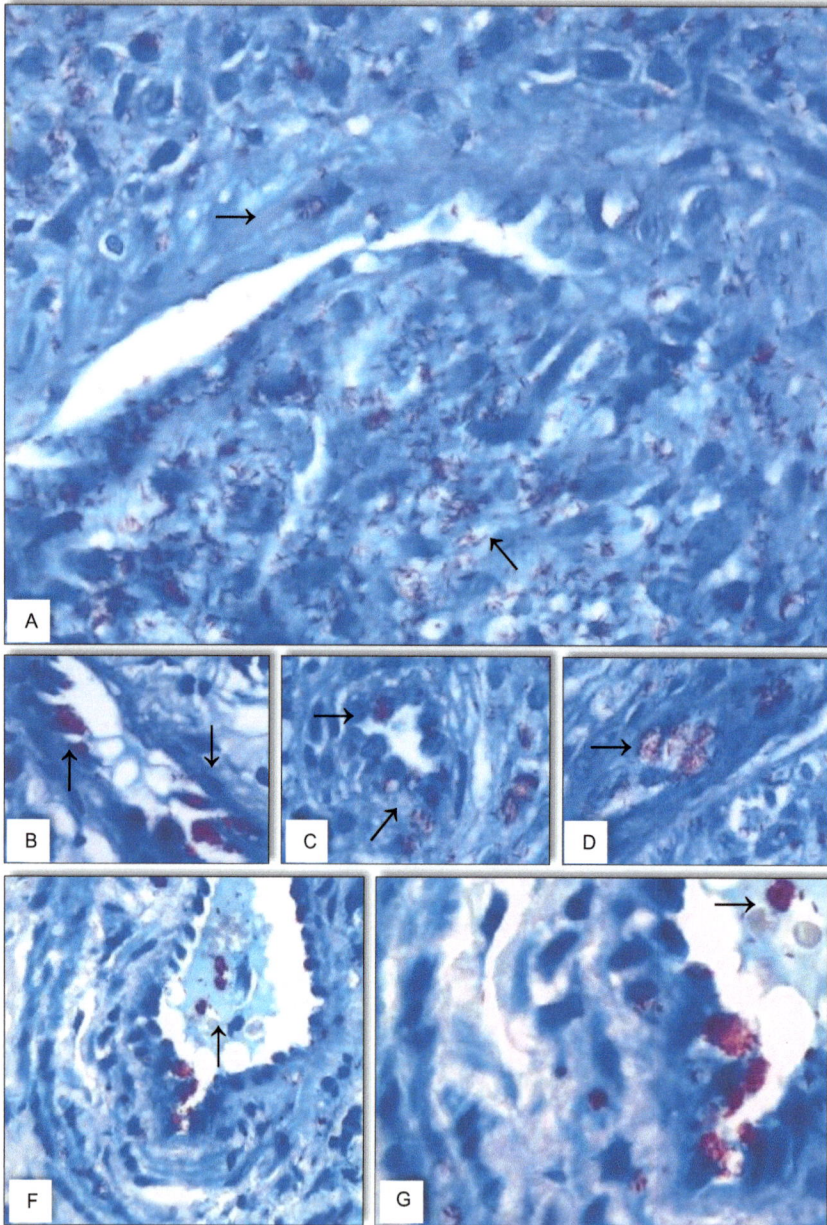

Fig. (20). (A-D) In lepromatous leprosy (LL) lesions, there is important parasitism of the smooth muscle cells of the vessel wall and also of the endothelium (→). (E and F) Moreover, it is possible to observe mononuclear cells parasitized by *M. leprae* in the vessel lumen (bacillaemia) (→). (A-F) Fite-Faraco staining.

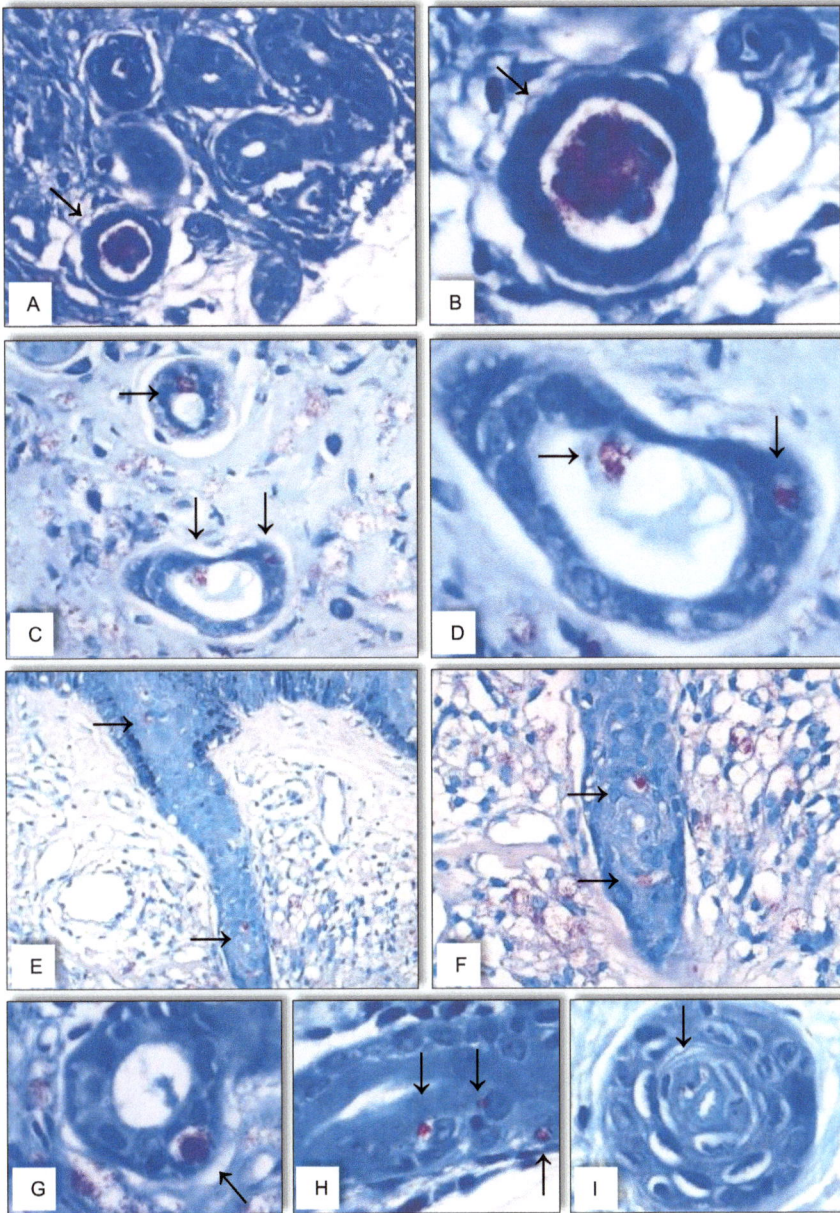

Fig. (21). Lepromatous leprosy (LL) lesion with bacilli parasitizing sweat glands. There is parasitism at different levels and types of glandular cells. (A-D) Parasitism of secretory epithelial cells and myoepithelial cells in the secretory portion of the glands, including cells parasitized inside the gland lumen (→). (E-I) Bacilli parasitizing the secretory and excretory portions of the glands (eccrine duct), with bacilli within myoepithelial and epithelial cells (→). (A-I) Fite-Faraco staining.

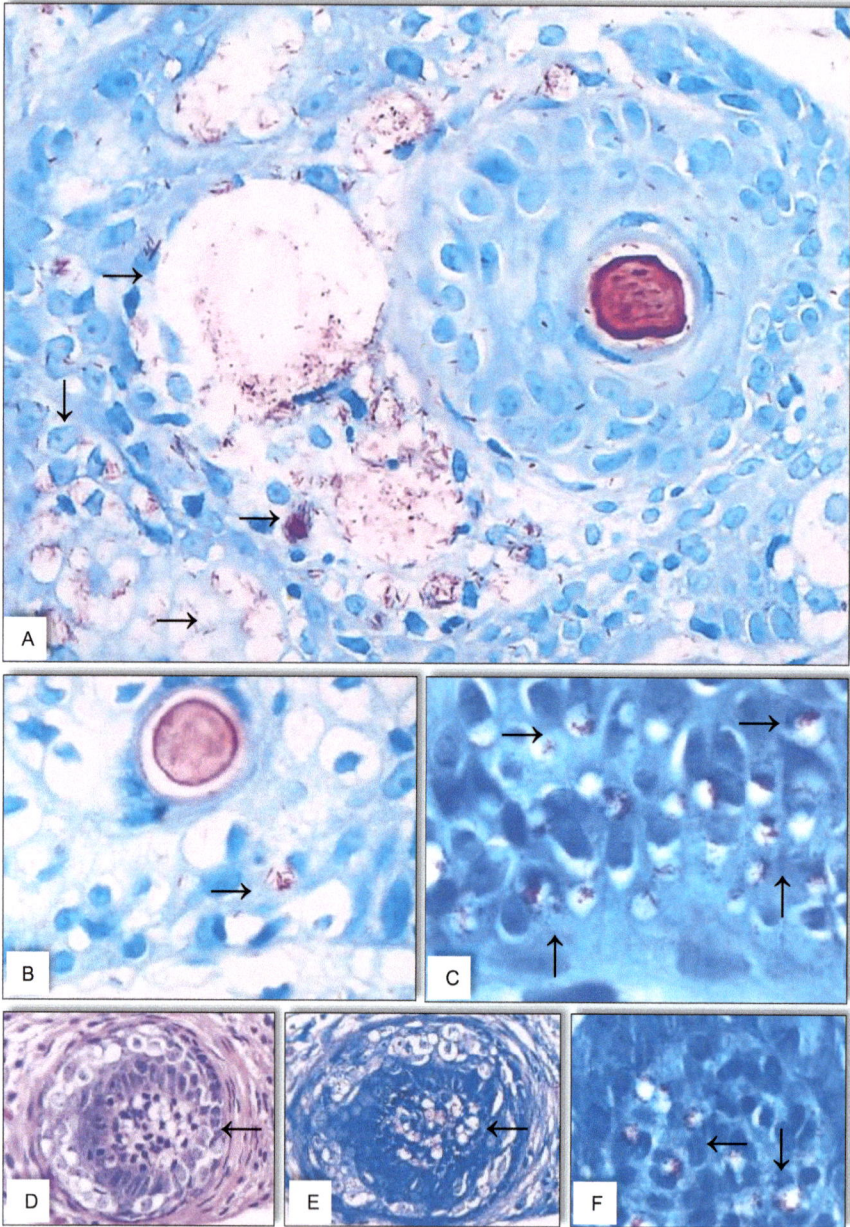

Fig. (22). Histopathological characteristics and bacilloscopic examination of lepromatous leprosy (LL) lesions with involvement of the pilosebaceous follicle. (A, B, and C) Bacilli parasitizing different cell types (sebaceous and squamous from the hair sheath) of the pilosebaceous unit (→). (D, E, and F) Parasitism of cells of the dermal papilla of the pilosebaceous follicle (→). (A, B, C, and E) Fite-Faraco staining. **(D)** Hematoxylin and eosin staining.

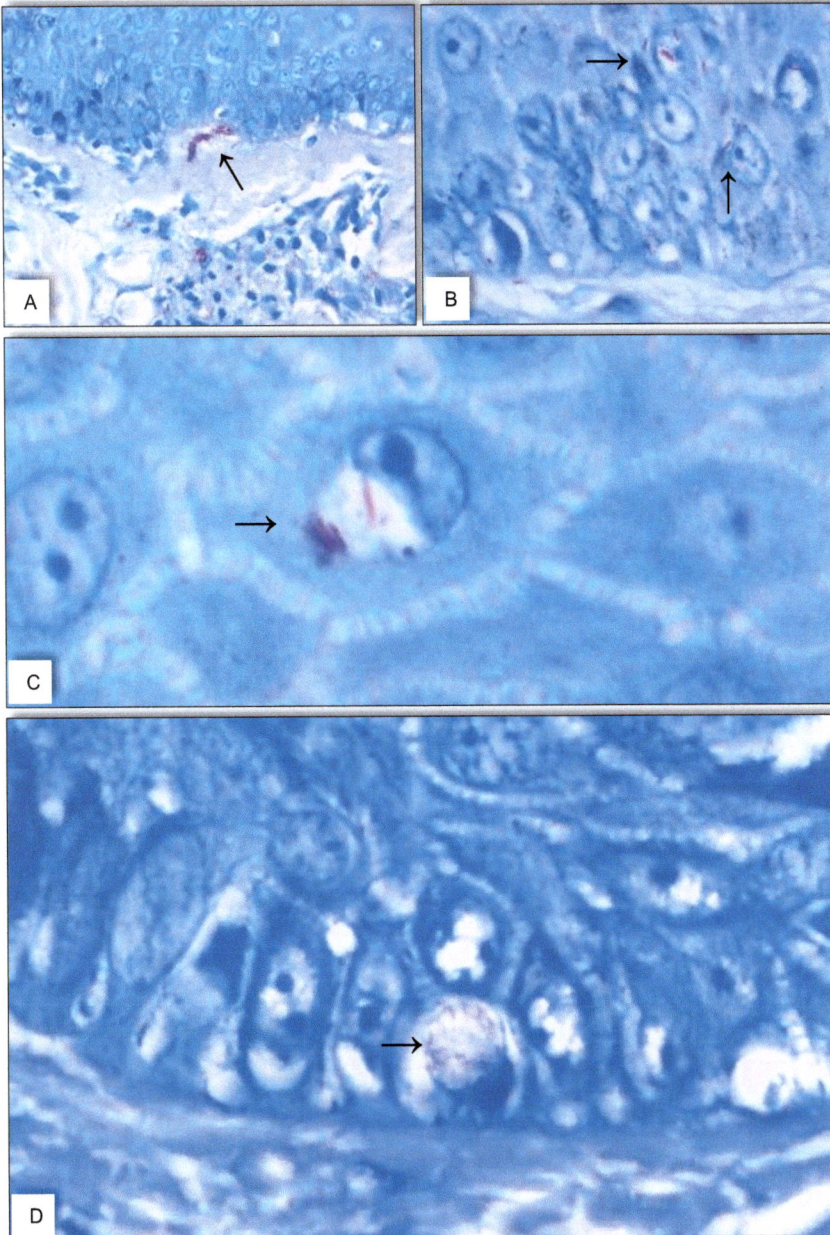

Fig. (23). Histopathological characteristics and bacilloscopic examination of lepromatous leprosy (LL) lesions with epidermal involvement. **(A)** Fusiform structure, probably neural filament, intensely parasitized at the dermo-epidermal junction (→). (B and C) Squamous epithelial cells of the epidermis parasitized by *M. leprae* (→). **(D)** A melanocytic cell in the basal layer of the epidermis containing fragmented bacilli (→). (A-D) Fite-Faraco staining.

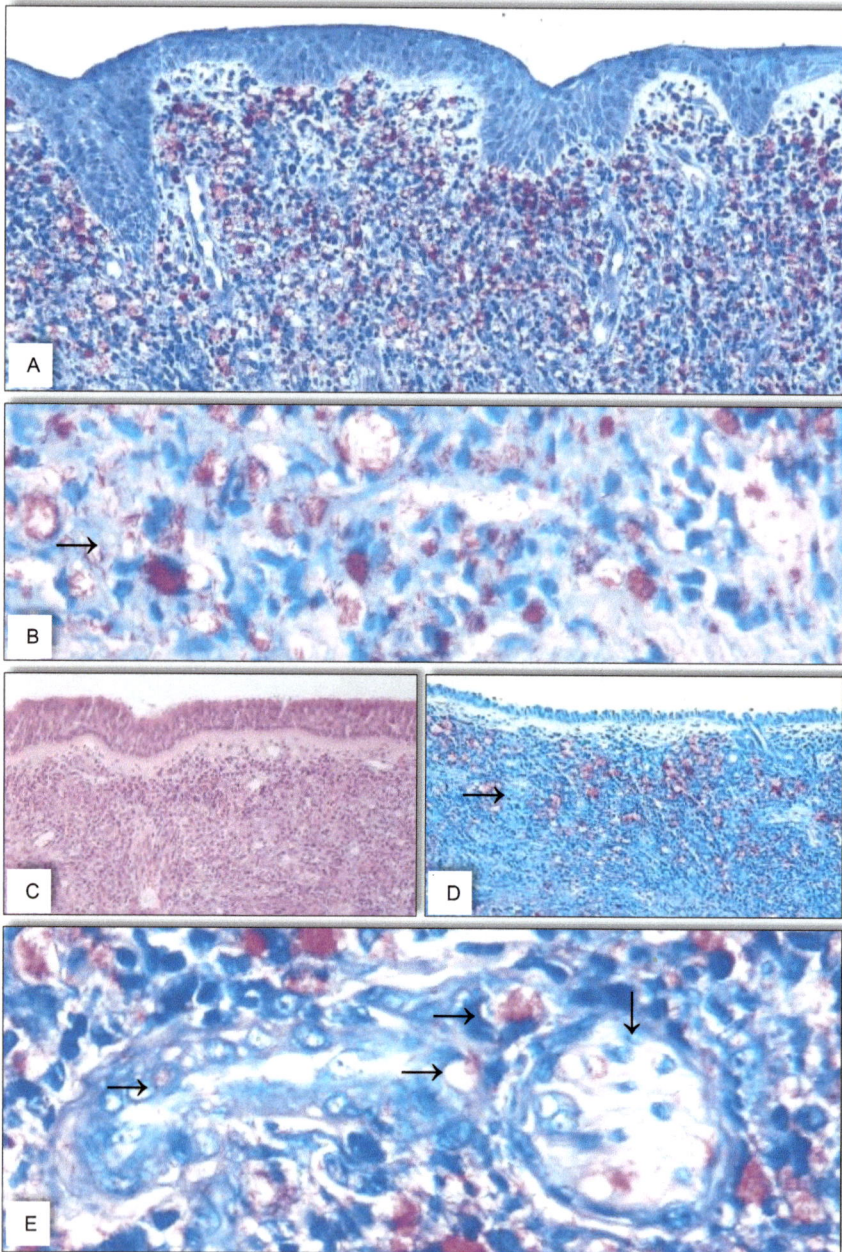

Fig. (24). Histopathological characteristics and bacilloscopic examination of lepromatous leprosy (LL) lesions with mucosal involvement. (A and B) Bacilli intensively parasitizing all components of the oral mucosa (→). (C, D, and E) Bacilli extensively parasitizing the mucosa of the nasal sinus, including macrophages, vessels, and neural branches of the mucosa (→). (A, B, D, and E) Fite-Faraco staining. **(C)** Hematoxylin and eosin staining.

The main differential clinical diagnoses of LL are secondary syphilis, drug reactions, anergic cutaneous leishmaniasis, lobomycosis, systemic lupus erythematosus, and neurofibromatosis, among others [8, 9]. The histological characteristics of the diffuse infiltrate of multivacuolated macrophages containing many bacilli (Fite-Faraco staining) allow the elimination of all of these clinical hypotheses. From a histopathological point of view, lesions containing xanthomatous macrophages or with histiocytic differentiation (xanthomatous or xanthogranulomatous lesions and fibrohistiocytic neoplasms) and granular cell tumor are the main differential diagnoses (Fig. **25**). The presence of bacilli in different cell types and the neural involvement observed in leprosy lesions are characteristic of leprosy and practically exclude other lesions or diseases.

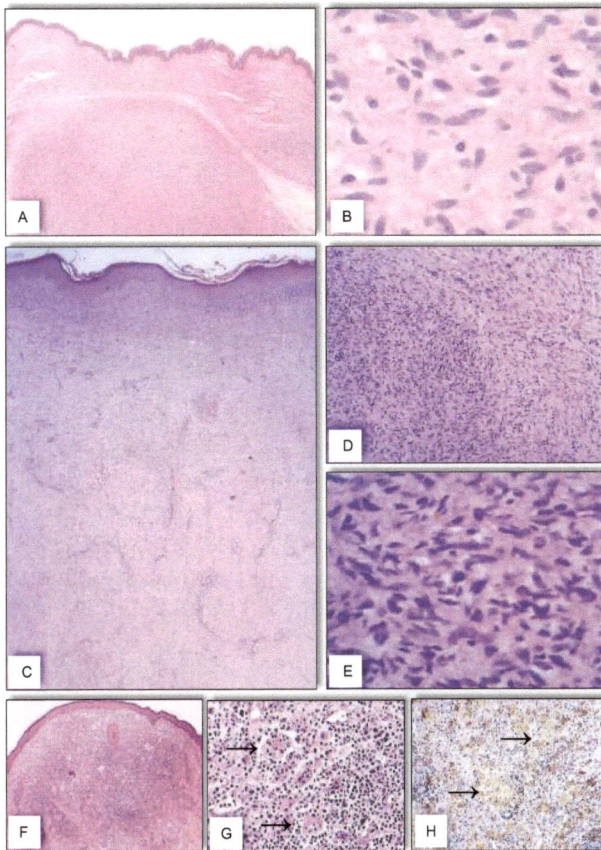

Fig. (25). Clinical-pathological differential diagnoses of lepromatous leprosy (LL). (A and B) Neurofibroma presenting papular lesions consisting predominantly of fibroblasts and Schwann cells. (C-E) Dermatofibrosarcoma protuberans consisting of fusiform mesenchymal cells with atypia, storiform pattern, and compromising the entire dermis and subcutaneous cellular tissue. (F-H) Rosai-Dorfman disease consisting of modified macrophages, expressing S-100 and with emperipolesis, permeated by lymphocytes and plasma cells (→). (A-G) Hematoxylin and eosin staining. (H) Immunohistochemistry (S-100). None of these lesions present significant neural involvement, and the bacilloscopic examination is negative (BI 0).

CONCLUSION

The polar forms of leprosy (TT and LL) are two presentations of the disease with completely different clinical, histopathologic, and bacilloscopic characteristics. Identifying these forms is crucial for determining the appropriate treatment protocol. Furthermore, understanding the characteristics of these intermediate forms (Chapter 4) and the reaction phenomena they can develop on leprotic lesions is also essential for patient management.

REFERENCES

[1]   Modlin RL. Cytokine responses in leprosy lesions. Nippon Rai Gakkai Zasshi 1995; 64(2): 85-8.
       [http://dx.doi.org/10.5025/hansen1977.64.85] [PMID: 7592165]

[2]   Fleury RN. Patologia e manifestações viscerais. In: DVA Opromolla, Hansenologia Noções de, Eds. Bauru, Centro de Estudos "Dr Reynaldo Quagliato,". 2nd ed. 2000; pp. 63-71.

[3]   Opromolla DVA, Ed. Bauru, Centro de Estudos "Dr Reynaldo Quagliato,". DVA Opromolla, Hansenologia Noções de, Eds. 2000.

[4]   Hastings RC, Gillis TP, Krahenbuhl JL, Franzblau SG. Leprosy. Clin Microbiol Rev 1988; 1(3): 330-48.
       [http://dx.doi.org/10.1128/CMR.1.3.330] [PMID: 3058299]

[5]   Fachin LR, Soares CT, Belone AF, *et al.* Immunohistochemical assessment of cell populations in leprosy-spectrum lesions and reactional forms. Histol Histopathol 2017; 32(4): 385-96.
       [PMID: 27444702]

[6]   Fleury RN, Bacchi CE. S-100 protein and immunoperoxidase technique as an aid in the histopathologic diagnosis of leprosy. Int J Lepr Other Mycobact Dis 1987; 55(2): 338-44.
       [PMID: 3298479]

[7]   Azevedo MC, Ramuno NM, Fachin LR, *et al.* qPCR detection of *Mycobacterium leprae* in biopsies and slit skin smear of different leprosy clinical forms. Braz J Infect Dis 2017; 21(1): 71-8.
       [http://dx.doi.org/10.1016/j.bjid.2016.09.017] [PMID: 27888674]

[8]   Talhari C, Talhari S, Penna GO. Clinical aspects of leprosy. Clin Dermatol 2015; 33(1): 26-37.
       [http://dx.doi.org/10.1016/j.clindermatol.2014.07.002] [PMID: 25432808]

[9]   Kundakci N, Erdem C. Leprosy: A great imitator. Clin Dermatol 2019; 37(3): 200-12.
       [http://dx.doi.org/10.1016/j.clindermatol.2019.01.002] [PMID: 31178103]

CHAPTER 4

Intermediate or Borderline Forms (BT, BB, and BL)

Abstract: Leprosy is a long-term spectrum disease and can present various clinical and histopathological aspects. Between the two poles of leprosy, there is a wide range of types, consisting of intermediate or borderline forms. In this chapter, the clinical, histopathological, and bacilloscopic characteristics of the intermediate forms (borderline-tuberculoid [BT], borderline-borderline [BB], and borderline lepromatous [BL]) are presented and discussed. The main clinical and pathological characteristics that allow the diagnosis and classification of leprosy among the different borderline forms are described and illustrated in panel form, as well as their most significant clinical and histopathological differential diagnoses are also discussed. The clinical-pathological classification of this disease has important implications in the choice of the correct treatment, the understanding of the pathophysiology, and the development of the reaction phenomena typical of leprosy.

Keywords: Borderline lepromatous, Borderline tuberculoid, Hansen's disease, Leprosy, Mid-borderline.

INTRODUCTION

Between the pole of maximum resistance (TT) and minimum resistance (LL), there is a wide range of individuals with partial immunity to *Mycobacterium leprae*. These individuals who have partial immunity when they develop leprosy, present forms of the disease with clinical-pathological and bacilloscopic characteristics between the two poles which are also known as borderline leprosy (Fig. **1**). When the bacilli parasitize and proliferate in the cells, the cellular immune system detects the bacterial antigens and produces a reaction that is characteristic for defining the location of the individual in the spectrum of resistance to bacilli. This partial resistance to *M. leprae*, which presents in borderline individuals, allows a portion of bacilli to continue to proliferate. The progressive intracellular proliferation of bacilli can cause structural changes in macrophages, granulomas, and different parasitized cells and tissues. This proliferation also causes changes in the morphology, number, and extent of cutaneous-neural lesions. As the disease progression is slow and gradual, there may be changes in the individual's cellular immune response during the long course of the disease progression; therefore, the majority of patients in the borderline group tend not to heal spontaneously. Moreover, after many years or decades of disease progression, patients' histopathological, bacilloscopic, and clinical characteristics also change gradually and progress towards the lepromatous pole, to the point that they can present clinicopathological characteristics notably similar to lepromatous leprosy (LL) (Fig. **2**) [1 - 3]. However, when treated, patients may gradually return to present their original characteristics. Ridley and Jopling (R&J) divided the borderline group into three subgroups: tuberculoid borderline (BT), borderline-borderline or mid-borderline (BB), and lepromatous borderline (BL), with defined clinical, bacilloscopic, and histopathological criteria [4]. They also introduced the concepts of degradation ("downgrading"), defined as the evolutionary worsening towards the lepromatous pole and reversion ("upgrading") when there is an evolutionary improvement towards the tuberculoid pole (Fig. **1**) [4].

It is sometimes difficult to classify an individual among the three borderline forms (BT, BB, or BL). The main causes that can hinder the classification are (1) inadequate or insufficient samples of the biopsy, with a small representation of tissues containing nerves, (2) insufficient or absent clinical information, (3) variations in the extension of the inflammatory leprosy process between different skin lesions from different locations, and (4) associated reaction phenomena (described in Chapters 5 and 6). In these situations, the precise diagnosis of the subgroup is less important than the classification of the individual as borderline, without specifying whether it is BT, BB, or BL, as borderline patients are considered to be multibacillary, as well as lepromatous patients, and the treatment used will be the same (currently between 12 and 24 months with conventional polychemotherapy-MDT) [5]. Bacilloscopic evaluation is essential because it usually demonstrates the bacilli parasitizing different tissues and cells (bacilloscopic index [BI] ≥ 2 +) and detects the presence of morphologically solid bacilli, which indicates that the disease is active.

TUBERCULOID BORDERLINE LEPROSY (BT)

BT patients histologically present a granulomatous reaction notably similar or equal to that observed in tuberculoid leprosy (TT). When compared to TT lesions, BT lesions commonly have more preserved neural branches, and the BI can vary up to about 2+. This indicates a lower bacillary clearance capacity of these individuals and skin lesions with a lower degree of neural impairment, that is, requiring fewer anesthetics. However, in some cases, it is difficult, if not impossible, to differentiate between TT and BT only using histopathological and bacilloscopic characteristics as a close correlation with clinical data for the correct classification is required [2, 3].

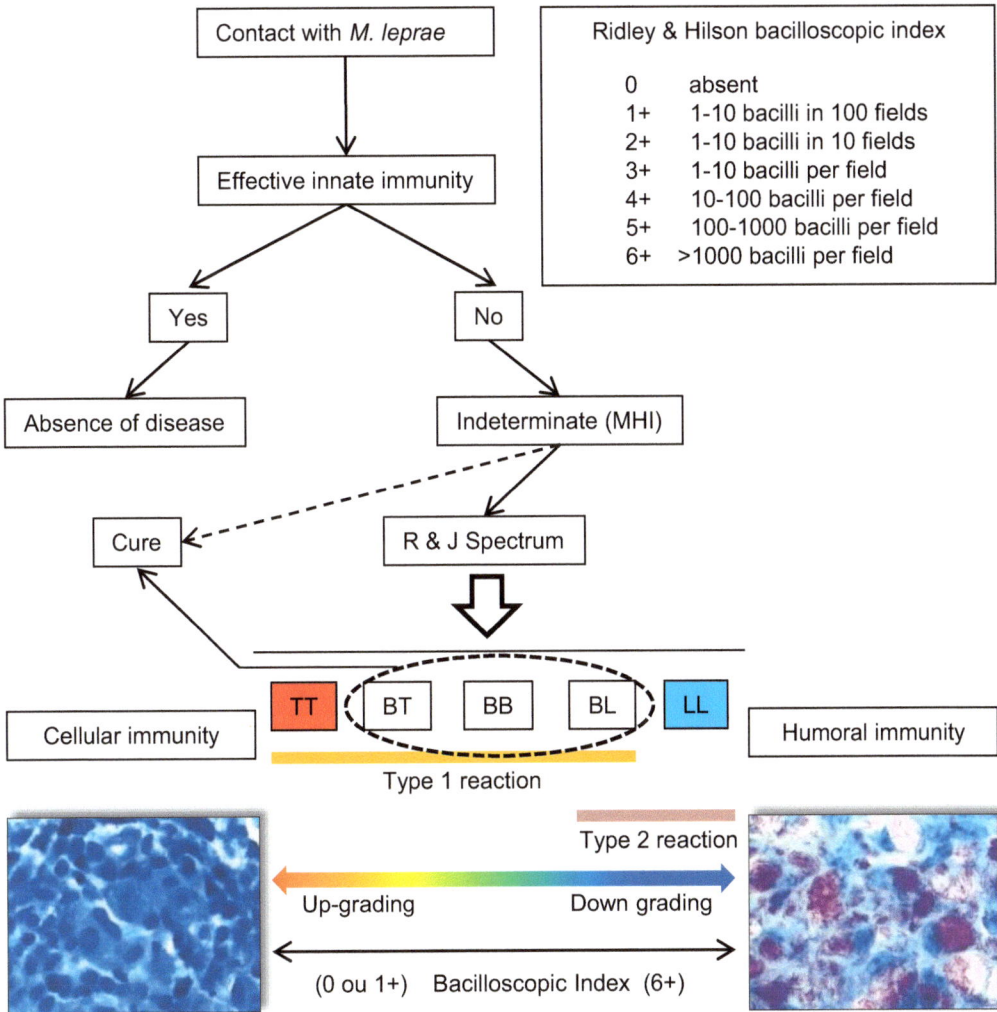

Fig. (1). The clinical spectrum and bacilloscopic index of leprosy forms and reactions. Patients who are exposed to *Mycobacterium leprae* can eliminate the bacilli through the mechanisms of the primary immune response and do not develop the disease. If the primary immune defense cannot contain the proliferation of the bacilli, the patient develops indeterminate leprosy (I), the early stage of the disease preceding the polarized forms of the Ridley and Jopling (R&J) classification: tuberculoid (TT); borderline-tuberculoid (BT); borderline-borderline (BB); borderline lepromatous (BL); and lepromatous or virchowian (LL). Late recognition of bacillary antigens by the individual may result in an intense and effective immune response (TT and BT pattern), which may lead to the destruction of the bacilli and a spontaneous cure. TT individuals have effective cellular immunity; however, if cellular immunity is not effective, proliferation and dissemination of the bacilli persist, and the disease progresses toward the lepromatous pole. LL individuals are anergic and react to the bacilli through humoral immunity. Type 1 reactions (T1R) affect patients in the range from TT to BL. Type 2 reactions (T2R) affect patients on the lepromatous side (BL and LL). The bacilloscopic index ranges from 0-6+.

The clinical characteristics of BT lesions are varied. In general, they are erythematous-hypochromic plaques with partially well-defined limits; that is, part of the lesion has well-defined limits, while in other parts, the limits are imprecise [1, 2]. Small papules may be seen at the edge of the lesion (Fig. **3**) but are not as evident as in TT lesions. The presence of a satellite lesion is relatively common (Fig. **3**) [1, 2]. The number of lesions is small (less than five lesions); however, in some cases, several lesions can be observed (Fig. **4**) [1, 2]. The size of the lesions can also vary, and they are typically small lesions (up to 5.0 cm), but in some cases, they can be extensive (Fig. **4**). The slit-skin smear on the border of BT lesions can be both negative and positive, containing a small number of bacilli [1].

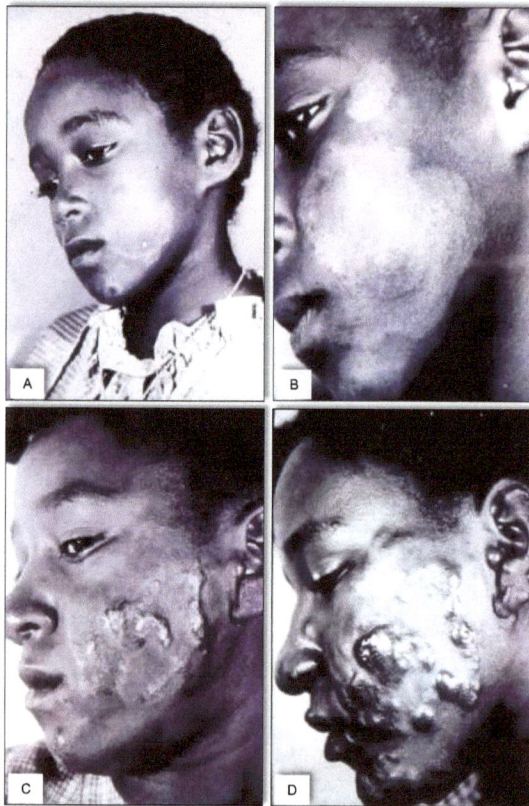

Fig. (2). An example of the clinical evolution of Leprosy. Photographs of a patient with borderline leprosy, diagnosed in the pre-sulfonic era, with a disease progression for decades, towards the lepromatous pole. Observe the change in the clinical characteristics of the lesions. Initially, two plaque lesions **(A)** were progressively increasing in size and becoming more infiltrative **(B** and **C)**. Finally, the patient has numerous lesions, with the appearance of lepromas involving the entire face, nose, and ear **(D)**. Photos belong to the archives of the Instituto Lauro de Souza Lima (ILSL).

The histopathological characteristics of BT are an inflammatory process consisting of a tuberculoid granulomatous reaction (epithelioid macrophages and lymphocytes) involving the neural branches and pili muscle and papillary dermis tissues. Like TT, granulomas in-depth are more organized, with a center formed by macrophages surrounded by a thick lymphocytic mantle (Fig. **5**). Certain neural branches are completely destroyed by the granulomatous reaction, to the point of observing only rare neural fragments within granulomas. However, it is most common that the neural branches are better preserved than those in TT lesions (Chapter 3). Commonly neural segments are usually identified within the granulomas. This indicates that the immunocellular reaction capacity of BT is less than that of TT. Moreover, this translates into a significant loss of sensitivity in skin lesions, although less intense than in TT (Fig. **6**). Additionally, bacilli are more easily found (BI of up to 2+) and can be seen in the center of the tuberculoid granulomas, which is uncommon in TT and in mononucleated cells, in the papillary dermis (Fig. **7**). Other areas of the skin are preserved, sometimes with discrete foci of aggression to the basal layer of the epidermis associated with epithelial hyperplasia and hyperkeratosis. The pili muscle is also commonly permeated by granulomas, and bacilli can be found inside (Fig. **8**). Bacilli are not detected in the vessel walls, endothelium, interstitial fibroblasts, or other skin components. The immunohistochemical profile of the cell composition of BT granulomas is similar to that of TT, with epithelioid macrophages of the M1 pattern located in the center and surrounded by a mantle of "T" lymphocytes, "B" lymphocytes, plasma cells, and other rare cells (Chapter 3) (Fig. **9**) [6].

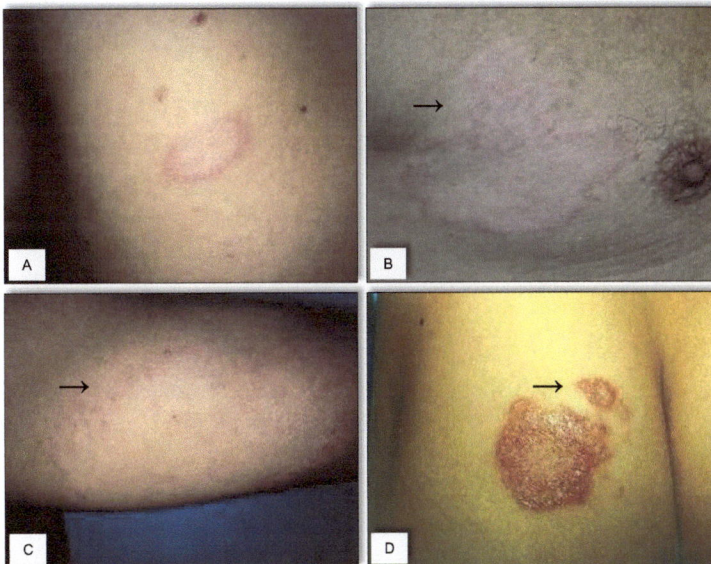

Fig. (3). Borderline-tuberculoid leprosy (BT). Lesions consisting of erythematous and hypochromic plaques with partially well-defined limits (A, B, and C), with part of the lesion presenting well-defined limits while in the other part, the limits are imprecise. Small papules (→) are seen at the edge of the lesions. The presence of a satellite lesion (→) is relatively common **(D)**. Courtesy of Dr. Cássio C. Ghidella.

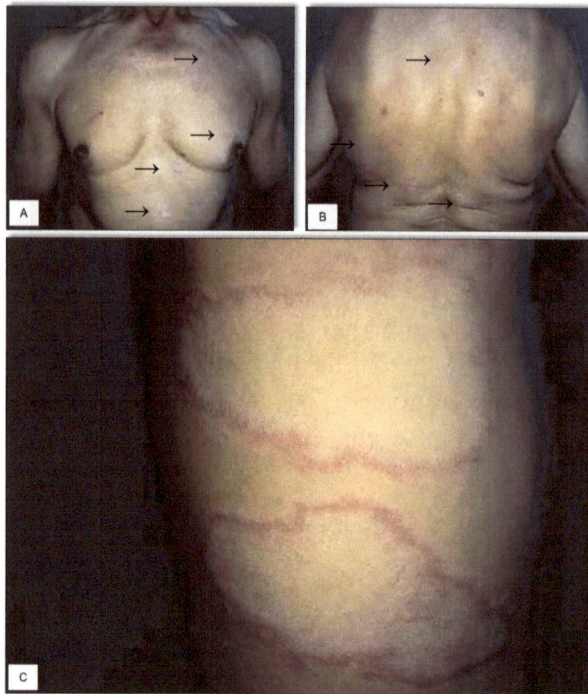

Fig. (4). Borderline-tuberculoid leprosy (BT). The number of lesions is generally small (<5 lesions), but in some cases, several lesions can be seen (→) (A and B). Lesions that are commonly small (up to 5.0 cm) can be extensive, as in this case, occupying almost the entire flank (**C**). Courtesy of Dr. Cássio C. Ghidella.

The main differential diagnoses of BT leprosy are similar to those of tuberculoid leprosy (TT). Among the clinical differential diagnostics are tinea corporis, pityriasis rosea, granuloma annulare, erythema annulare centrifugum, hypohidrotic eczema, secondary syphilis, urticaria, pityriasis versicolor, facial granuloma, sarcoidosis, paracoccidioidomycosis, cutaneous tuberculosis, discoid lupus erythematosus, and especially, leprosy borderline (BB or BL) with type 1 reaction (T1R) associated [1, 7, 8]. The histopathological examination of most of these entities is not granulomatous (tinea corporis, pityriasis rosea, centrifugal annular erythema, hypohidrotic eczema, urticaria, pityriasis versicolor, and systemic lupus erythematosus), which allows for the ability to differentiate them from the BT form relatively easily. Other diseases with a granulomatous reaction (annular granuloma, secondary syphilis, facial granuloma, sarcoidosis, paracoccidioidomycosis, cutaneous tuberculosis) do not have tuberculoid pattern granulomas involving and destroying neural branches. Consequently, such lesions do not typically present changes in sensitivity upon clinical examination (Fig. **10**). Histopathologically, the main differential diagnosis of BT lesions is leprosy TT and type 1 reaction (T1R), affecting lesions of leprosy BB and BL. The T1R outlines the tuberculoid pattern of granulomas, which are morphologically similar to tuberculoid granulomas form of BT, which can lead to misclassification. In these cases, the histological characteristics of tuberculoid granulomas and a BI of 4+ or 5+ help to differentiate BT from BB-BL with associated T1R (Figs. **4 - 11**). The histopathological characteristics of tuberculoid-like granulomas of type 1 reaction (T1R) and their differentiation from tuberculoid granulomas of leprosy lesions in the T side (TT and BT) are detailed in Chapter 5.

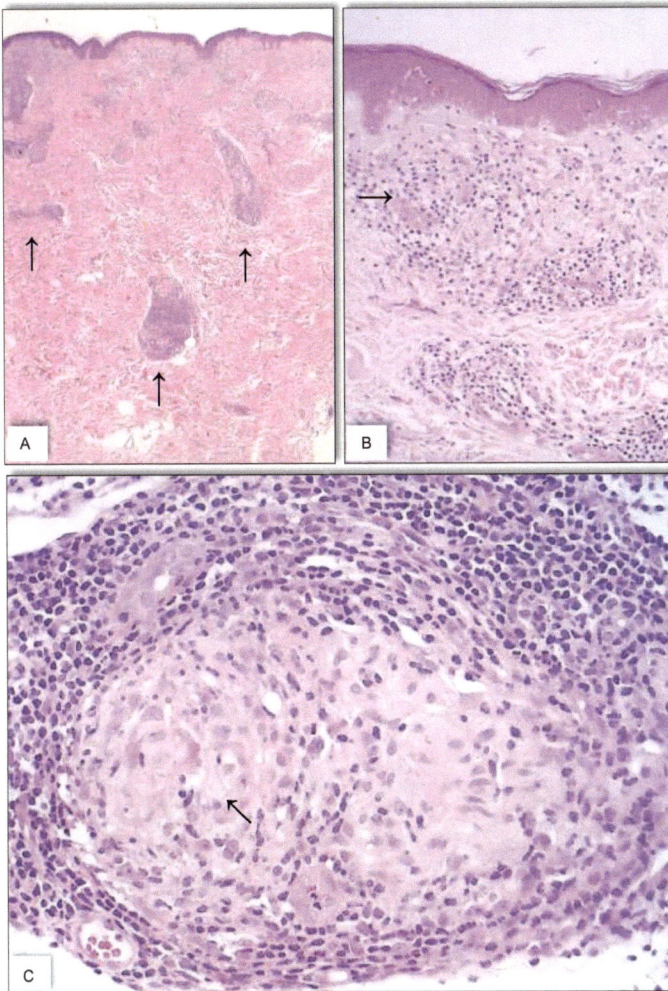

Fig. (5). Borderline-tuberculoid leprosy (BT). **(A)** Tuberculoid granulomas follow the neural ramifications, giving an ascending and arboriform appearance (→). **(B)** In general, granulomas in the papillary dermis are poorly organized, with lymphocytes permeating the macrophages (→). **(C)** The granulomas in depth are organized, with a center formed by epithelioid macrophages surrounded by a thick lymphocytic mantle (→). HE staining.

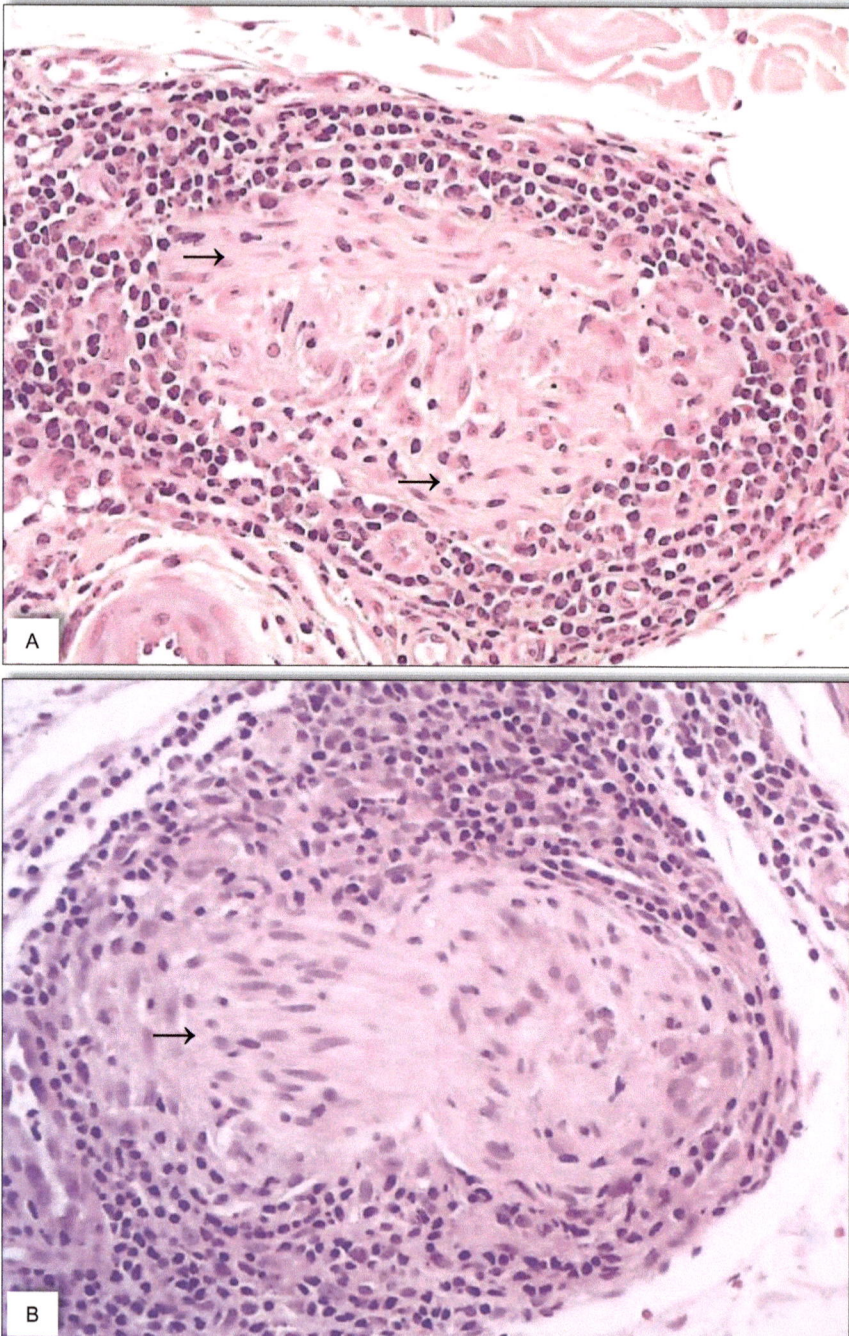

Fig. (6). Borderline-tuberculoid leprosy (BT) (A and B). The neural branches are involved and permeated by an intense inflammatory infiltrate. Usually, there is no complete destruction of the neural branches, and part of it can be identified within the granulomas (→). HE staining.

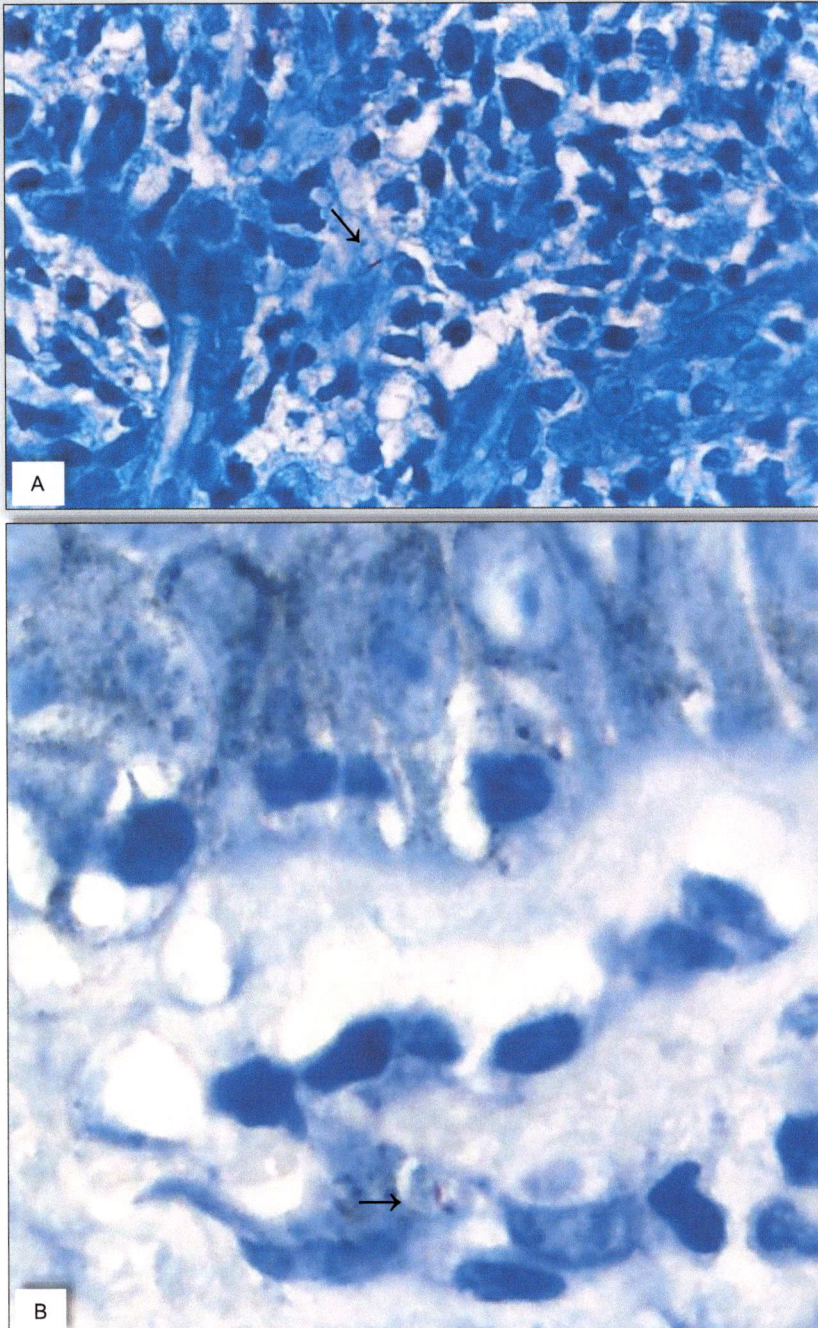

Fig. (7). Borderline-tuberculoid leprosy (BT). There is a bacillus in the center of the tuberculoid granuloma **(A)** (→) and in the papillary dermis **(B)** (→). Fite-Faraco staining.

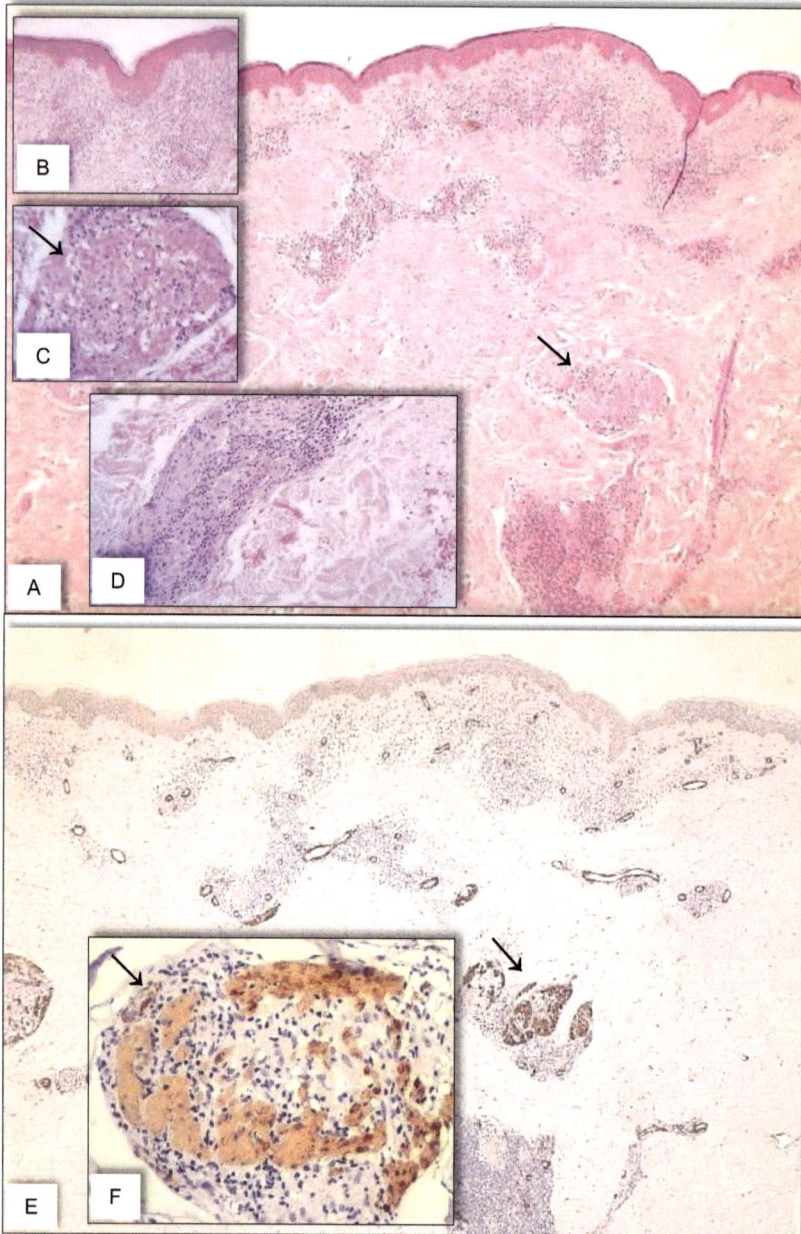

Fig. (8). Borderline-tuberculoid leprosy (BT). There is an inflammatory process with granuloma formation affecting the neural branches, pili muscle (→), and papillary dermis (A, B, C, and D). Other areas of the skin are preserved. Foci of aggression to the basal layer of the epidermis associated with mild epithelial hyperplasia and hyperkeratosis **(B)**. Immunohistochemistry demonstrates the pili muscle (→) partially destroyed by the granuloma (E and F). A, B, C, and D stained by HE. E and F by Immunohistochemistry (smooth muscle actin-1A4).

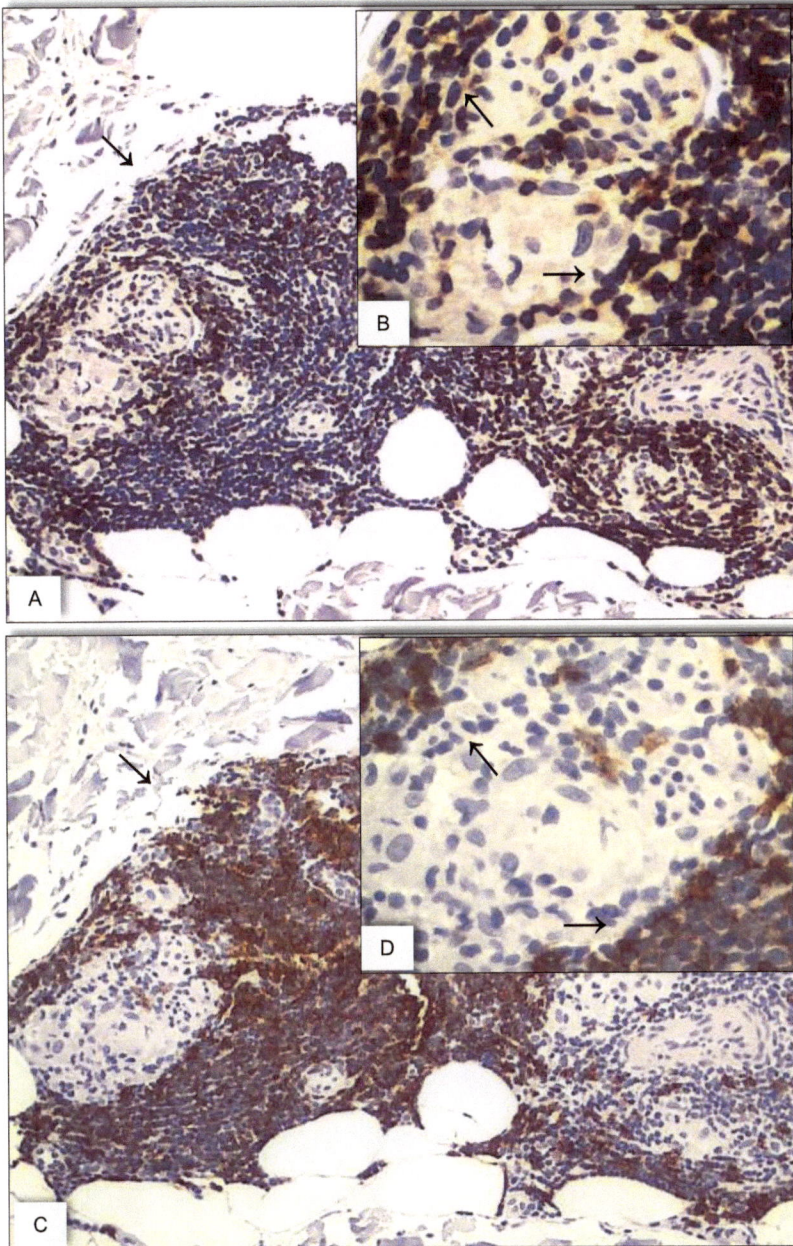

Fig. (9). Borderline-tuberculoid leprosy (BT). The immunohistochemical profile of the cell composition of BT granulomas is similar to that of TT, with epithelioid macrophages located in the center, with few lymphocytes permeating the macrophages, and surrounded by a thick mantle of "T" lymphocytes CD3+ (→) and "B" lymphocytes CD20+ (→), sometimes with a predominance of "B" lymphocytes. Immunohistochemistry for CD3 (A and B) and CD20 (C and D).

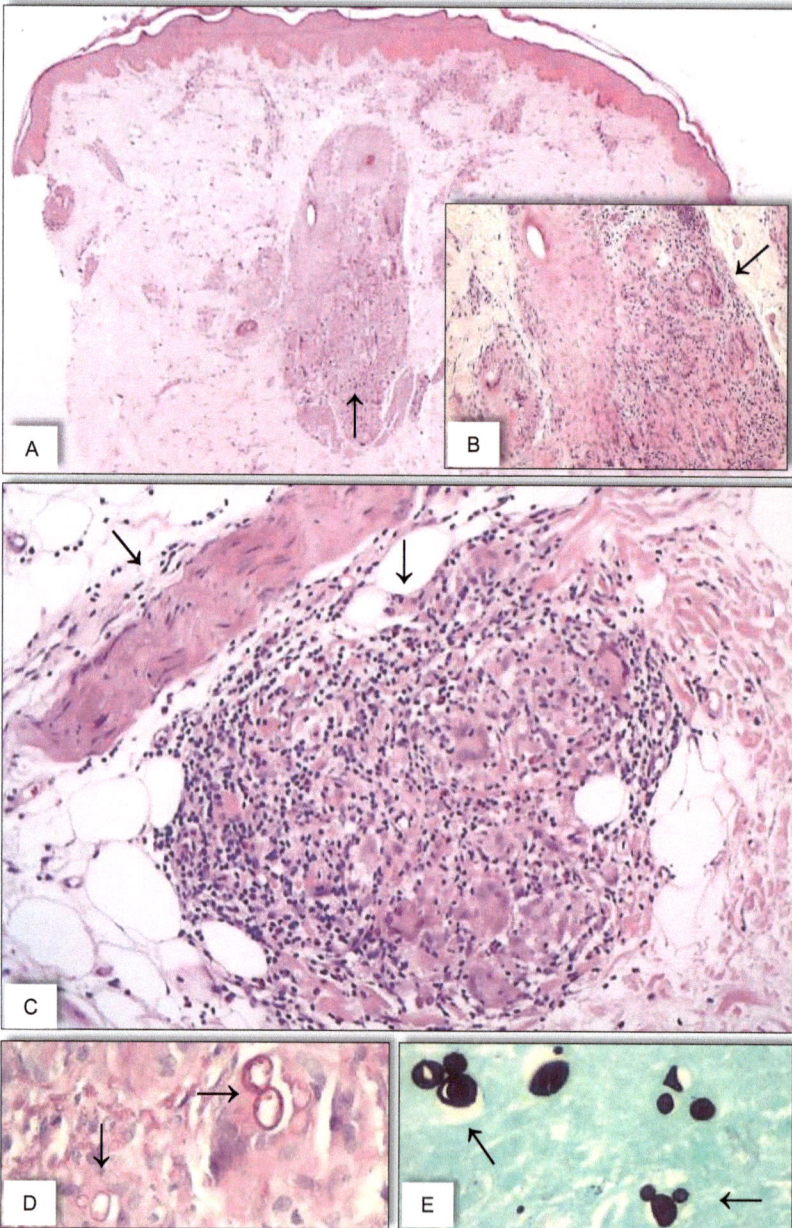

Fig. (10). Differential diagnosis of borderline-tuberculoid leprosy (BT). Lesion on the face clinically suspected for BT with histopathological features of paracoccidioidomycosis. Periadnexal granulomatous infiltrate without characteristics of involvement of neural branches (→) (A, B, and C). Granuloma poorly organized and without involvement of the adjacent neural branch (→) **(C)**. Presence of multinucleated giant cells permeated with numerous lymphocytes and eosinophils (→) **(C)**. Fungi with the appearance of "mickey mouse" (→) inside the granulomas (D and E). HE staining (A, B, and C), PAS with diastasis **(D)**, and silver methenamine **(E)**.

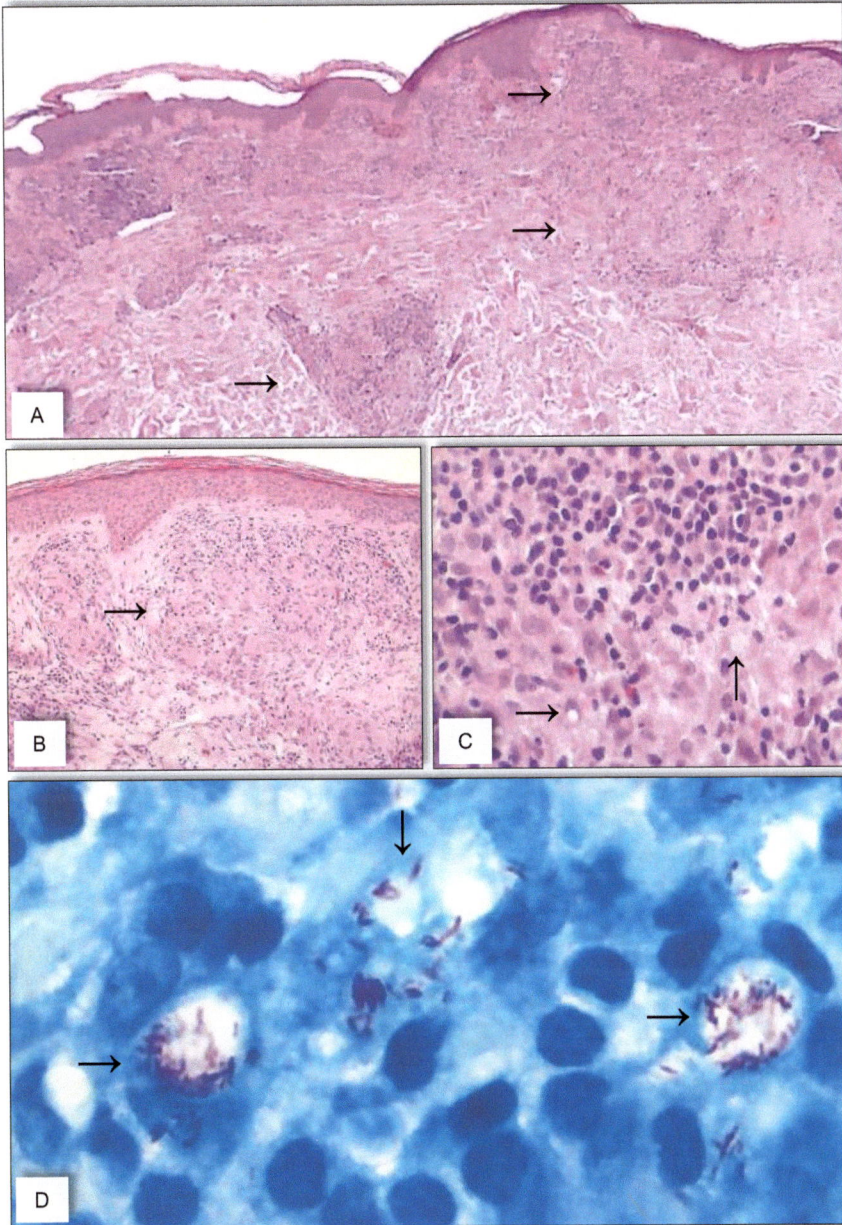

Fig. (11). Differential diagnosis of borderline-tuberculoid leprosy (BT). Case of borderline leprosy (BB-BL) with an associated type 1 reaction (T1R) initially diagnosed as BT. The type 1 reaction causes the outline of granulomas with a tuberculoid pattern on pre-existing BB / BL lesions, but without the lymphocyte mantle on the periphery (→) (A and B). There are lymphocytes and plasmocytes permeating several epithelioid macrophages at the center of the granulomas **(C)**. Macrophages have intracytoplasmic vacuoles (→) that are filled with a large number of bacilli (C and D). HE staining (A, B, and C) and Fite-Faraco **(D)**.

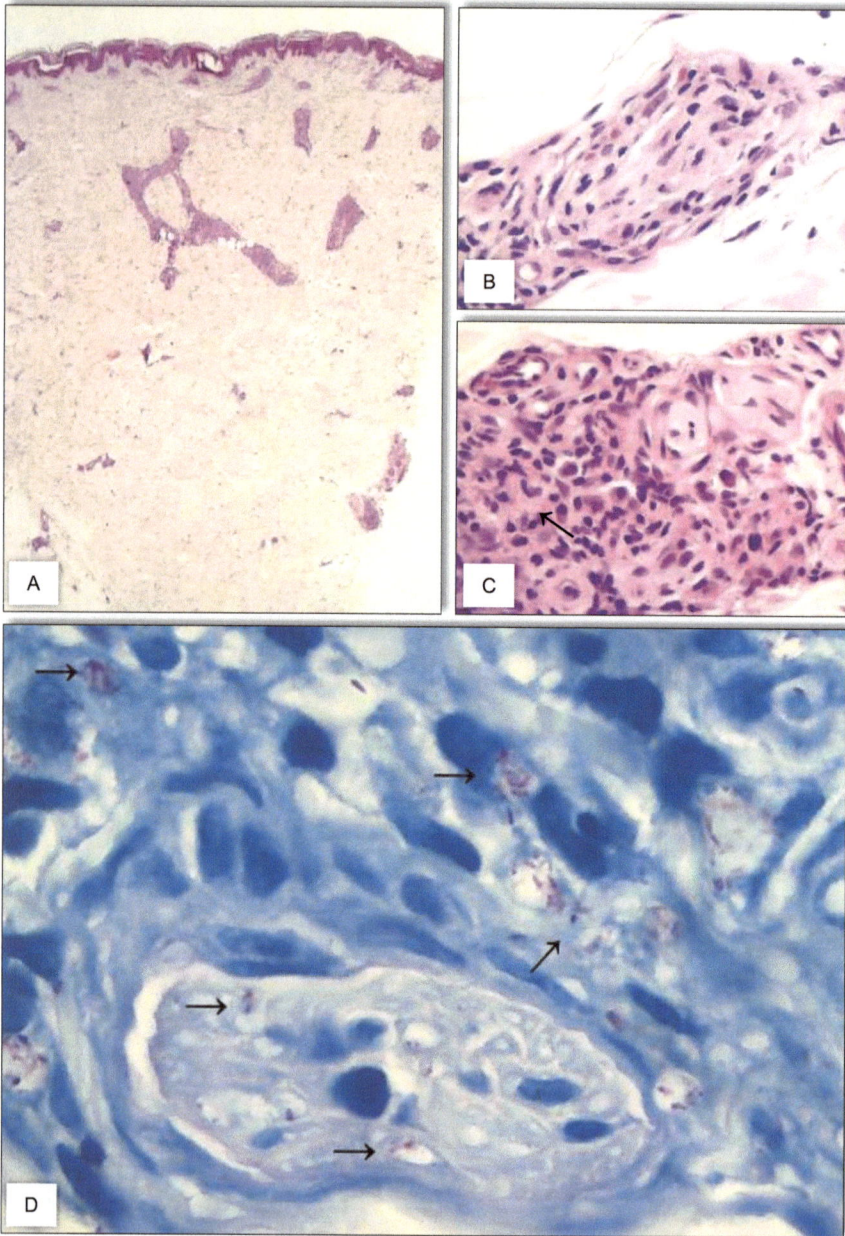

Fig. (12). Borderline-borderline leprosy (BB). A lymphohistiocytic and plasmacytic infiltrate with a granuloma outline following the vasculoneural bundles and penetrating the neural branches (A, B, and C). Several macrophages are epithelioids (→) **(C)**. The bacilloscopic examination shows numerous bacilli (bacilloscopic index of 4+ or 5+), solid or fragmented, within the neural branches and in the adjacent macrophages (→) **(D)**. HE staining (A, B, and C). Fite-Faraco **(D)**.

BORDERLINE-BORDERLINE OR MID-BORDERLINE LEPROSY (BB)

Patients who develop BB leprosy have a low capacity to efficiently identify and process mycobacterial antigens. Inflammatory infiltrates are characterized histologically by granulomas consisting of a predominance of multivacuolated macrophages (M2 pattern), associated with rare macrophages with epithelioid characteristics (M1 pattern), sometimes outlining a tuberculoid arrangement (Fig. **12**) [6]. There are lymphocytes, plasma cells, and spindle-shaped macrophages on the periphery of the granulomas (Fig. **12**) [6]. The inflammatory infiltrate with a granuloma outline is discrete, following the vasculoneural bundles, and involving and penetrating the neural branches (Fig. **12**). The nerves are slightly affected by the inflammatory process, but their destruction is not observed. The inflammatory infiltrate surrounds and penetrates several neural branches, forming a concentric delamination and giving the appearance of an "onion" or "target" (Fig. **13**). There are no tuberculoid granulomas with an intense lymphocytic infiltrate in the periphery, as seen in the TT and BT forms. The non-destructive impairment of the neural branches translates into a slight loss of sensitivity in the skin lesions. Schwann cells and parasitic macrophages inside the neural branches have intracytoplasmic vacuoles filled with grayish amorphous material when stained by HE. This grayish material inside the vacuoles consists of solid and fragmented bacilli when stained by Fite-Faraco (Fig. **14**).

A consequence of the low ability to block proliferation and bacillary dissemination in BB patients is that the BI is higher, ranging from 3+ to 5+, with a more frequent BI of 4+. Parasitism is also more comprehensive in the skin tissues of these patients, when compared to TT and BT patients. The presence of bacilli is common in macrophages within the granulomas, in neural branches, the pili muscle, in interstitial macrophages, fibroblasts, and rarely, in the vessel wall (Fig. **15**). Bacilloscopic examination can show the parasitism of different types of skin cells and tissues even though they do not present histopathological changes (Fig. **15**). In general, bacilli are absent in the endothelial cells, epithelial cells (epidermis, pilosebaceous follicle, and glands), myoepithelial cells, and melanocytes.

The clinical characteristics of BB lesions are annular plaques, irregular in outline, unclear boundaries, and an erythematous-brown color. The center of the lesion is smooth and hypochromic (Fig. **16**). Certain lesions present with a circular, hypochromic, flat, well-defined central area and with the infiltrated periphery forming a thick border that gradually spreads to the adjacent skin. These lesions are also known as "Swiss cheese type" lesions (Fig. **16**) [1, 2]. BB patients commonly present with multiple lesions, but in rare cases, only one or a few lesions are noticed. Slit-skin smears collected from the edge of BB lesions are invariably positive. It is important to note that the skin adjacent to the edge of BB lesions may be parasitized by *M. leprae*, even though clinically, it is apparently normal; however, this phenomenon is most frequently seen in BL and LL lesions (Fig. **17**).

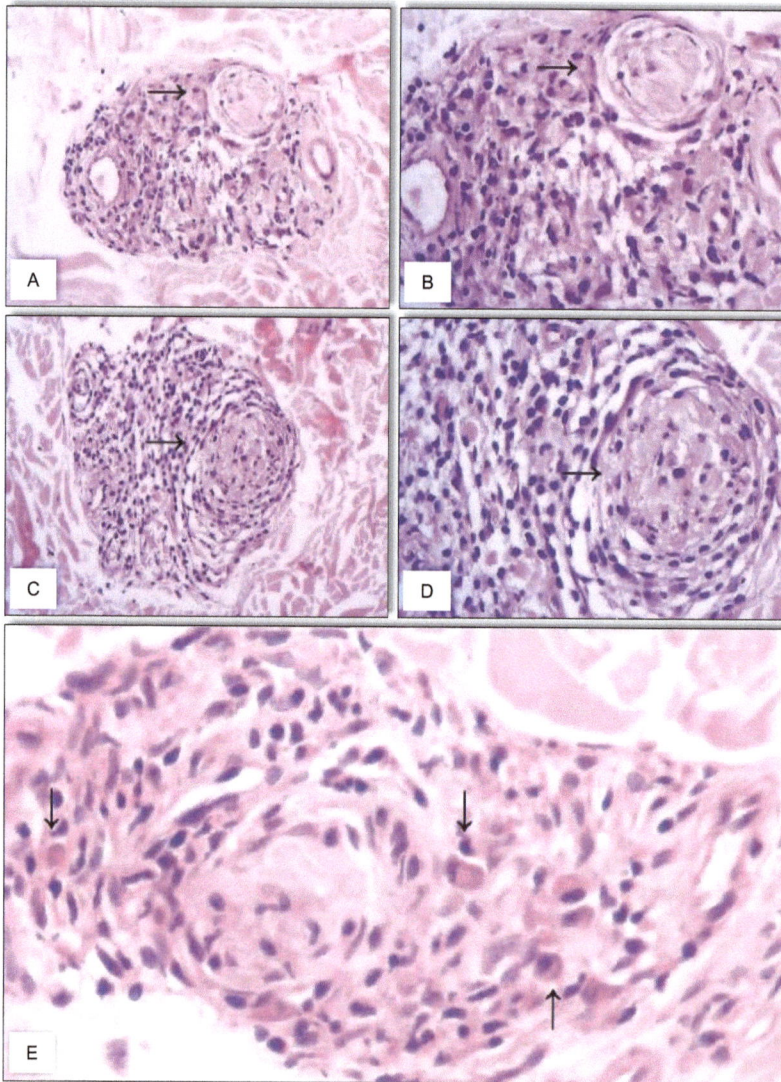

Fig. (13). Borderline-borderline leprosy (BB). The inflammatory process that affects the neural branches does not have tuberculoid granulomas as seen in TT and BT (A, B, C, D, and E). The lymphohistiocytic infiltrate surrounds and penetrates the neural branches without destroying them, forming, in some, a concentric delamination with the appearance of an "onion" or "target" (→) (A, B, C, and D). Plasma cells are common in BB infiltrates permeating macrophages and lymphocytes (→) **(E)**. HE staining.

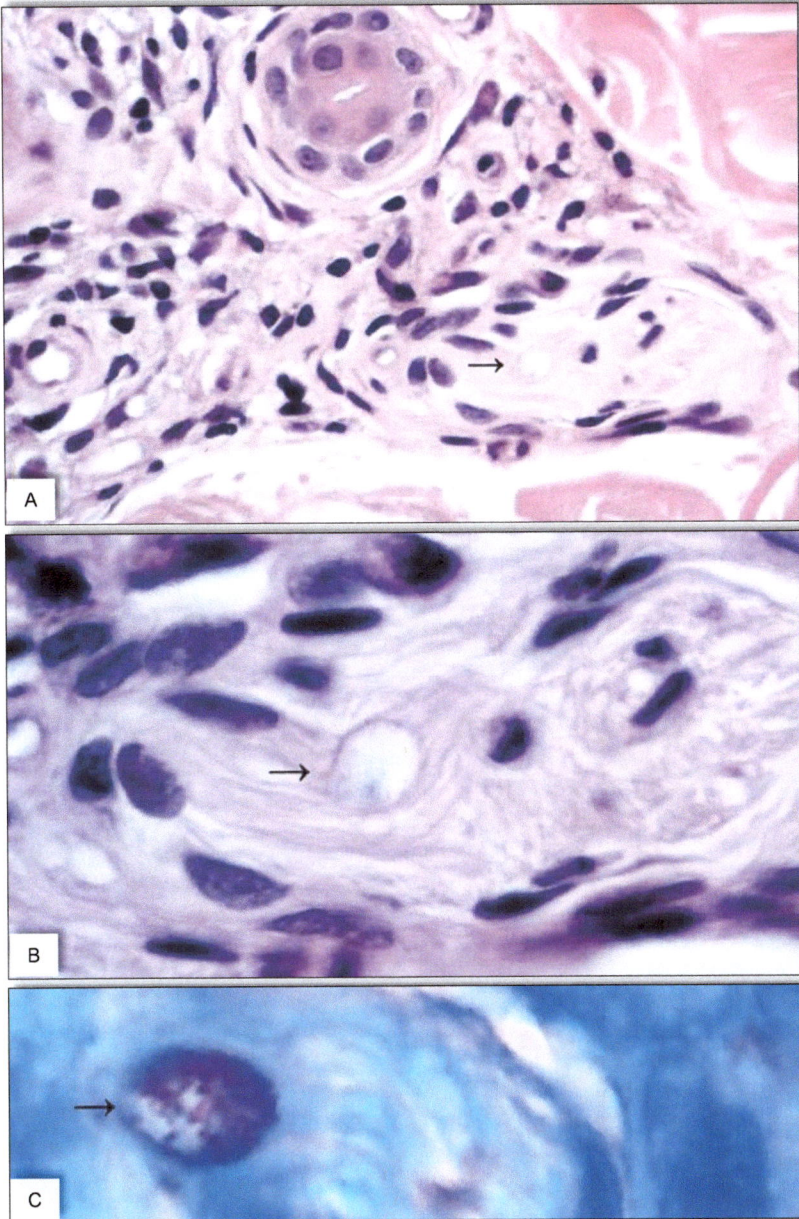

Fig. (14). Borderline-borderline leprosy (BB). Within the neural branches, there are parasitized Schwann cells presenting intracytoplasmic vacuoles filled with grayish amorphous material when stained with HE (→) (A and B). This amorphous material that fills the vacuoles consists of solid and fragmented bacilli when stained with Fite-Faraco (→) (**C**).

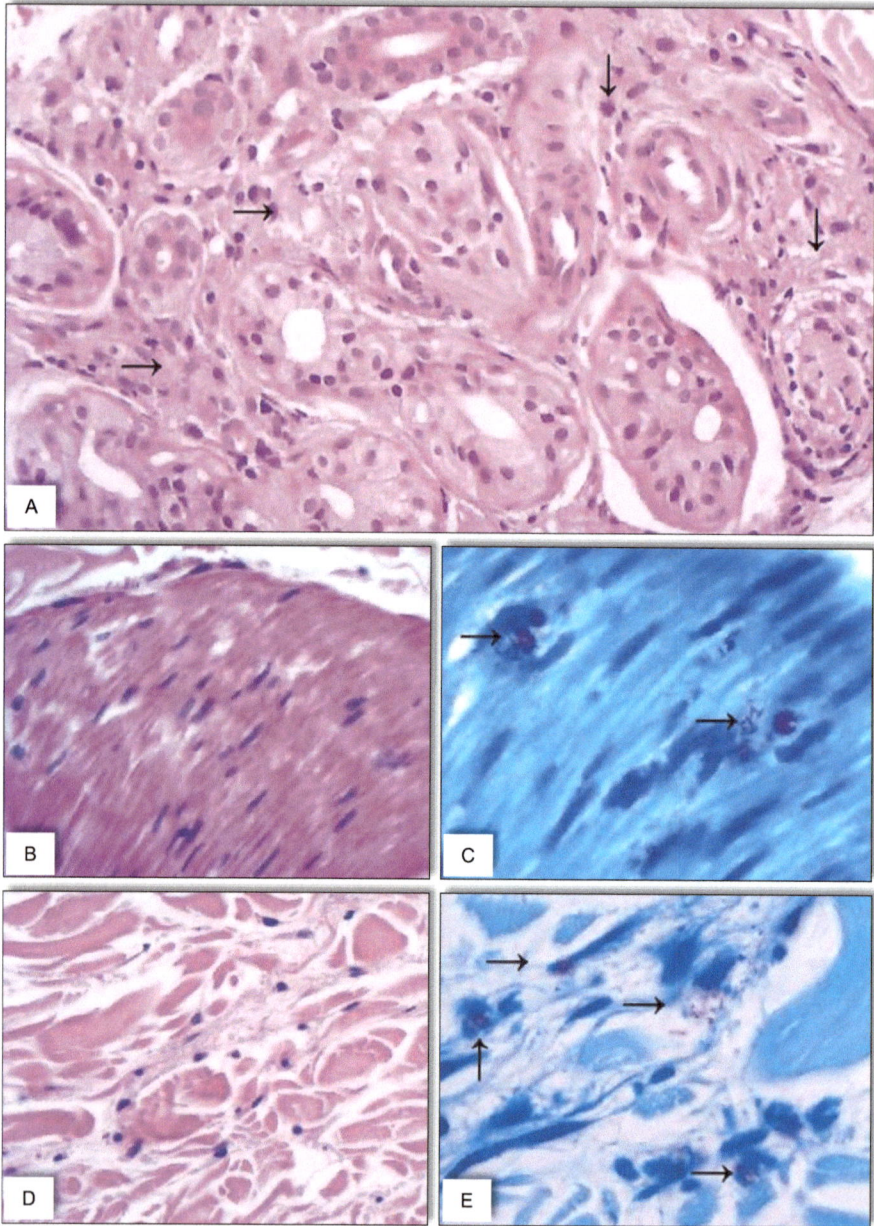

Fig. (15). Borderline-borderline leprosy (BB). The inflammatory process involving neural branches and periglandular tissues (→) **(A)**. Parasitism of the pili muscle (→) (B and C). Macrophages and interstitial mononucleated cells containing bacilli in the cytoplasm (→) (D and E). HE staining (A, B, and D) and Fite-Faraco (C and E).

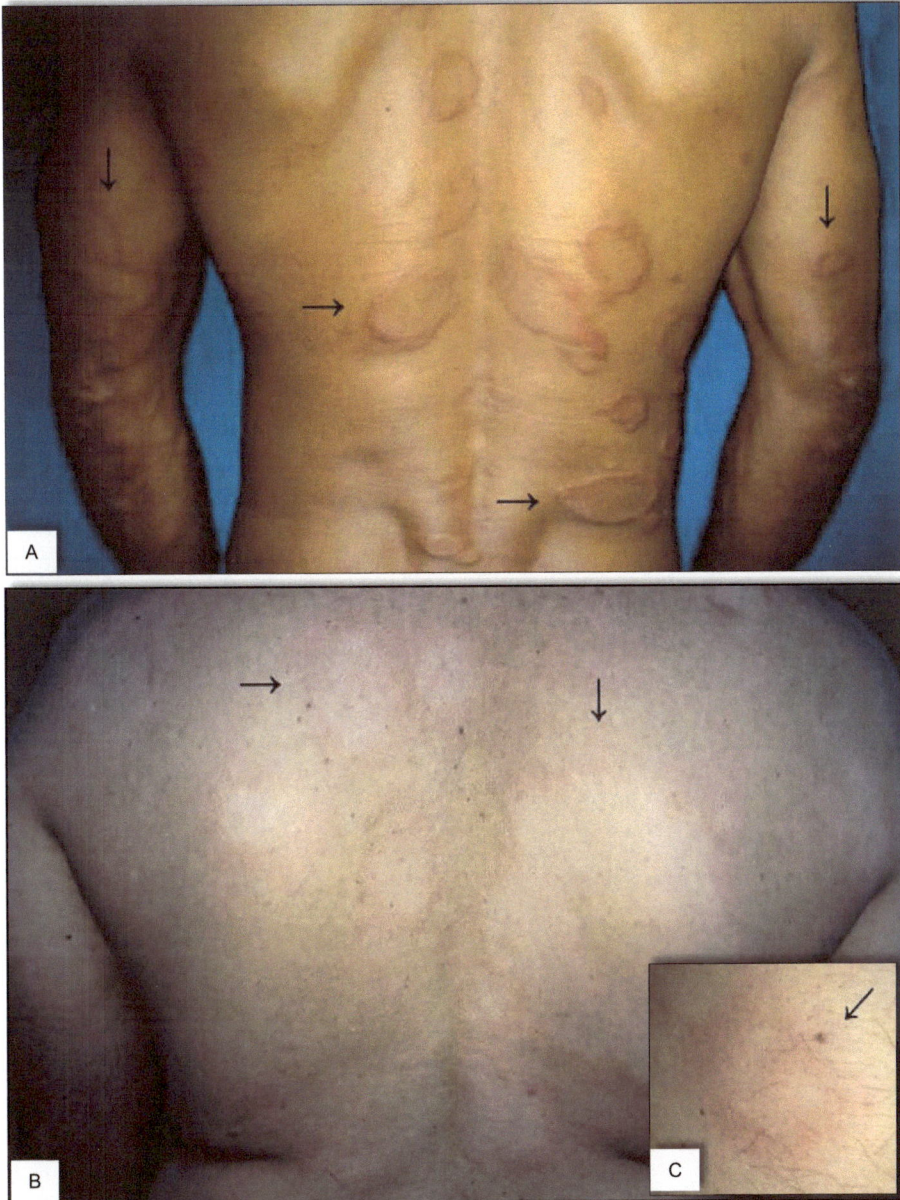

Fig. (16). Borderline-borderline leprosy (BB). BB lesions usually present as annular plaques with irregular edges and unclear borders and with an erythematous-brown color. The center of the lesion is smooth and hypochromic (A, B, and C). Some lesions have a circular, hypochromic, flat, well-defined central area with an infiltrated periphery forming a thick border that gradually spreads to the adjacent skin (B and C). Courtesy of Dr. Cássio C. Ghidella.

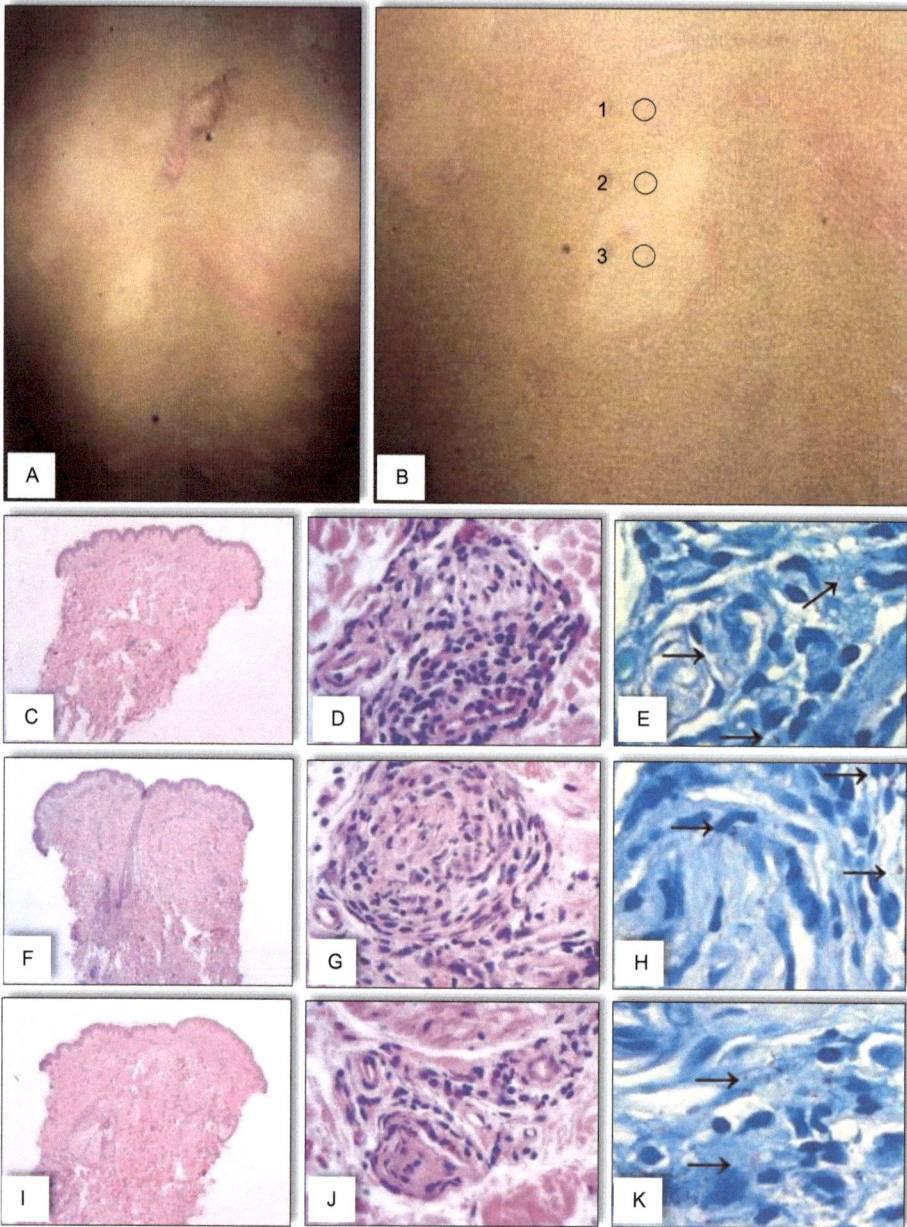

Fig. (17). Borderline-borderline leprosy (BB). Some BB patients have parasitism of the skin adjacent to the lesions (**A** and **B**). Histological sections of skin adjacent to the lesion and considered normal (**B1, C, D,** and **E**). The lesion border (**B2, F, G,** and **H**) and the lesion center (**B3, I, J,** and **K**) show a lymphohistiocytic infiltrate, compromising the neural branches of the BB pattern, present in all samples. The bacilloscopic exam (Fite-Faraco) shows bacilli ($\rightarrow$) (BI 4+) in all samples (**E, H,** and **K**). (**A** and **B**). Courtesy of Dr. Cássio C. Ghidella.

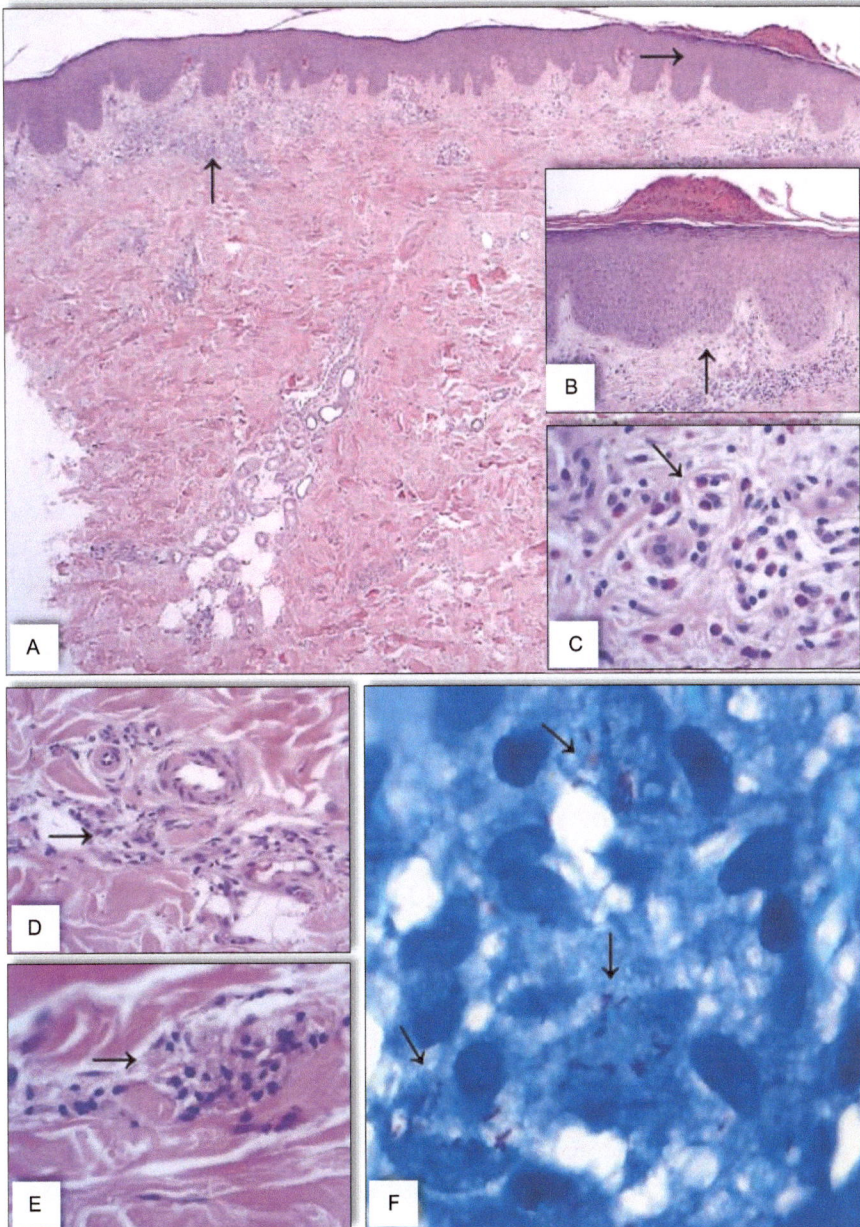

Fig. (18). Borderline-Borderline Leprosy (BB) and associated chronic eczema. A 45-year-old patient with eczematous plaques throughout the body and changes in sensitivity in the lesions. Histological characteristics demonstrate a lymphohistiocytic and eosinophilic infiltrate in the papillary dermis with aggression to the epidermis associated with hyperplasia, hyperkeratosis, and parakeratosis of the epidermis (probable drug reaction) (→) (A, B, and C) and in-depth the inflammatory infiltrate of BB pattern involving neural branches (→) (D and E) with a positive smear of 4+ (→) **(F)**. HE staining (A-E) and Fite-Faraco **(F)**.

The main differential clinical and histopathological diagnoses of leprosy BB include all those referring to BT, adding drug reactions, mycosis fungoides, indeterminate leprosy (I), and borderline lepromatous leprosy (BL) [3, 7, 8]. Rarely, drug reaction and mycosis fungoides lesions have a granulomatous pattern. When both have granulomas, there is no impairment of the neural branches. The bacilloscopic exam is important in differentiation because, in these situations, it is negative, and in BB lesions, it varies from 3+ to 5+. A relatively common situation is the presence of non-leprosy lesions (chronic eczema, drug reaction, lichenoid lesions, *etc.*) concomitant with BB, BL, or LL lesions. In these cases, the histological sections show characteristics of these lesions and of the specific leprosy lesion (Fig. **18**). The pathologist needs to be aware of the involvement of the neural branches that is characteristic of leprosy. If there is an inflammatory infiltrate involving the neural branch, it is recommended to request special staining for *M. leprae* (Fite-Faraco). The presence of different types of diseases or conditions that manifest on skin with leprosy damage is a relatively frequent finding in endemic countries and likely makes it difficult or masks the identification of concomitant leprosy damage, delaying its diagnosis and treatment.

Moreover, indeterminate leprosy (I) can clinically simulate BB leprosy. Parasitism of different types of skin cells and tissues (BI of +4) detected in BB lesions excludes I. The histopathological and bacilloscopic characteristics that differentiate I from BB, and vice versa, are described in detail in Chapter 2. BL leprosy, as a differential diagnosis of BB, will be discussed below.

BORDERLINE LEPROMATOUS LEPROSY (BL)

Patients with borderline lepromatous leprosy (BL) have cutaneous lesions with histopathological changes characterized by clusters of non-epithelioid multivacuolate macrophages permeated by lymphocytes and plasma cells. Inflammatory infiltrates are notably similar to those seen in BB lesions; however, they are more extensive and have a greater number of cells (macrophages, lymphocytes, and plasma cells). It is common to have small clusters of lymphocytes outlining lymphoid nodules, without a follicular center, and a perivascular plasmacytic infiltrate that is quite evident (Fig. **19**). Like BB, BL commonly presents neural branches with concentric delamination of the perineurium, giving the appearance of an "onion" or "target" (Fig. **20**). In general, the neural branches are preserved, with macrophages, lymphocytes, and plasma cells permeating the perineurium and Schwann cells (Fig. **20**). There are no tuberculoid granulomas involving the neural branches or any other skin component. Certain Schwann cells, macrophages, and several other parasitized cells have intracytoplasmic vacuoles containing grayish amorphous material that are bacilli when stained by Fite-Faraco (globi) (Fig. **20**). The same histopathological characteristics observed in the skin are observed in any organ or tissue parasitized by *M. leprae*, such as the lymph nodes, liver, spleen, bone marrow, mucous membranes, testis, and deep nerves (Fig. **21**). The inflammatory infiltrate of BL does not destroy the nerves, as observed in TT and BT, but it can cause important demyelination of the nerves, and consequently, cause disturbances in the conduction of electrical impulses. The demyelination process of the neural branches occurs in all forms of leprosy (Fig. **22**). The bacilloscopic examination of BL lesions shows solid and fragmented bacilli inside different types of skin cells and tissues. The BI ranges from 4+ to 6+, more often around 5+. The presence of bacilli is common in the neural branches, macrophages, vessel walls, endothelium, and interstitial cells (macrophages and fibroblasts) (Fig. **23**). Bacilli are less frequently seen inside the epithelial cells of the pilosebaceous follicle or in the epithelial and myoepithelial cells of the sweat glands (Fig. **24**). Patients in the BL form with many years or decades of disease progression may present with nodular or diffuse macrophage infiltrates, consisting of multivacuolated macrophages permeated by a small number of lymphocytes and plasma cells. In this situation, patients have clinical and histopathological characteristics very similar to LL (Chapter 3), with diffuse parasitism, and bacilli can be found in virtually all skin components (BI of 6+) (Fig. **25**). It is important to note that BL does not present a granulomatous reaction with a tuberculoid pattern. If the histological sections show a lymphohistiocytic infiltrate containing granulomas, outlining a pattern similar to those of TT and BT, and a BI of 4 or 5+, the patient is likely presenting an associated type 1 (T1R) reaction (Fig. **26**). BL cases with an associated T1R may erroneously be classified as TT or BT, resulting in improper treatment. The histopathological and bacilloscopic characteristics of a T1R affecting borderline forms are described in detail in Chapter 5.

Clinically, BL lesions are more similar to LL lesions than to BB lesions. In general, there are several infiltrative plaques with a rust or brownish color. In addition to plaques, there are papules or nodules (lepromas). The auricular pavilions are often compromised by lesions, and madarosis is discreet (Fig. **27**) [1, 2]. Slit-skin smears collected from the edge of the BB lesions are always positive, with numerous bacilli. Nasal mucosa involvement is common, and there may be lesions in the ocular mucosa. Parasitism of the skin adjacent to the edge of BL lesions is more common than in BB lesions (Fig. **17**), even though clinically, the adjacent skin is apparently normal.

The main differential clinical and histopathological diagnoses of BL leprosy include all those referring to BB, mainly drug reaction and mycosis fungoides, adding secondary syphilis, onchocercosis, and neurofibromatosis [1, 7, 8]. The histopathological and bacilloscopic characteristics that differentiate leprosy from drug reactions and mycosis fungoides are discussed above in the BB section. Secondary syphilis can simulate a BL lesion, mainly due to the loose lymphohistiocytic infiltrate with plasmocytes permeating the vessels and neural branches (Fig. **28**). In these cases, neural involvement with concentric delamination and intracytoplasmic vacuoles in Schwann cells and macrophages indicates leprosy. The bacilloscopic examination (Fite-Faraco) showing numerous bacilli (BI of 5+) parasitizing different types of tissues and the use of immunohistochemistry for treponema (negative) are notably useful for establishing the diagnosis of BL. Solitary neurofibromas and neurofibromas associated with von Recklinghausen's disease (neurofibromatosis) can present as papules and spots on the body, simulating BL lesions. The histological characteristics of a neurofibroma characterized by a proliferation of Schwann cells, collagen fibers, myxoid matrix, and mast cells are histologically different from those of a leproma (Fig. **29**). Additionally, the bacilloscopic examination showing a large number of bacilli, excludes neurofibromatosis. BL and LL patients may develop papulonodular neoplastic lesions (neurofibroma, neurilemoma, melanocytic nevus, basal cell carcinoma, among others) on skin parasitized by *M. leprae*. In these cases, due to the long interaction of the bacillus with these neoplasms, it is possible to observe the parasitism of neoplastic cells by *M. leprae* (Fig. **30**) [9].

Among the forms of leprosy, the indeterminate (I), BB, and LL types can present clinical and histopathological characteristics similar to BL. The histopathological and bacilloscopic characteristics that differentiate "I" from other forms of leprosy are described in detail in Chapter 2, with bacilloscopic examination being of fundamental importance in differentiating between the types (BI of 0 or 1+ in "I" and 5+ in "BL"). In certain cases, differentiating between BL and BB or BL and LL based only on morphological and bacilloscopic characteristics can be difficult, if not impossible. The inflammatory infiltrates of BB are similar to BL, varying mainly in their extension and the parasitism of the tissues that are greater in BL (Fig. **31**). In relation to LL, BL can also show great similarity, especially in patients with a long evolution of the disease, also called subpolar (LLsp), where the formation of lepromas is observed, as well as diffuse infiltration of the entire skin, presence of a collagenized band in the papillary dermis (Unna band), and bacilloscopic examination showing parasitism of different types of skin cells and tissues associated with a BI of 6+ (Figs. **25** and **31**) [7]. In these cases of uncertainty between BB and BL or BL and LL, clinical information fundamentally important to ensure the correct clinical-pathological classification. However, the exact classification is more academic than practical, as these cases will be treated identically [5]. An alternative for the histopathological report of these uncertain cases is to define it as borderline leprosy and add that it is likely

BB/BL or define it as leprosy in the lepromatous side (BL/LL). In our experience, most patients classified as LL are, in fact, BL and have had a long disease evolution. Additionally, certain BL patients may have leprosy constituted predominantly by spindle macrophages, containing a large number of bacilli, which can be confused with histoid leprosy, a special presentation of lepromatous leprosy (BL and LL). This presentation of lepromatous leprosy affects patients who were previously treated, mainly by dapsone, and is clinically characterized by lesions with a keloid aspect and histopathological picture of fusiform histiocytes, simulating a dermatofibroma, with a large number of bacilli (Fig. **32**) [10]. The histopathological characteristics of histoid leprosy are described in Chapter 8.

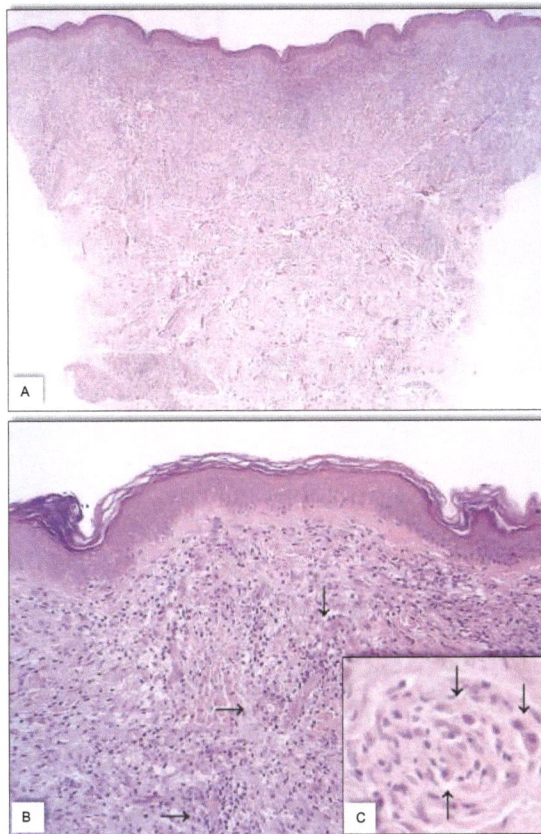

Fig. (19). Borderline lepromatous leprosy (BL). Cutaneous lesions present clusters of multivacuolated, non-epithelioid macrophages, permeated by lymphocytes and plasma cells (A and B). Inflammatory infiltrates are notably similar to those observed in BB lesions; however, they are more extensive and with a greater number of lymphocytes and plasma cells that are increasingly evident in the perivascular spaces (B and C). HE staining.

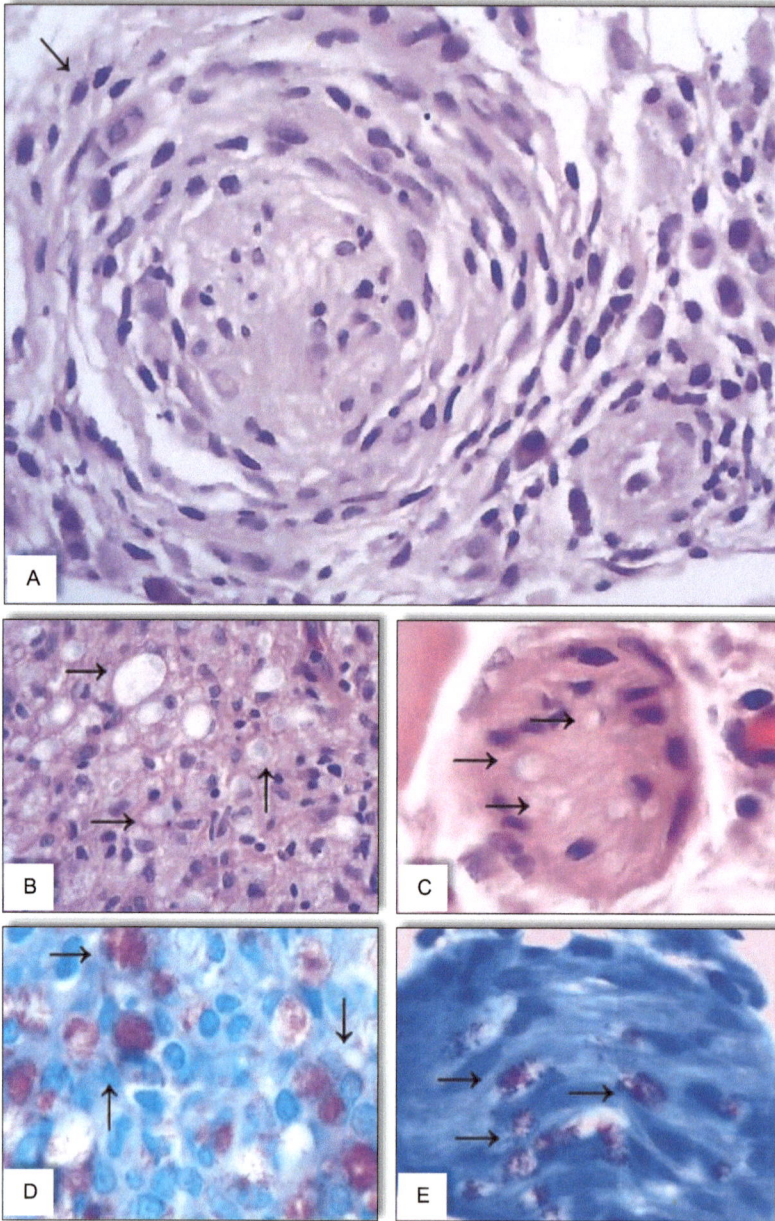

Fig. (20). Borderline lepromatous leprosy (BL). BL commonly presents neural branches with concentric delamination of the perineurium, giving the appearance of an "onion" or "target" (→) **(A)**. The neural branches are preserved, with macrophages, lymphocytes, and plasmocytes permeating Schwann cells (→) **(A)**. Macrophages (→) **(B)** and Schwann cells (→) **(C)** with intracytoplasmic vacuoles containing gray amorphous material that are bacilli, solid, and fragmented when stained by Fite-Faraco (→) (D and E).

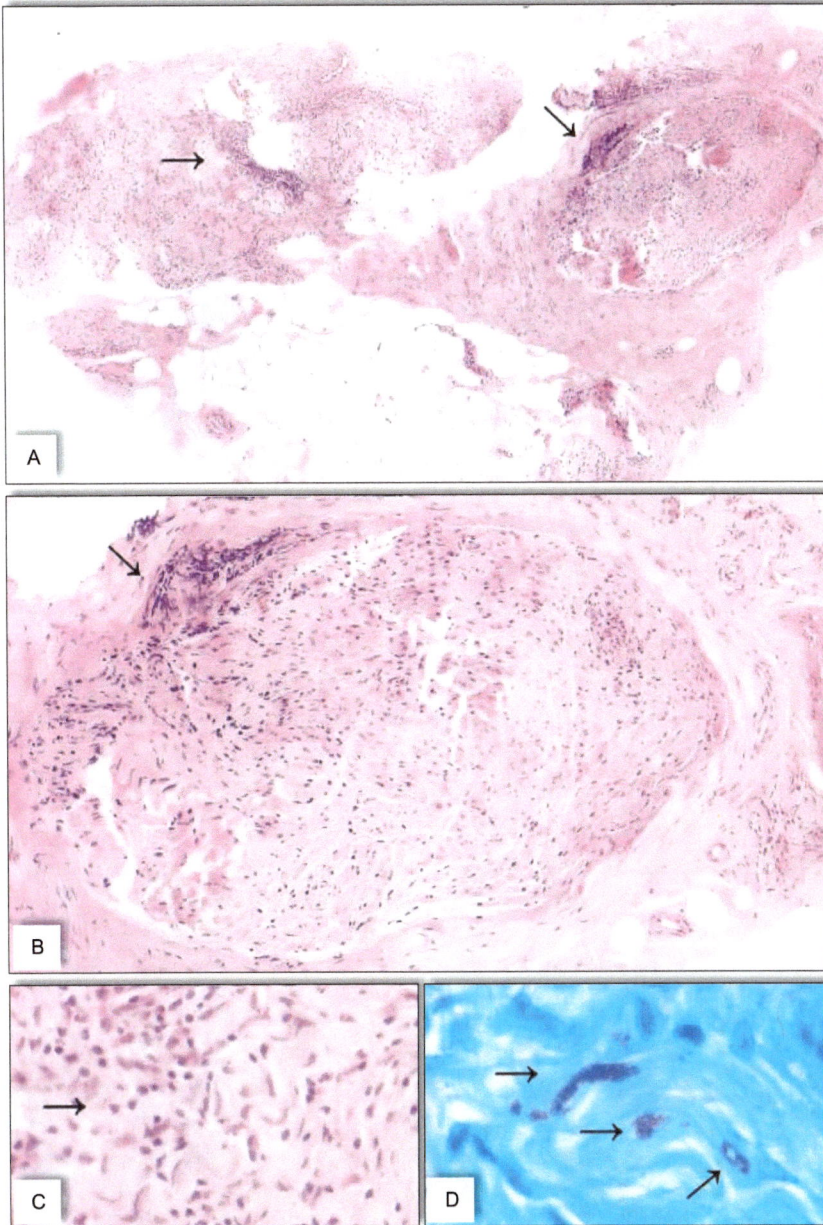

Fig. (21). Borderline lepromatous leprosy (BL). Biopsy of the sural nerve with a BL inflammatory process (→) characterized by lymphocytes, macrophages, and plasmocytes permeating the perineural and endoneural tissues, without nerve destruction (→) (A, B, and C). Bacilloscopy shows numerous bacilli in Schwann cells (→) **(D)**. HE staining (A, B, C, and D) and Fite-Faraco **(E)**.

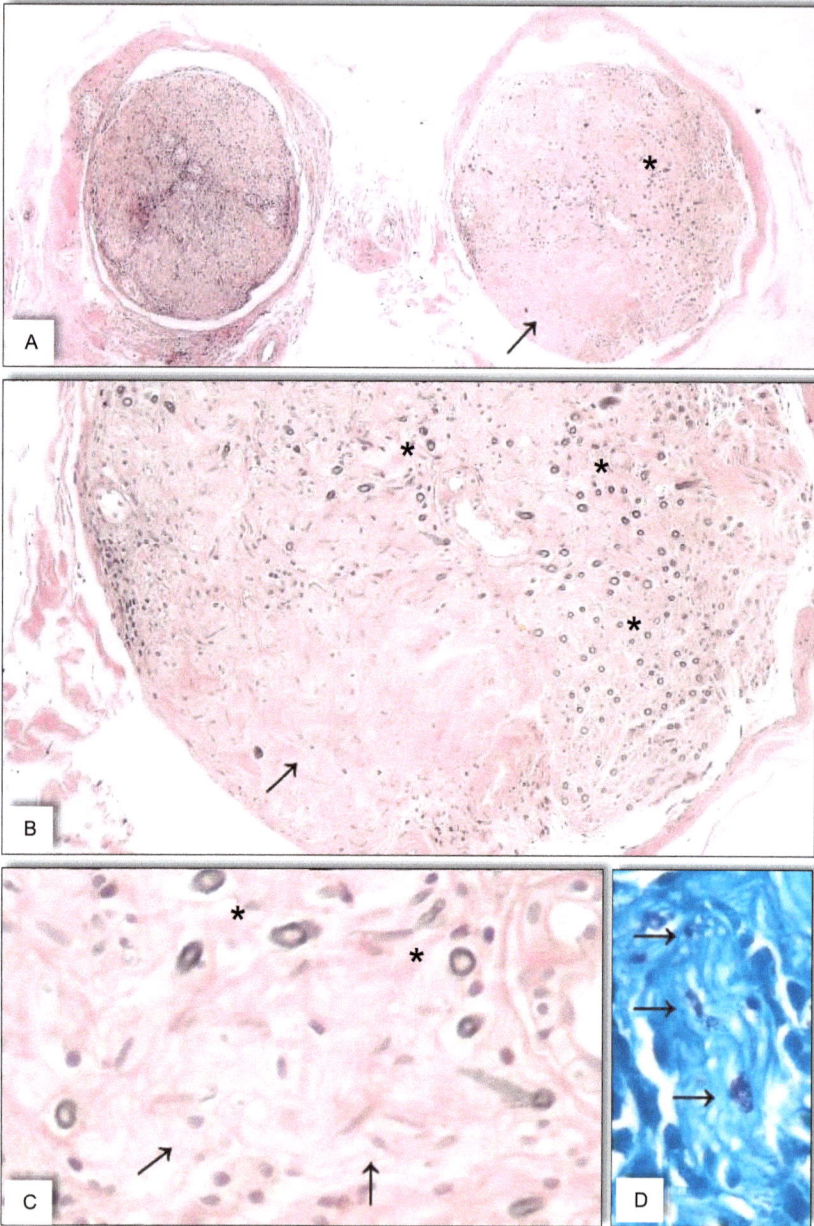

Fig. (22). Borderline lepromatous leprosy (BL). Biopsy of the sural nerve with BL pattern inflammatory process showing myelinated (*) and demyelinated (→) (A, B, C, and D) areas. Post-fixed biopsy with osmium tetroxide shows the dark gray myelin sheath present in some parts of the neural branch (*) and absent in the demyelinated areas (→) (B and C). Bacilloscopy shows numerous bacilli in Schwann cells (→) **(D)**. HE staining (A, B, C, and D) and Fite-Faraco **(E)**.

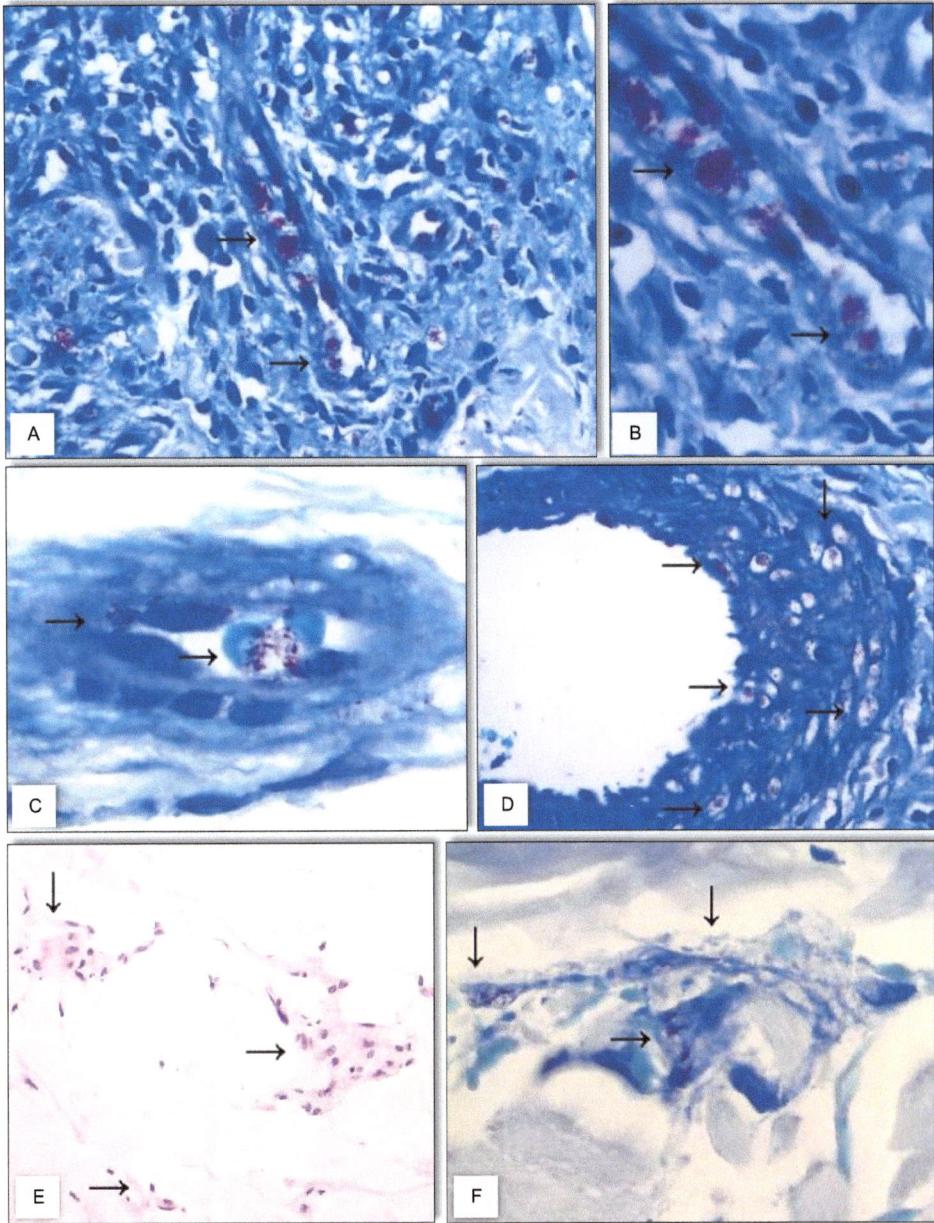

Fig. (23). Borderline lepromatous leprosy (BL). Presence of bacilli inside endothelial cells (→) (A, B, and C), the entire thickness of the vessel wall (→) **(D)**, and cells in the interstitium (→) (E and F). HE staining **(E)** and Fite-Faraco (A, B, C, D, and F).

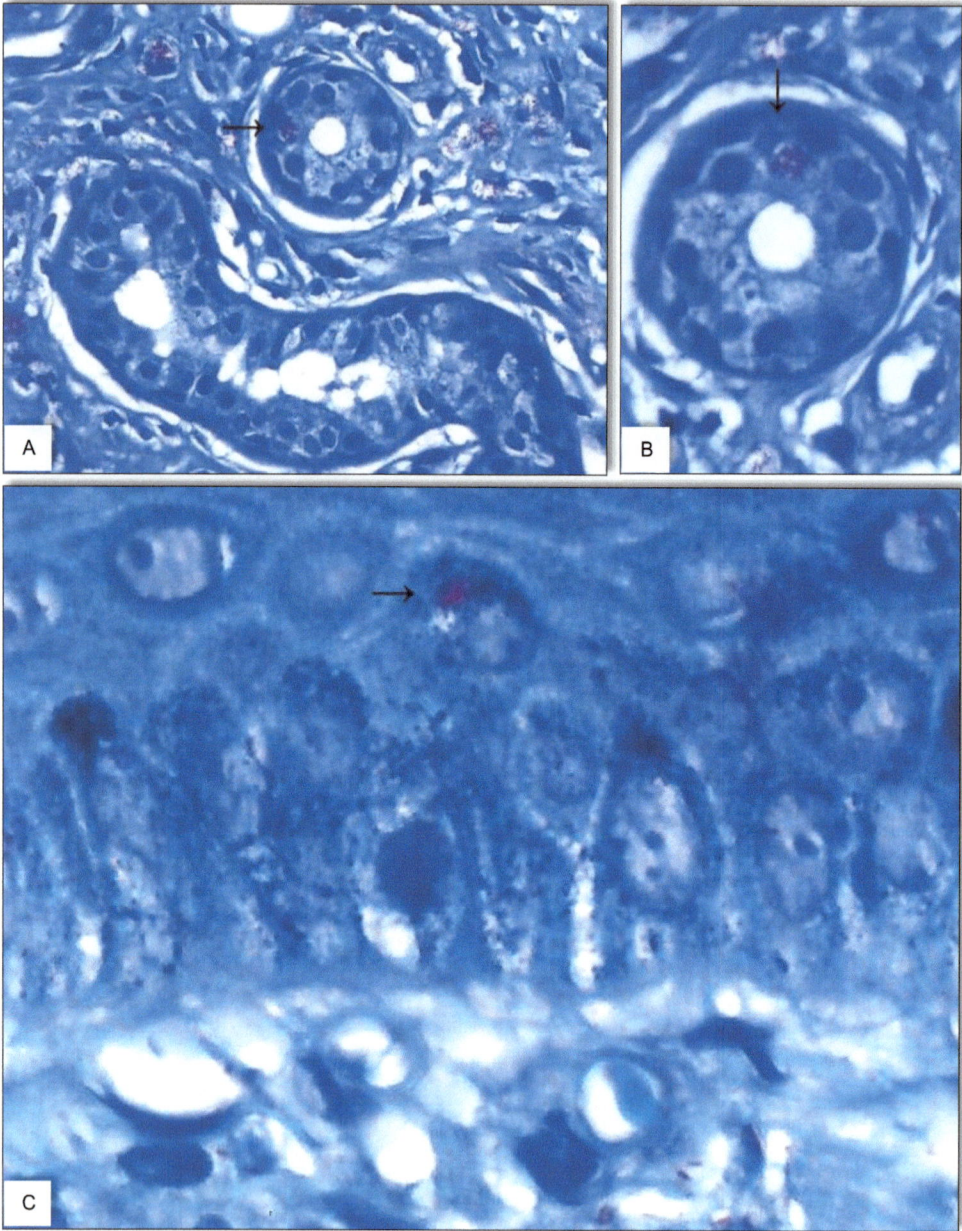

Fig. (24). Borderline lepromatous leprosy (BL). Presence of bacilli in the cytoplasm of sweat gland secreting cells (→) (A and B) and squamous epithelial cells of the epidermis (→) **(C)**. Fite-Faraco staining.

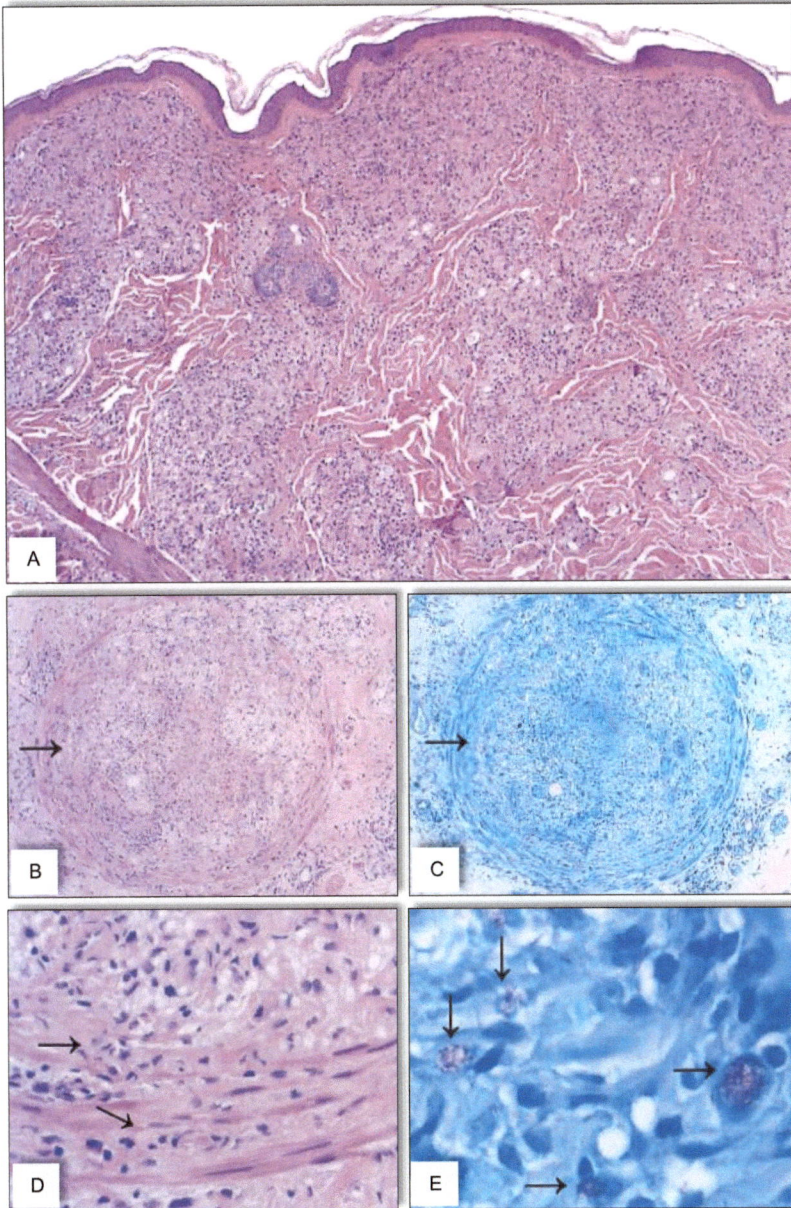

Fig. (25). Borderline lepromatous leprosy (BL). Long-term BL lesion with impairment of all skin components. Confluent macrophage infiltrates, consisting of multivacuolated macrophages permeated by a small number of lymphocytes and plasma cells. Infiltrate affecting all layers of a vein (→) (B and D). Bacilloscopy with numerous bacilli in all layers (→) (C and E). HE staining (A, B, and D) and Fite-Faraco (C and E).

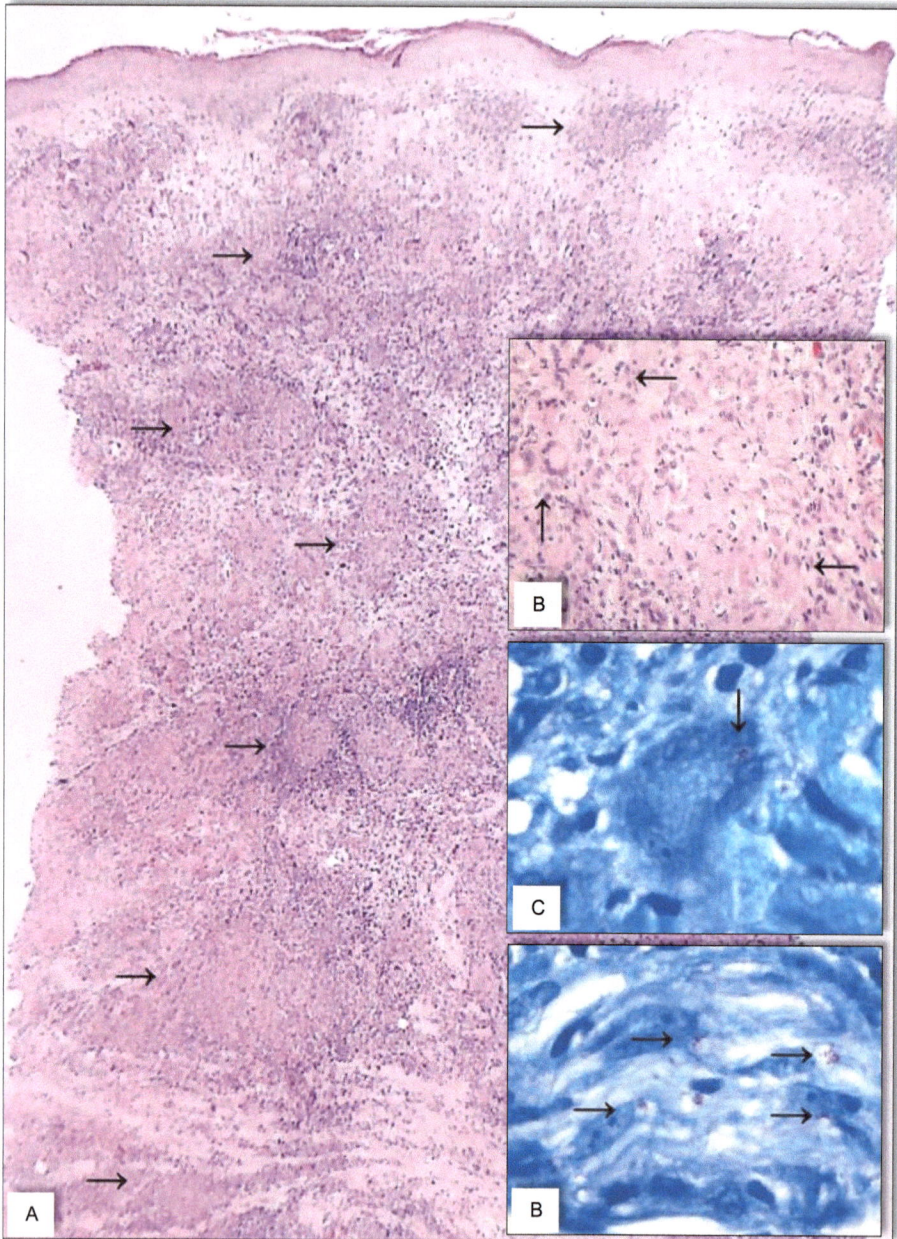

Fig. (26). Borderline lepromatous leprosy (BL) with a type 1 reaction (T1R). **(A)** An extensive lymphohistiocytic infiltrate with an outline of tuberculoid granulomas (→). Granulomas of poorly defined limits containing multinucleated giant cells (→) **(B)**. Bacilloscopy (4+) showing numerous bacilli in multinucleated giant cells (→) **(C)** and neural branches (→) **(D)**. HE staining (A and B) and Fite-Faraco (C and D).

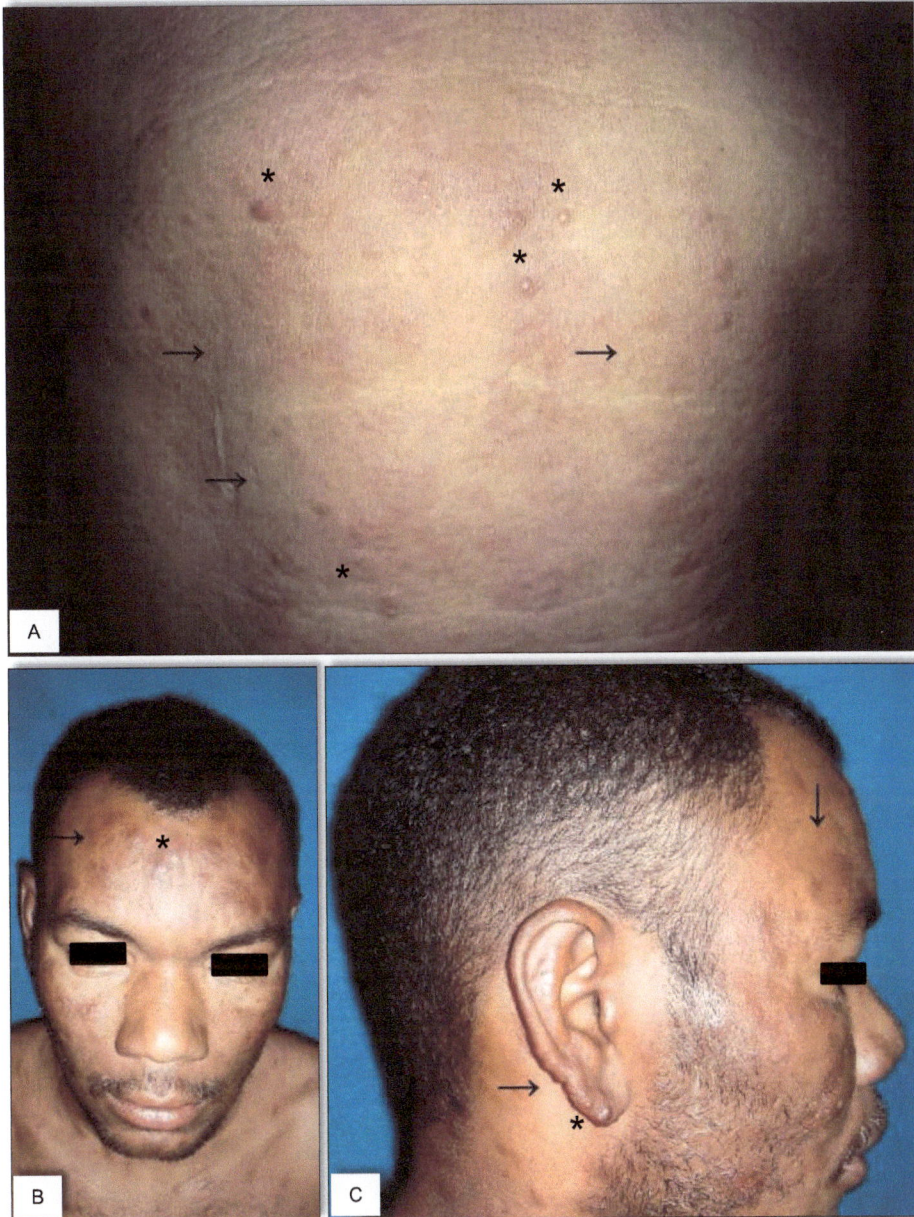

Fig. (27). Clinical features of borderline lepromatous leprosy (BL). Infiltrating plaques in a ferruginous or brownish tone (→) and papules or nodules (*) that are lepromas (A, B, and C). The auricular pavilion is often compromised, and the madarosis is discreet **(C)**. Courtesy of Dr. Cássio C. Ghidella.

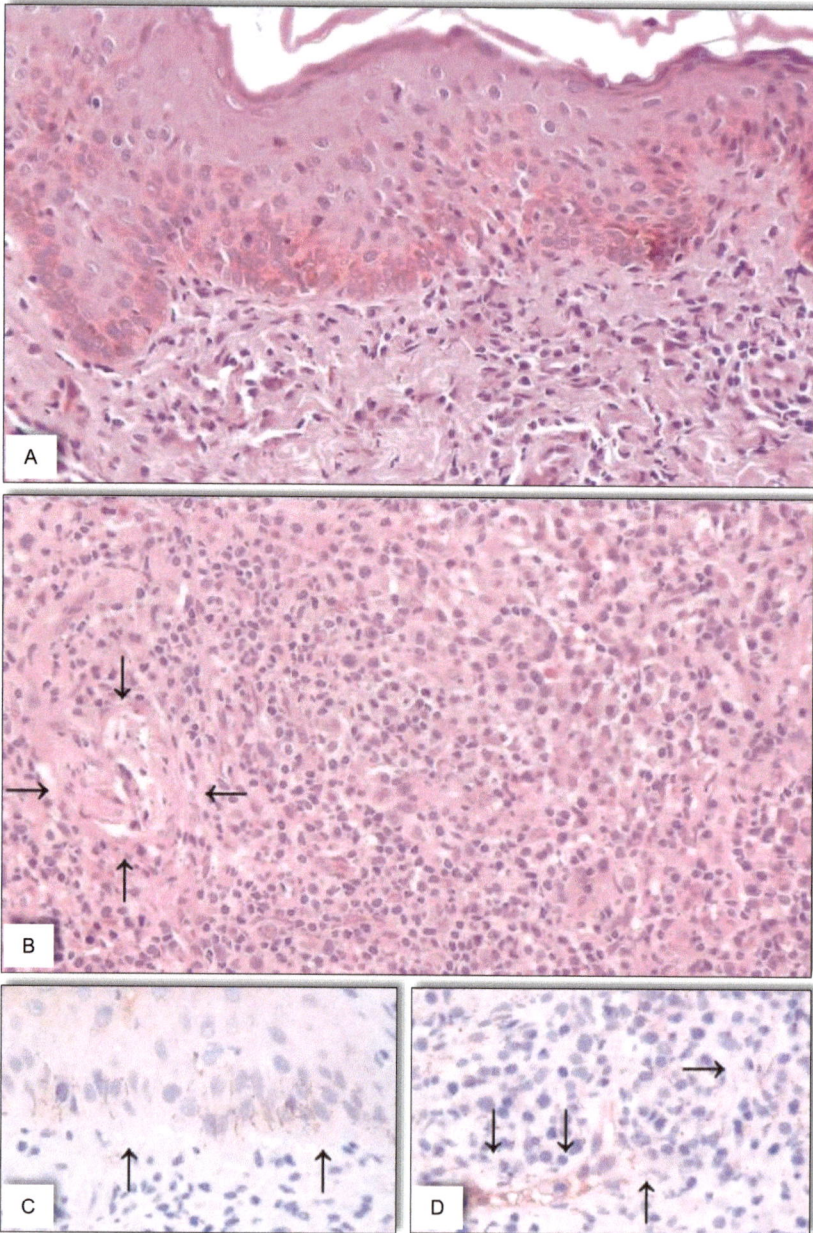

Fig. (28). Differential diagnosis of borderline lepromatous leprosy (BL). Secondary syphilis with an intense lymphohistiocytic and plasmacytic infiltrate at the dermoepidermal junction **(A)** and permeating neural branches (→) and vessels **(B)**. Immunohistochemistry demonstrates numerous treponemas at the dermoepidermal (→) **(C)** and perivascular (→) **(D)** interface. HE staining (A and B) and anti-treponema immunohistochemistry (C and D).

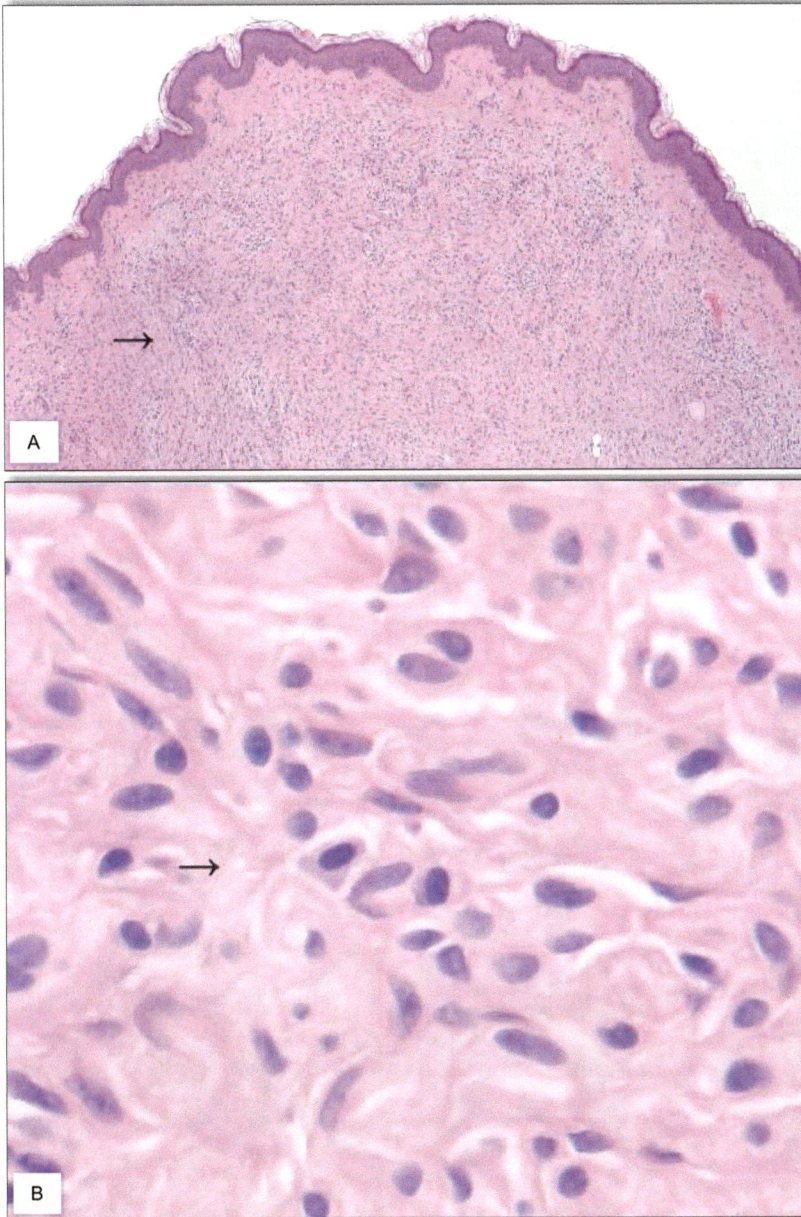

Fig. (29). Differential diagnosis of borderline lepromatous leprosy (BL). Neurofibroma (→) characterized by a proliferation of spindle cells in short fascicles and consisting of Schwann cells, collagen fibers, myxoid matrix, and mast cells (A and B). HE staining.

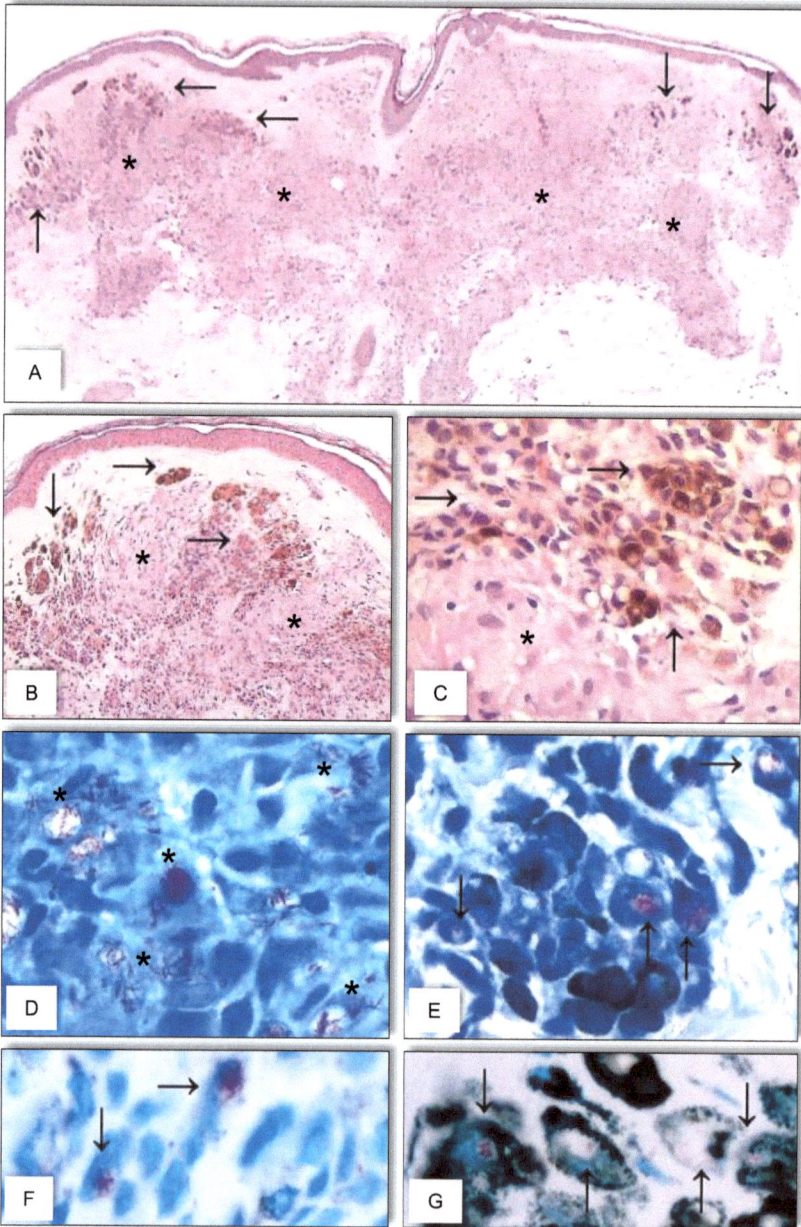

Fig. (30). Melanocytic nevus parasitized by *Mycobacterium leprae* in a BL patient. Skin papule consisting of a melanocytic nevus (→) and BL leprosy lesion (*) permeating the nevus (A, B, and C). Macrophages from leprosy lesions (*) **(D)** and parasitic nevus cells (→) **(E)**. Double staining (IHC + Fite-Faraco) demonstrates nevus cells (→) [CD68 negative **(F)** and melan A positive **(G)**] containing bacilli in the intracytoplasmic vacuoles. HE staining (A, B, and C), Fite-Faraco (D and E), and double staining (IHC + Fite-Faraco) (F and G).

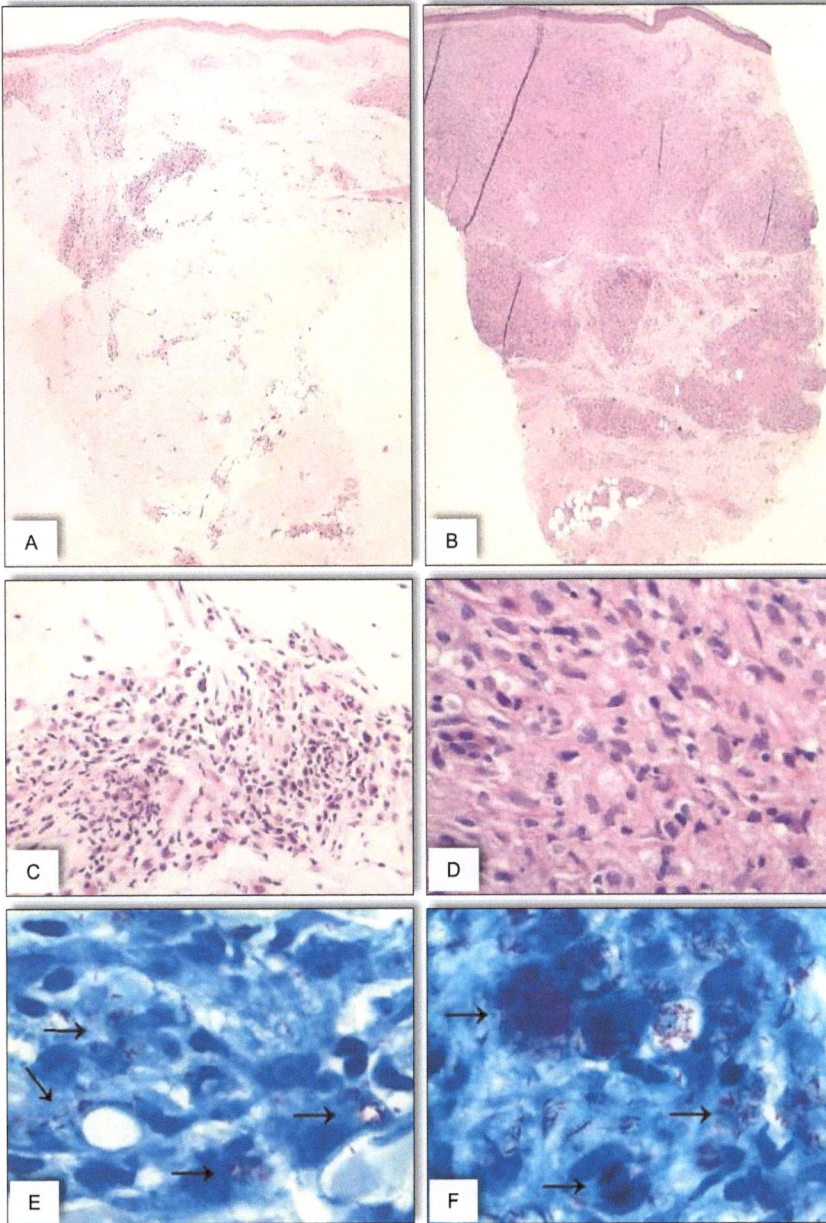

Fig. (31). Borderline Lepromatous Leprosy (BL). Two cases with clinical, histopathological, and bacilloscopic characteristics of BL resembling BB and LL. In A, C, and E, the infiltrate is similar to that observed in BB lesions with a bacilloscopic index of 5+ (→) **(E)**. In B, D, and F, the infiltrate is similar to that observed in LL lesions with a bacilloscopic index of 6+ (→) **(F)**. HE staining (A, B, C, and D) and Fite-Faraco (E and F).

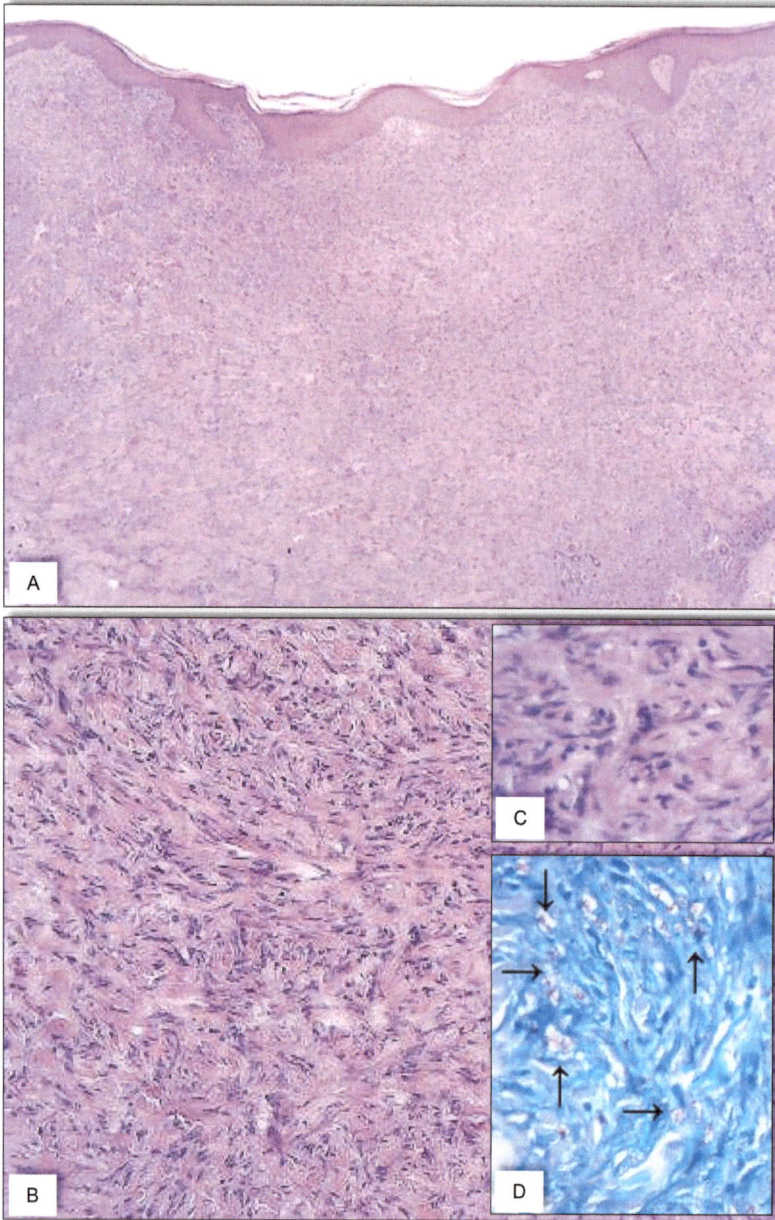

Fig. (32). Borderline Lepromatous Leprosy (BL). Some BL lesions in the form of a papule or nodule (leproma) may have diffuse infiltration of the dermis and subcutaneous tissue by spindle-shaped macrophages (A, B, and C). Bacilloscopy shows numerous bacilli in macrophages (→) **(D)**. HE staining (B, C, and D) and Fite-Faraco **(E)**.

CONCLUSION

The intermediate or borderline forms of leprosy (BT, BB, and BL) are variants of the disease within the spectrum of its polar forms (TT and LL). Recognition of the histopathologic and bacilloscopic characteristics of these forms is important for determining the correct classification, choice of treatment, and type of reaction phenomenon that may develop post-treatment initiation (Chapters 5 and 6).

REFERENCES

[1]   Opromolla DVA. Manifestações clínicas e reações. Noções de Hansenologia. 2nd ed. Bauru, Brazil: Centro de Estudo Dr Reynaldo Quagliato, Instituto Lauro de Souza Lima 2000; pp. 51-8.

[2]   Lima LS. Sobre a classificação Sul Americana das formas da lepra / On the classification of South American forms of leprosy. Rev Bras Leprol 1945; 13: 135-42.

[3]   Fleury RN. Patologia e manifestações viscerais.Noções de Hansenologia. 2nd ed. Bauru, Brazil: Centro de Estudo Dr Reynaldo Quagliato, Instituto Lauro de Souza Lima 2000; pp. 63-71.

[4]   Ridley DS, Jopling WH. Classification of leprosy according to immunity. A five-group system. Int J Lepr Other Mycobact Dis 1966; 34(3): 255-73.
       [PMID: 5950347]

[5]   Lazo-Porras M, Prutsky GJ, Barrionuevo P, *et al.* World Health Organization (WHO) antibiotic regimen against other regimens for the treatment of leprosy: a systematic review and meta-analysis. BMC Infect Dis 2020; 20(1): 62.
       [http://dx.doi.org/10.1186/s12879-019-4665-0] [PMID: 31959113]

[6]   Fachin LRV, Soares CT, Belone AF, *et al.* Immunohistochemical assessment of cell populations in leprosy-spectrum lesions and reactional forms. Histol Histopathol 2017; 32(4): 385-96.
       [PMID: 27444702]

[7]   Talhari C, Talhari S, Penna GO. Clinical aspects of leprosy. Clin Dermatol 2015; 33(1): 26-37.
       [http://dx.doi.org/10.1016/j.clindermatol.2014.07.002] [PMID: 25432808]

[8]   Kundakci N, Erdem C. Leprosy: A great imitator. Clin Dermatol 2019; 37(3): 200-12.
       [http://dx.doi.org/10.1016/j.clindermatol.2019.01.002] [PMID: 31178103]

[9]   Teixeira CS, Montalvão PP, de Oliveira IT, Wachholz PA. Neoplastic cells parasitized by *Mycobacterium leprae*: report of two cases of melanocytic nevus and one of basal cell carcinoma. Surg Exp Pathol 2019; 2: 26.
       [http://dx.doi.org/10.1186/s42047-019-0051-x]

[10]   Andrade TCPC, Itimura G, Vieira BC, *et al.* Hanseníase históide símile: desafio diagnóstico. Hansenol Int 2014; 39: 66-9.

CHAPTER 5

Type 1 Reaction (T1R)

Abstract: A type 1 reaction (T1R) is also known as a reversal reaction. This phenomenon involves exacerbation of the immune system or delayed-type hypersensitivity in response to the antigens of *Mycobacterium leprae* present in parasitized tissues. It occurs in most patients of the tuberculoid and borderline forms of the Ridley & Jopling classification for leprosy. It is an important phenomenon that can occur before, during, or after leprosy treatment and can be destructive, causing tissue damage mainly in the nerves, as well as irreversible sequelae. The recognition of T1R in histological sections may be notified prior to clinical presentation. Histopathological recognition is vital in defining or confirming the presence of T1R, guiding the treatment of the reaction process, avoiding or reducing the possibility of serious sequelae, correcting possible mistakes in the classification of patients within the spectrum of leprosy, and ruling out other diseases that can clinically simulate a T1R. In this chapter, the histopathological characteristics that allow the recognition of T1R, various histopathological aspects of the common forms of leprosy, and histopathological differential diagnoses are discussed.

Keywords: Downgrading, Hansen's disease, Leprosy, Reaction type 1, Reversal reaction, Upgrading.

INTRODUCTION

Leprosy is a slow and progressive disease noted by inflammatory signs on the skin as lesions and in the peripheral nervous system. Granulomas develop slowly, allowing endoneural structures and other parasitic tissues to adapt to the immune response. Functional changes are noticed after long-term disease progression as a result of the low antigenicity of *M. leprae* that limits an acute, intense, or destructive immunocelluar reaction. However, highly intense and destructive episodes involving the abrupt onset of cutaneous-neural lesions may appear during the course of the disease. These episodes are called leprosy reactions.

Reactions are important events that occur throughout the progression or regression of leprosy. To date, there is no specific treatment to prevent the occurrence of these epiphenomena, nor an effective treatment protocol for all cases [1 - 3]. Generally, during these episodes, neurological lesions can worsen and cause permanent functional disabilities [1, 2]. There are two main types of reactions identified in leprosy: type 1 reaction (T1R) and type 2 reaction (T2R). In this chapter, the histopathological characteristics of T1R will be discussed.

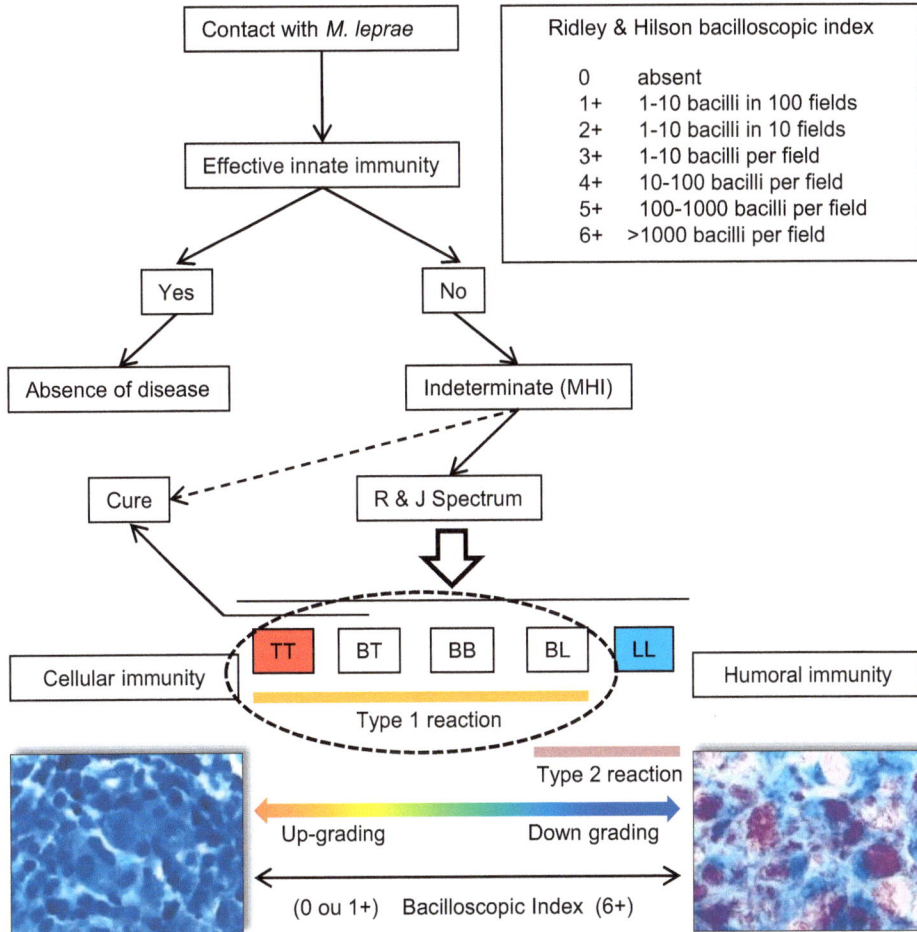

Fig. (1). Clinical spectrum and bacilloscopic index of leprosy forms and reactions. Patients who are exposed to *M. leprae* can eliminate the bacilli through mechanisms of primary immune response and do not develop the disease. If the primary immune defense cannot contain the proliferation of the bacilli, the patient develops indeterminate leprosy (I), the early stage of the disease preceding the polarized forms of the Ridley & Jopling (R&J) classification: tuberculoid (TT), borderline-tuberculoid (BT), borderline-borderline (BB), borderline-lepromatous (BL) and lepromatous or virchowian (LL). Late recognition of bacillary antigens by the individual may result in an intense and effective immune response (TT and BT pattern), which may lead to the destruction of the bacilli and spontaneous cure. TT individuals are those with effective cellular immunity. If cellular immunity is not effective, proliferation and dissemination of the bacilli persist, and the disease progresses toward the lepromatous pole. LL individuals are anergic and react to the bacilli through humoral immunity. Type 1 reactions (T1R) affect patients in the range from TT to BL. Type 2 reactions (T2R) affect patients on the lepromatous side (BL and LL). The bacilloscopic index ranges from 0-6+.

Histopathological and Bacilloscopic Characteristics of T1R

T1R is an exacerbation of the immunocellular response that occurs in patients in the TT, BT, BB, and BL forms (Fig. **1**). The clinical signs of the reaction are swelling and erythema over pre-existing lesions (Fig. **2**). Some skin lesions that are difficult to identify or clinically imperceptible may become evident during the reaction process (Fig **2**). T1R can occur at different locations on the skin and other parasitic tissues with varying intensity (Fig. **3**). Necrosis and ulceration of lesions are characteristics of intense T1Rs, especially when it occurs in patients in the tuberculoid side (TT and BT) (Figs. **4 - 5**) [4]. T1Rs are represented histologically by a tuberculoid granuloma, similar to those observed in TT and BT granulomas ("TT/BT-like granuloma"), consisting mainly of M1-pattern epithelioid macrophages, permeated by T lymphocytes and followed by M2-pattern macrophages, B and T lymphocytes and other cells in the periphery (Fig. **6 - 7**) [5]. Macrophage fusion forming multinucleated giant cells is common. Granulomas are confluent and have inaccurate limits. Lymphocytes permeate epithelioid macrophages, which have intracytoplasmic vacuoles and intercellular edema. There may be deposition of interstitial fibrin, focal or confluent necrosis, and various degrees of aggression to the epidermis, with associated epithelial hyperplasia (Fig. **6**). These changes are due to the influx of new cells (macrophages, lymphocytes, plasma cells, and other cells) associated with changes that occur in existing cells, which constitutes the inflammatory process of pre-existing lesion leprosy [5]. Therefore, the histopathological and bacilloscopic characteristics of a histological section containing a type 1 reaction lesion are the sum of the histopathological characteristics of the lesion present before the reaction episode (TT, BT, BB, and BL) with the overlap of T1R histopathological characteristics.

Since T1R is an immunocellular reaction with an outline of tuberculoid granulomas, some cases of borderline leprosy with associated T1R can be confused with tuberculoid leprosy (TT). Although similar, the tuberculoid granulomas of T1R can be differentiated from those of the TT and BT forms. Some histological features are present in T1R tuberculoid granulomas and rare or absent in TT/BT tuberculoid granulomas: (1) granulomas are of imprecise and confluent limits; (2) they do not have a lymphocyte mantle on the periphery, especially those located in the reticular dermis or adipose tissue; (3) there are several lymphocytes permeating the epithelioid macrophages in the center of the granulomas; (4) there are important intercellular and intracellular edema in the macrophages in the center granulomas and in the interstitium and (5) fibrinoid or caseous necrosis is present in the center of the granulomas (Figs. **6 , 8 - 9**). The erroneous classification of a borderline patient with T1R as TT has important implications for the choice of appropriate treatment, since borderline with T1R patients follow a treatment protocol for multibacillaries and TT patients are treated for paucibacillaries (Figs. **10 - 11**) [6, 7]. If the histological sections show disorganized and confluent tuberculoid granulomas, significant edema, foci of necrosis within the granulomas, extension of the inflammatory process to the interstitium associated with stellated fibroblasts with evident nucleoli and a bacilloscopic index $\geq 2+$, this probably represents a T1R over a borderline lesion instead of leprosy in the tuberculoid side (TT/BT). The histopathological characteristics of tuberculoid granulomas of the TT and BT forms involving different skin tissues are detailed in chapters 3 and 4.

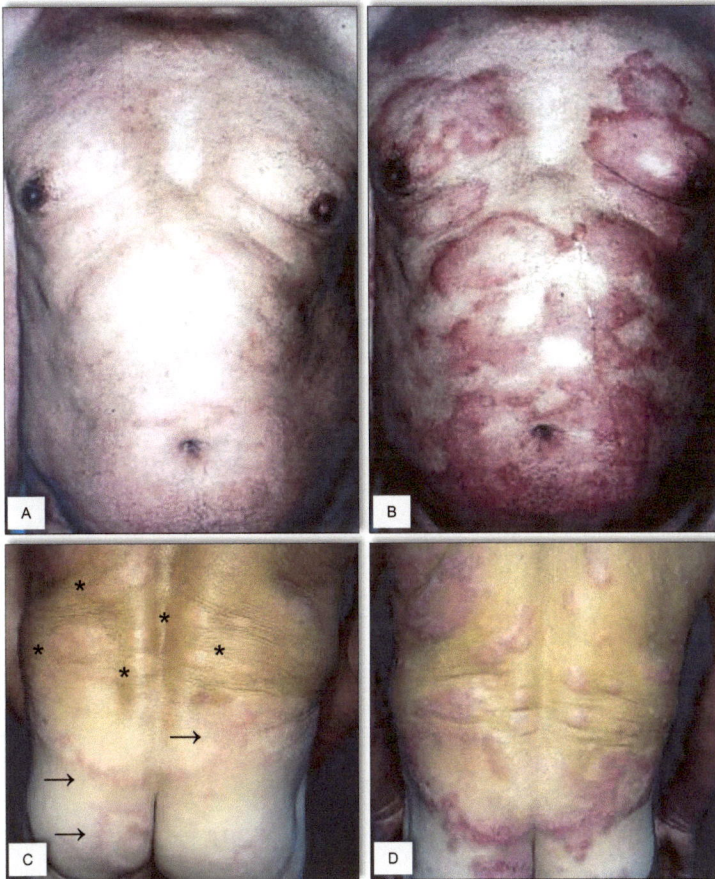

Fig. (2). Clinical characteristics of type 1 reaction (T1R) on borderline leprosy. Lesions affecting the skin of the chest and abdomen before the reaction process **(A)**. The reaction process develops on pre-existing lesions. T1R enhances pre-existing lesions by causing edema and hyperemia in them **(B)**. A borderline patient initiating the reaction process in part of the lesions (→) and in others, the reaction process is absent or initial (*) **(C)**. After a few days, T1R is established and active in all injuries **(D)**. Photos: A and B, archives of the Lauro de Souza Lima Institute (ILSL); C and D, courtesy of Dr. Cássio C. Ghidella.

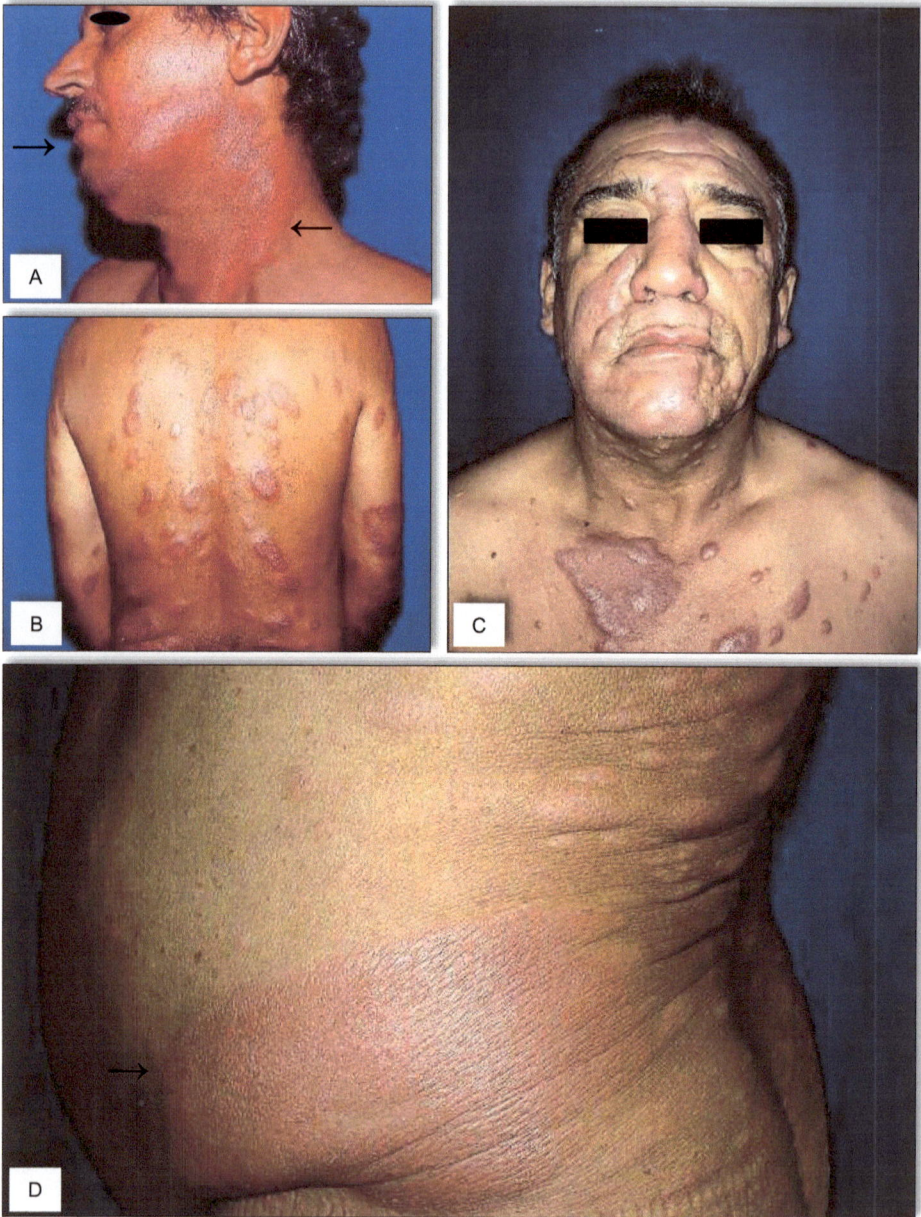

Fig. (3). Clinical characteristics of type 1 reaction (T1R). TT patient with T1R characterized by an erythematous plaque affecting the cervical region and face with raised surface and sharp limits, showing extension to the lips (→) **(A)**. Multiple borderline lesions with associated T1R consisting of annular erythematous plaques with flaking at the edges and partially defined limits (B and C). Several plaque lesions of different sizes with associated T1R, with one larger than the others (→) **(D)** ("motherboard"). Courtesy of Dr. Cássio C. Ghidella.

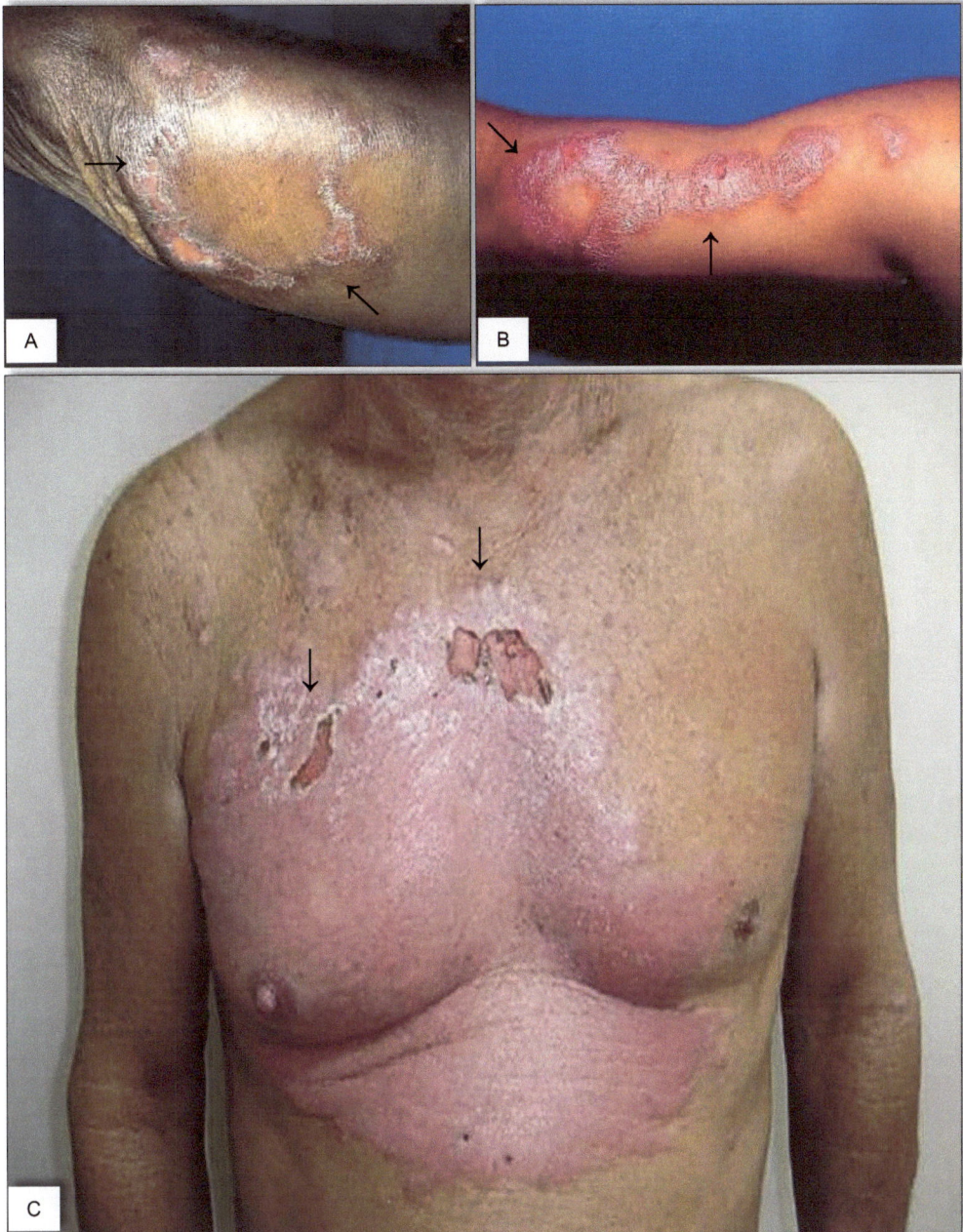

Fig. (4). Clinical characteristics of lesions in the tuberculoid side (TT/BT) with T1R associated with necrosis of the epidermis. Ulcerations start with an equimotic area and are mainly installed on the periphery of the lesions, forming an ulcerated ring (→) (A, B, and C). Courtesy of Dr. Cássio C. Ghidella.

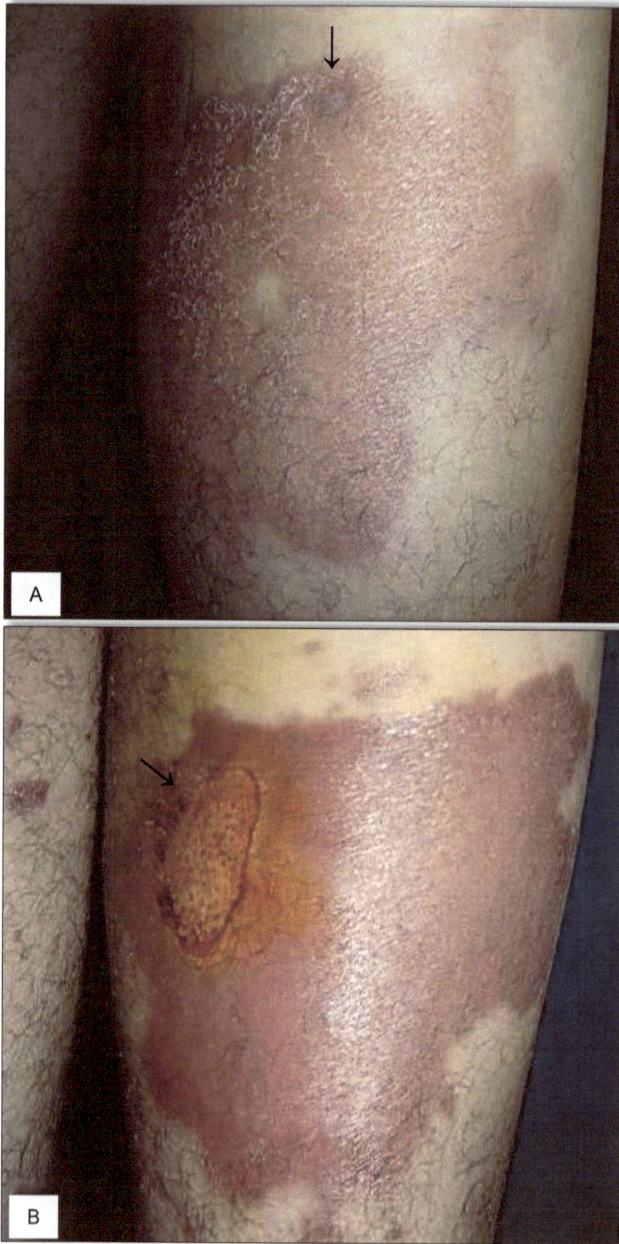

Fig. (5). Clinical characteristics of leprosy lesions with type 1 reaction (T1R) and associated necrosis. Erythematous plaque present at the reaction outbreak with a brownish and equimotic area at the top (→) **(A)**. Completely installed and intense T1R with an established necrotic area (→) **(B)**. Courtesy of Dr. Cássio C. Ghidella.

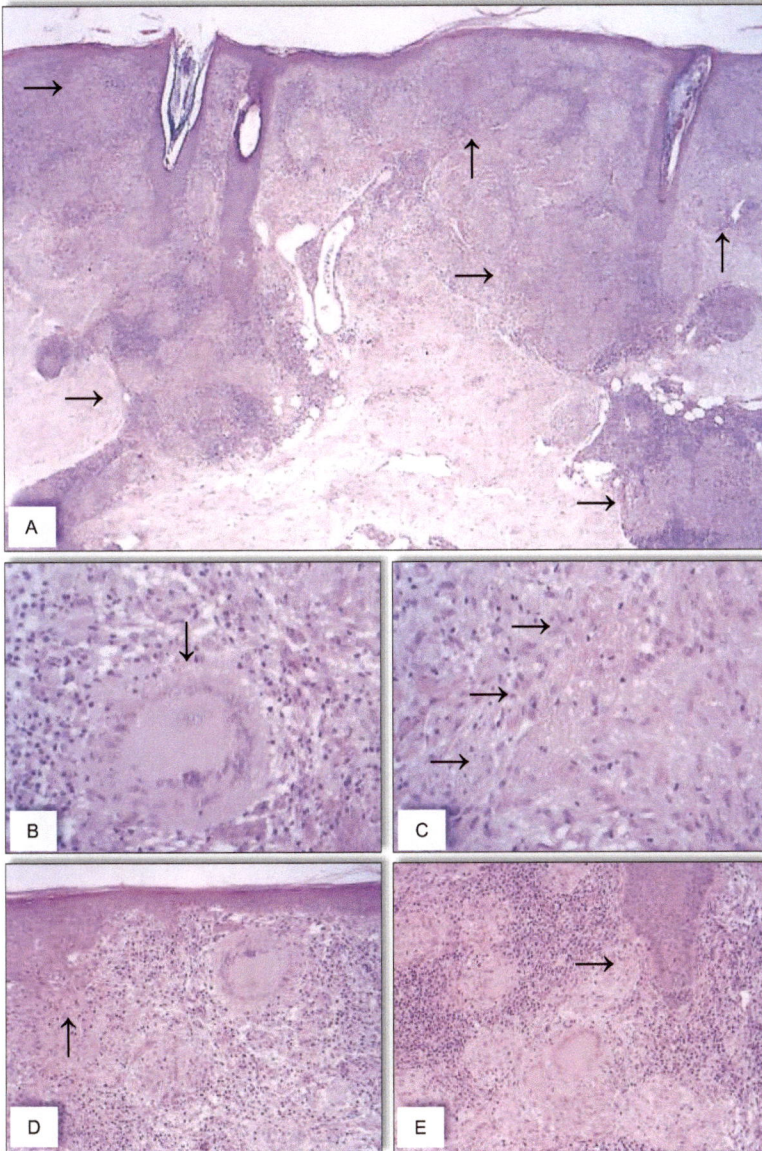

Fig. (6). Common histopathological characteristics of the type 1 reaction (T1R). Presence of more extensive, confluent, poorly defined granulomas that settle over pre-existing granulomas (→) **(A)**. Formation of multinucleated giant cells (→) **(B)**. Interstitial and intracellular edema with focal necrosis noted (→) **(C)**. Aggression to the epidermis with associated epithelial hyperplasia (→) (D and E). Hematoxylin and Eosin (HE) staining.

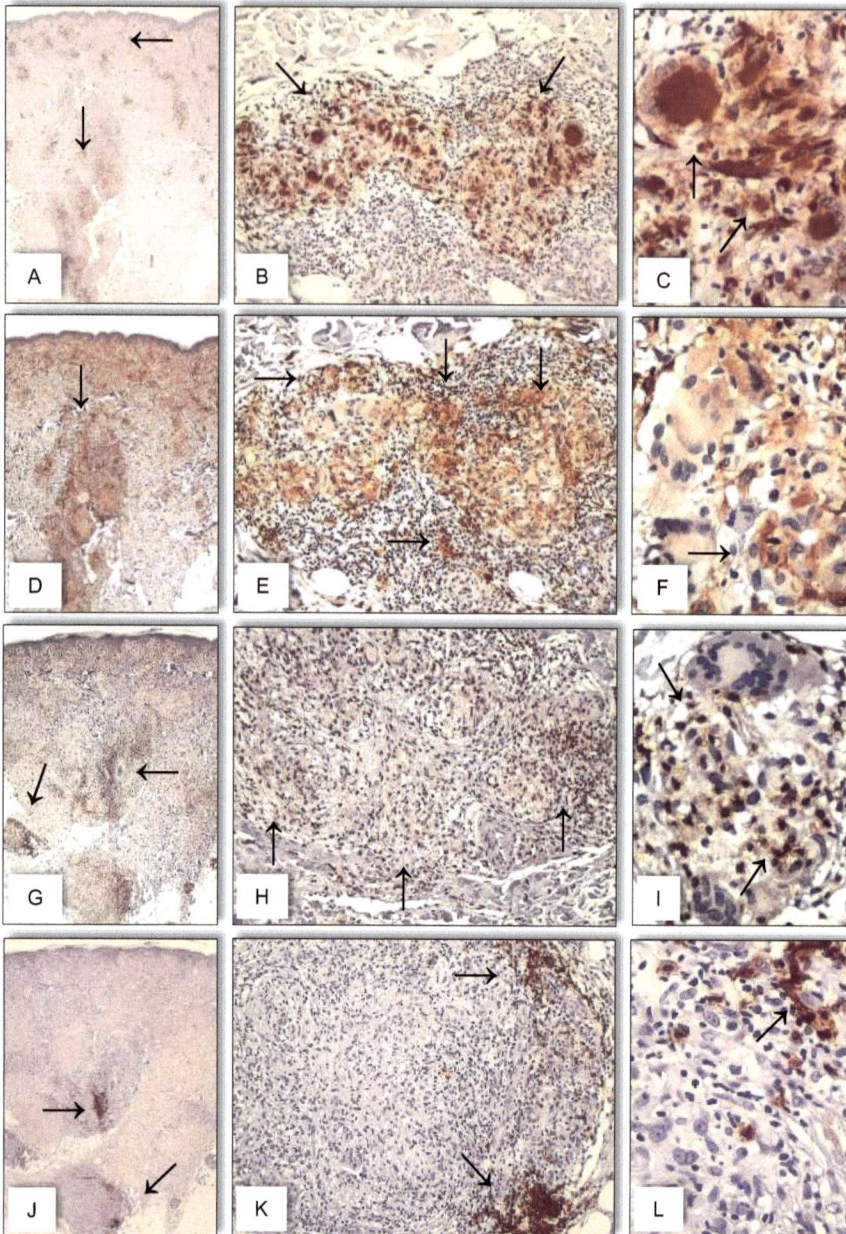

Fig. (7). Immunohistochemical profile characteristics of the T1R cell population. Epithelioid macrophages of M1 pattern (→) in the center of granulomas (A, B and C) surrounded by M2 macrophages (→) (D, E and F) and permeated by T lymphocytes (→) (G, H and I). Some granulomas may have a few B lymphocytes (→) in the periphery (J, K and L). Immunohistochemistry: CD68 (A, B and C), CD163 (D, E and F), CD3 (G, H and I) and CD20 (J, K and L).

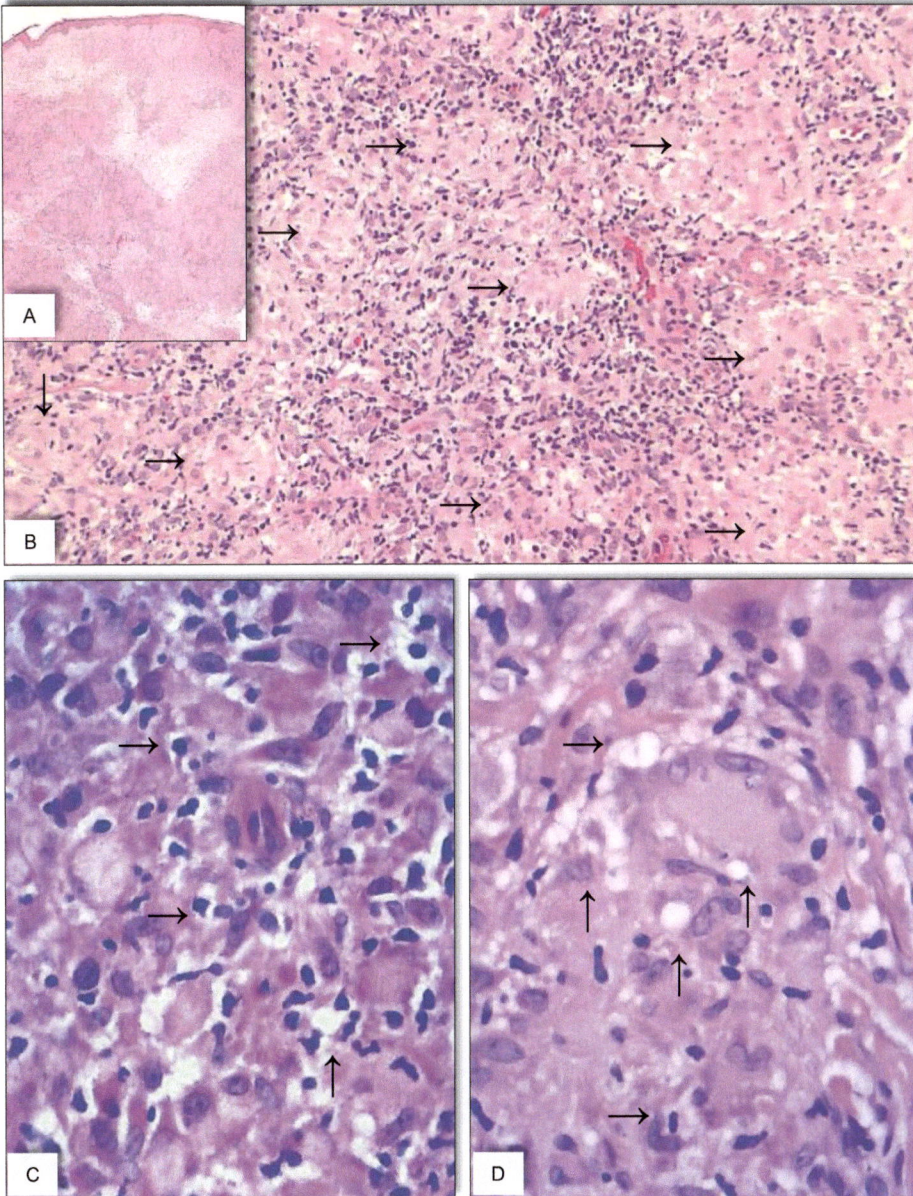

Fig. (8). Skin lesion in a BL patient with associated T1R presenting superficial and deep inflammatory infiltrate **(A)** with numerous confluent granulomas formed by epithelioid macrophages in the center and lymphocytes (→) **(B)**. Lymphocytes permeate macrophages in the center of granulomas (→) **(C)**. Intracellular and intercellular edema noted in the center of granulomas, with intracytoplasmic vacuoles in epithelioid macrophages and multinucleated giant cells (→) **(D)**. HE staining.

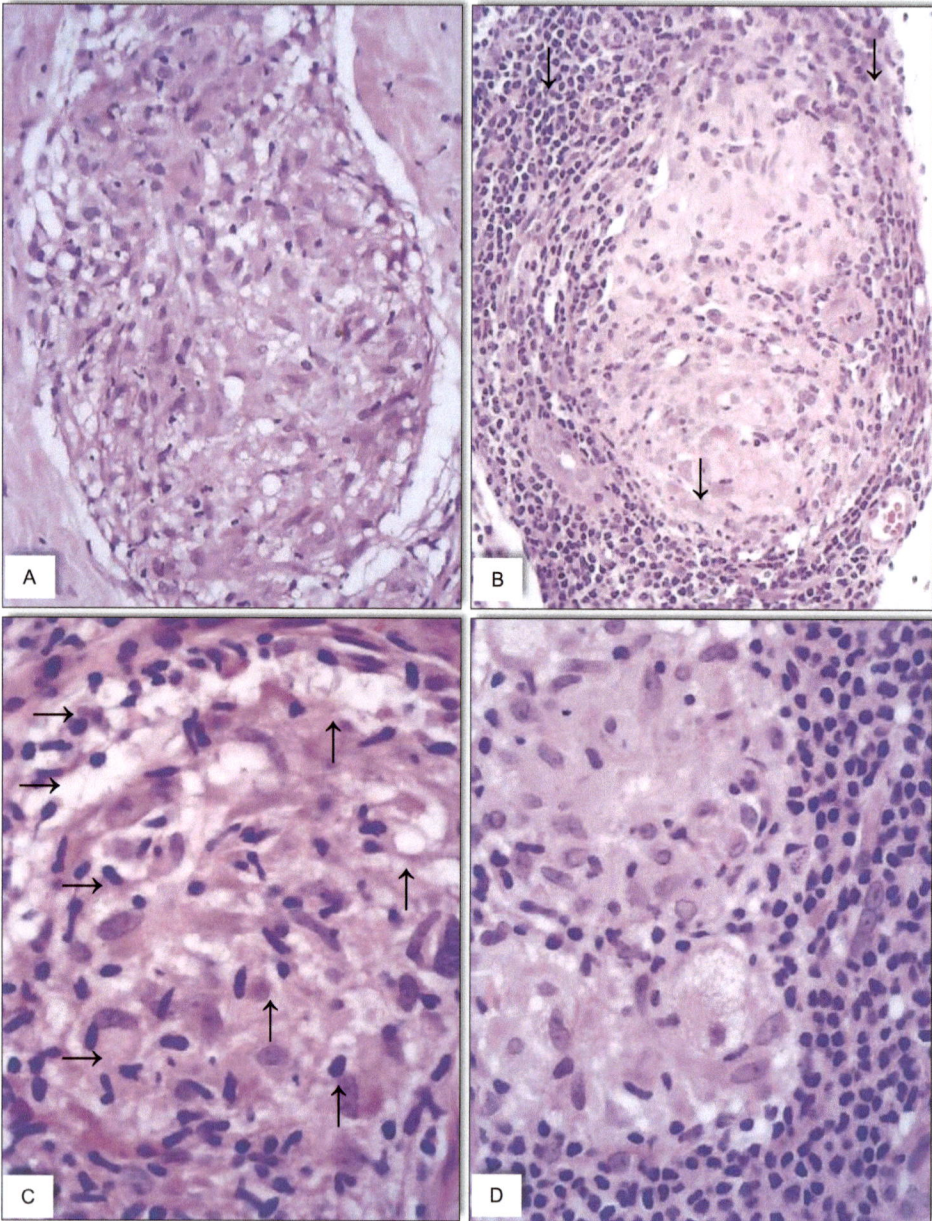

Fig. (9). Histopathological differences between T1R granulomas (A and C) and TT/BT forms (B and D). The "tuberculoid-like" granulomas of T1R **(A)** do not have a lymphocytic mantle in the periphery as in TT/BT (→) (B and D). There are many lymphocytes permeating the macrophages within the granulomas, and greater interstitial and intracellular edema in T1R granulomas (→) **(C)** than in TT/BT **(D)** granulomas. HE staining.

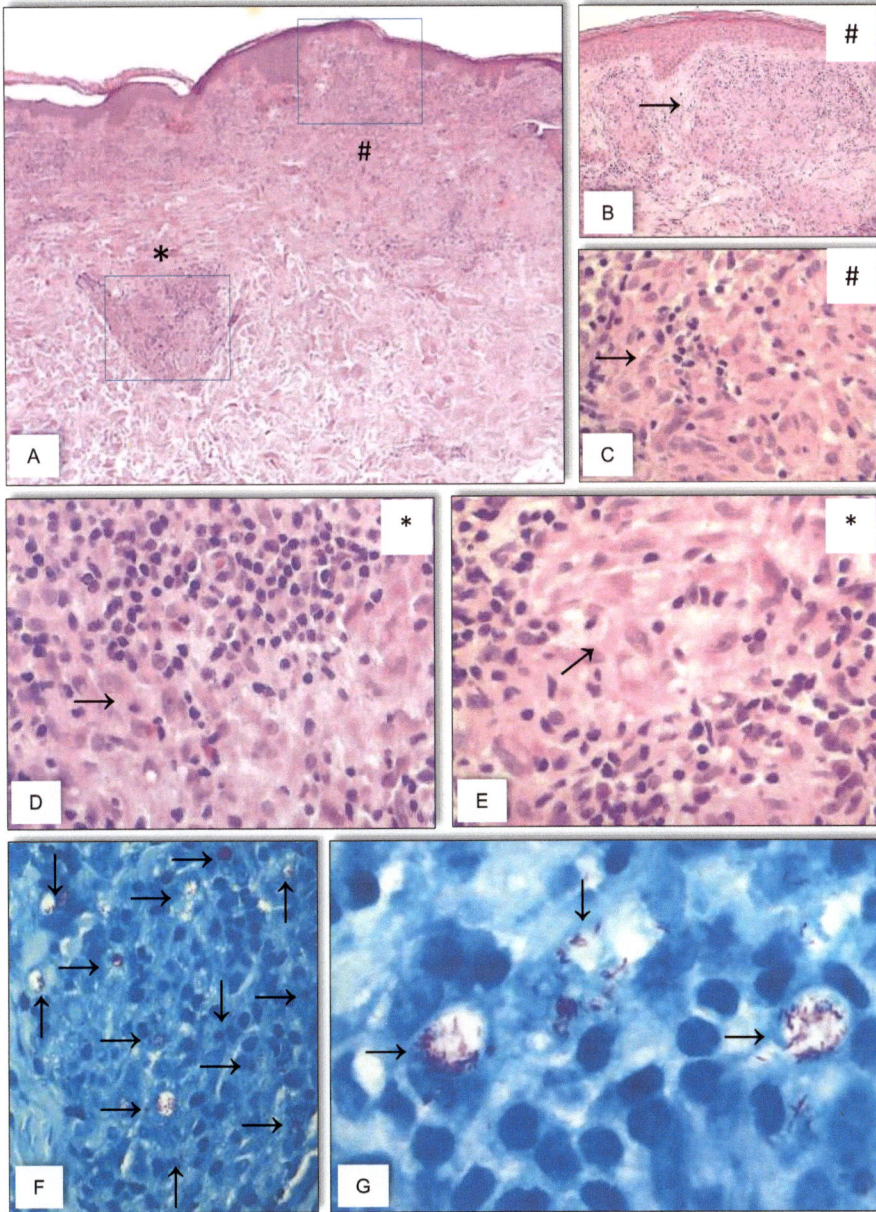

Fig. (10). Example of BB/BL with associated T1R, initially diagnosed as TT. A 35-year-old patient with an erythematous-hypochromic plaque with a clinical diagnosis of TT. Histopathological examination shows superficial (→) (#; A, B and C) and deep (→) (*; A, D and E) granulomas of the T1R. The bacilloscopic examination shows numerous solid and fragmented bacilli (→) (BI ≥ 5+) **(D)**. HE staining (A-E) and Fite-Faraco (FF) staining (F and G).

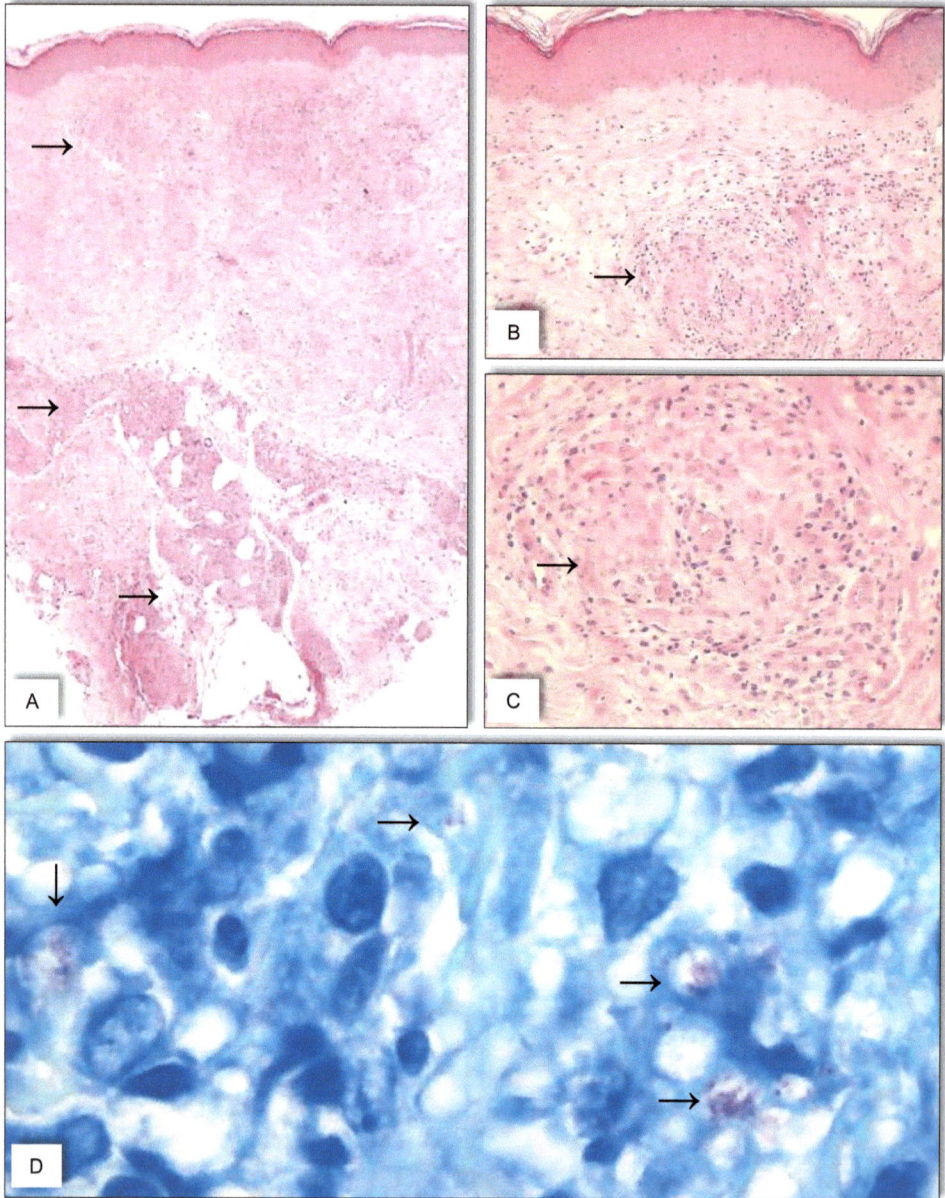

Fig. (11). Example of BB/BL with associated T1R, initially diagnosed as TT. A 77-year-old patient clinically diagnosed as TT and treated as paucibacillary. After treatment, he developed several erythematous plaques all over his body and lower limb edema. A biopsy was performed for reassessment, which showed an inflammatory infiltrate involving a large part of the skin tissue (→) **(A)**, presence of T1R granulomas (→) (B and C). A bacilloscopic exam showed numerous multifragmented and slightly colored bacilli (→) (BI ≥ 4+) **(D)**. HE staining (A-C) and FF staining **(D)**.

T1R episodes can occur during disease progression towards the lepromatous pole ("downgrading") before the treatment and in disease regression after the start of treatment ("upgrading"). T1R episodes that occur before, during or after treatment are histopathologically similar but with different bacilloscopic characteristics (Fig. **12**). The intensity and extent of T1R during upgrading is usually equal to or greater than that of T1R in downgrading. The mechanisms that trigger T1R are poorly understood, however there is a clear association between the development of reaction episodes and the presence of bacterial antigen in the tissues affected by T1R [2, 8]. In the absence of treatment, development of T1R in a patient at the disease progression phase can be explained by the occurrence of intense bacillary proliferation in some lesions, causing exposure of bacterial antigens and consequent immunocellular responses. Those patients in whom the disease has progressed and who are undergoing multidrug treatment (MDT), there is intense fragmentation of the bacilli, which results in modification of the mechanisms of bacillus-host interaction in the parasitized cells and tissues and exposure of the bacillary antigens to the host defense systems, thus triggering T1R. In this context, the bacilloscopic examination of T1R in patients with disease progression may show solid bacilli, in addition to fragmented ones, in different types of parasitized cells. This is observed mainly in BB and BL patients, where the bacilloscopic index ranges from 4+ to 6+. Further, there is a greater extent of parasitism than in those of the TT and BT forms (Fig. **12**). Conversely, in those patients who have T1R after the start of treatment, the reaction phenomenon commonly appears after the first three months of treatment, and the bacilli found are mostly fragmented (Fig. **12**).

Bacilloscopic examination is another important aspect in the assessment of reaction conditions. In the leprosy lesions of untreated patients, there are naturally fragmented bacilli and the predominance of solid bacilli. After starting MDT, fragmentation of the bacilli is intense, persisting throughout and beyond the treatment period. When T1R occurs over leprosy lesions, the reaction process itself fragments the bacilli, in addition to phagocyting and processing the bacillary antigens. This further decreases the bacilloscopic index (BI), making it difficult to classify patients within the Ridley & Jopling (R&J) spectrum (Chapters 3 and 4) (Fig **13**). In general, there is a decrease in the number of bacilli coupled with greater fragmentation within the reactional granulomas compared to other adjacent areas with leprosy injury but without T1R (Fig. **13**). A patient originally classified as BB or BL with BI of 4+ or 5+ before treatment may have a lower bacilloscopic index in lesions that develop T1R. In this situation, BI can decrease from 5+ to 1+ or 0 under the following conditions: (1) if the reaction process is more intense, (2) if there were repeated reaction episodes on the same injury, (3) if T1R occurred in long-term patients and those at the end of treatment, or (4) if it occurred many months or years after the end of treatment. Therefore, it is sometimes difficult to classify patients on basis of the form of leprosy using the R&J spectrum when an associated T1R is observed. In these cases, the clinical data and initial histopathological diagnosis are crucial for correct classification (Fig. **14**).

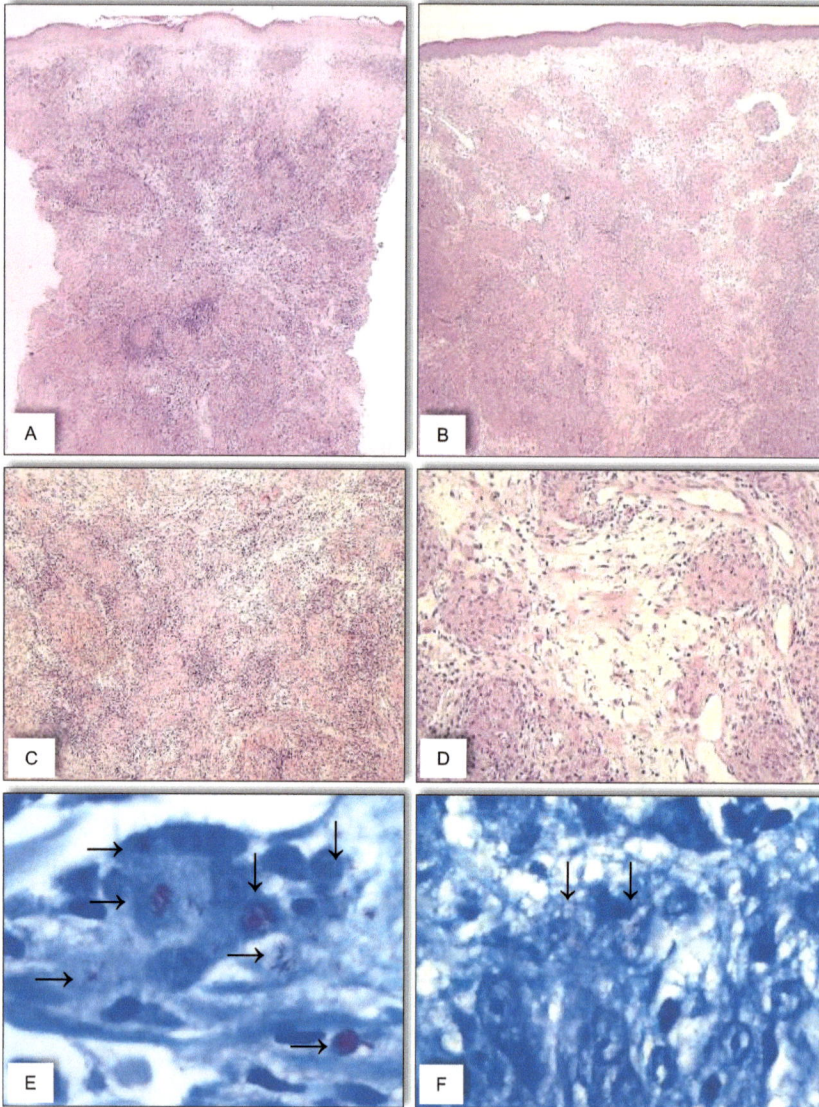

Fig. (12). Common histopathological characteristics of T1R. Two examples of BB/BL with T1R during disease progression (downgrading) (A, C and E) and after treatment (upgrading) (B, D and F). Reaction episodes of T1R in both are histopathologically similar, but with different bacilloscopic characteristics. Downgrading (**E**) shows solid and fragmented bacilli, well stained (→) in macrophages. In upgrading (**F**), the bacilli are multifragmented, poorly colored (→) and barely noticeable. HE staining (A-D) and FF staining (E and F).

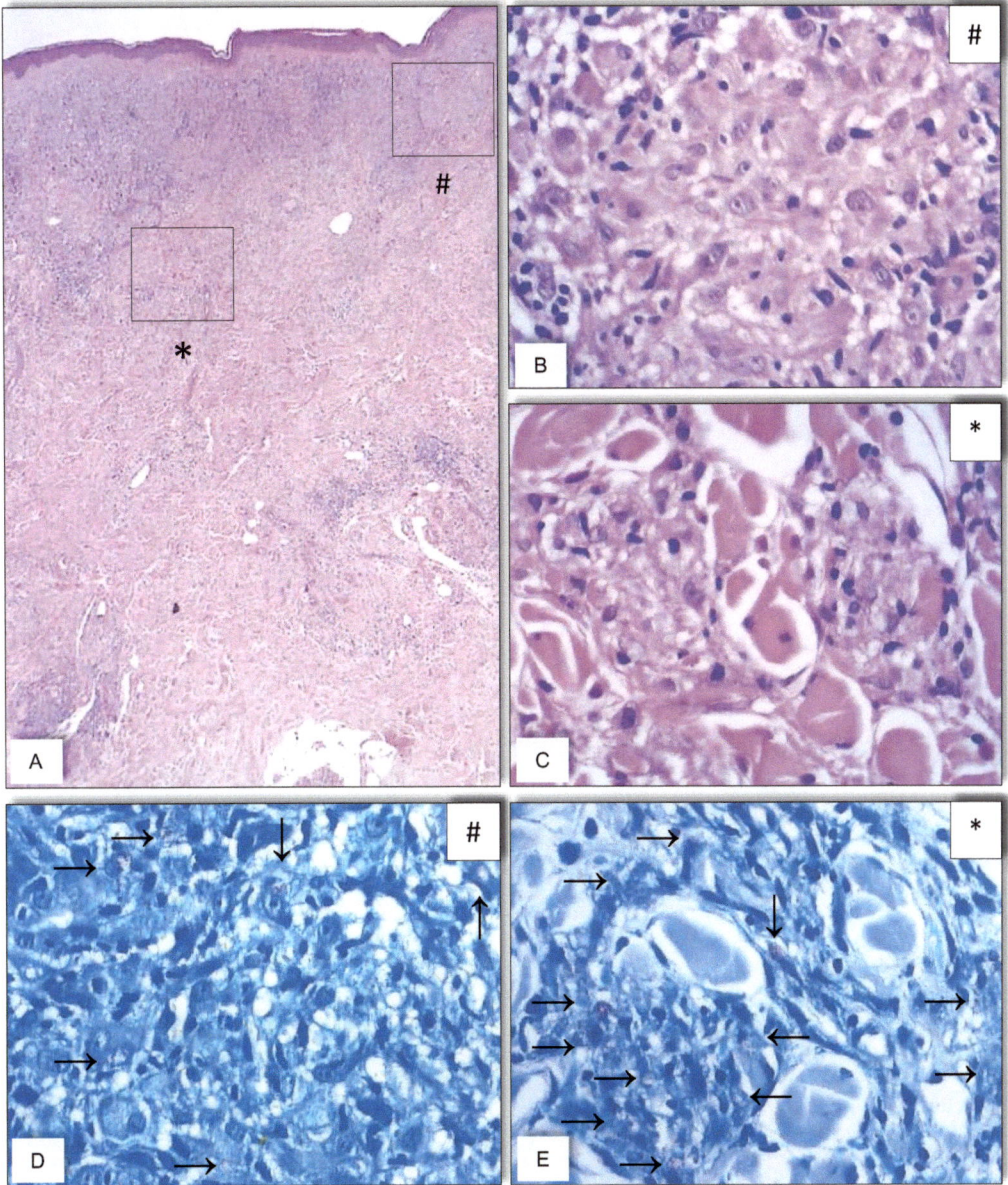

Fig. (13). Common histopathological characteristics of the type 1 reaction (T1R). BB patient who developed T1R two months after starting treatment. In areas with T1R (#; A, B and D), macrophages are epithelioids and the number of bacilli (→) is smaller, more fragmented and increasingly difficult to observe compared to adjacent areas without T1R (*; A, C and E), wherein macrophages are not epithelioids and fragmented bacilli (→) are numerous and easily observed. HE staining (A-C) and FF staining (D and E).

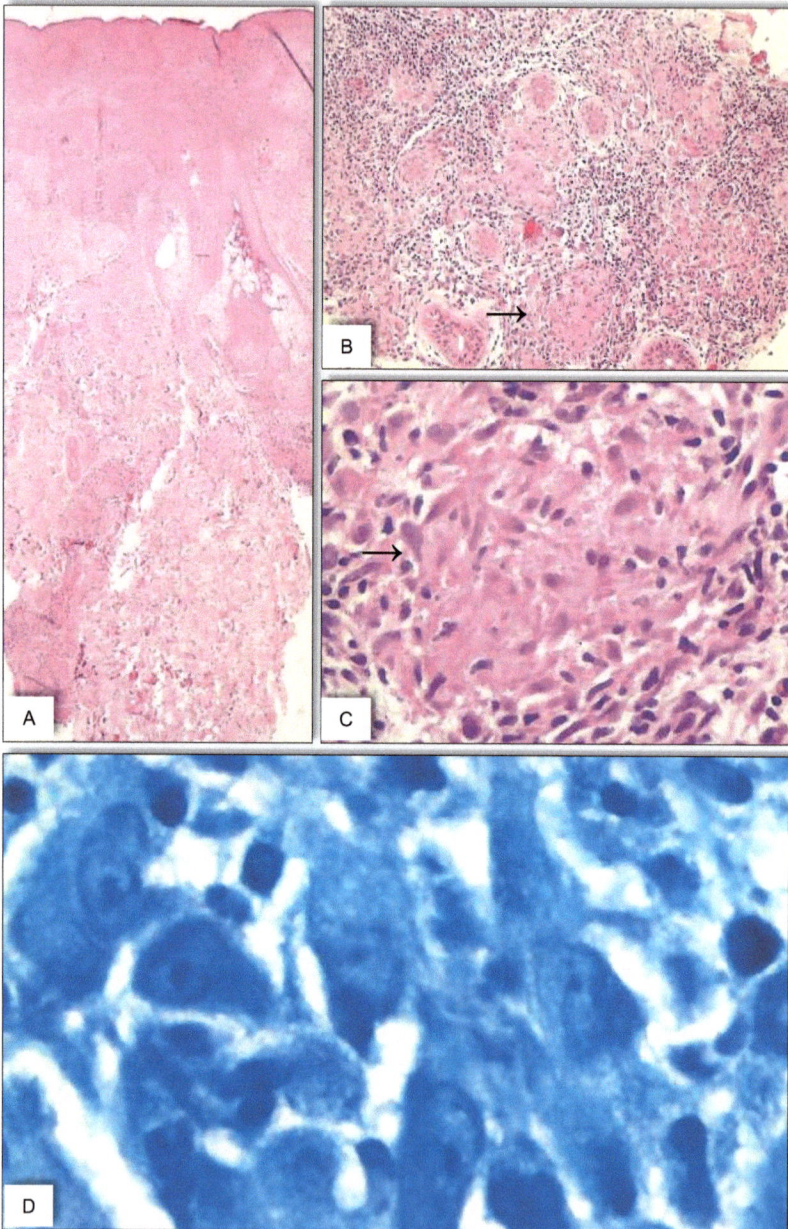

Fig. (14). Common histopathological characteristics of the type 1 reaction (T1R). Patient with previously confirmed clinical and histopathological diagnosis of BB developed T1R after the end of treatment. Presence of epithelioid macrophages forming well-defined T1R granulomas (→) (B and C) and absence of bacilli within granulomas (BI = 0) **(D)**.

In our experience, some patients develop T1R with intense fragmentation of the bacilli without having used specific treatment for leprosy. These cases are generally associated with patients who used antibiotics for a few months or years before developing episodes of T1R. It is common to use antibiotics to treat respiratory, urinary, neural or skin diseases that may or may not be associated with leprosy. These broad-spectrum antibiotics, some of which are part of treatment protocols for leprosy, have the ability to fragment *M. leprae*, which can trigger T1R (Fig. **15**) [6 - 8]. Additionally, there are reports in the literature that some patients with conditions such as pregnancy and AIDS that can alter their immune response capacity are likely to develop T1R in the postpartum period or after the beginning of anti-HIV treatment [9 - 11]. In some of these cases, T1R may also be associated with the use of prophylactic antibiotics during or after childbirth or for the treatment of AIDS-related opportunistic infections, leading to bacillary fragmentation and the triggering of T1R (Fig. **16**). Histopathological and bacilloscopic characteristics in these situations are similar to the cases of upgrading phase of T1R.

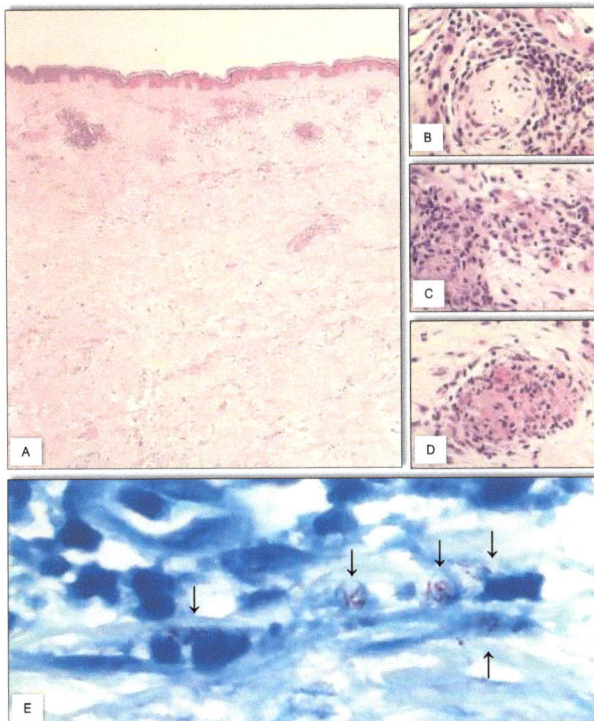

Fig. (15). Example of borderline leprosy with T1R associated post-treatment with non-specific antibiotics for leprosy. A 74-year-old man underwent eye surgery with prophylactic antibiotic therapy. After three months, he developed brownish erythematous plaques all over his body with clinical suspicion of a drug reaction or Sweet's syndrome. Histopathological examination showed a leprosy lesion, probably BB **(A)** with associated T1R, characterized by an inflammatory infiltrate involving neural branches **(B)**, T1R pattern granulomas (C and D) and a bacilloscopic examination with numerous fragmented and well-colored bacilli were observed (→) (BI = 4+) **(E)**. HE staining (A-D) and FF staining **(E)**.

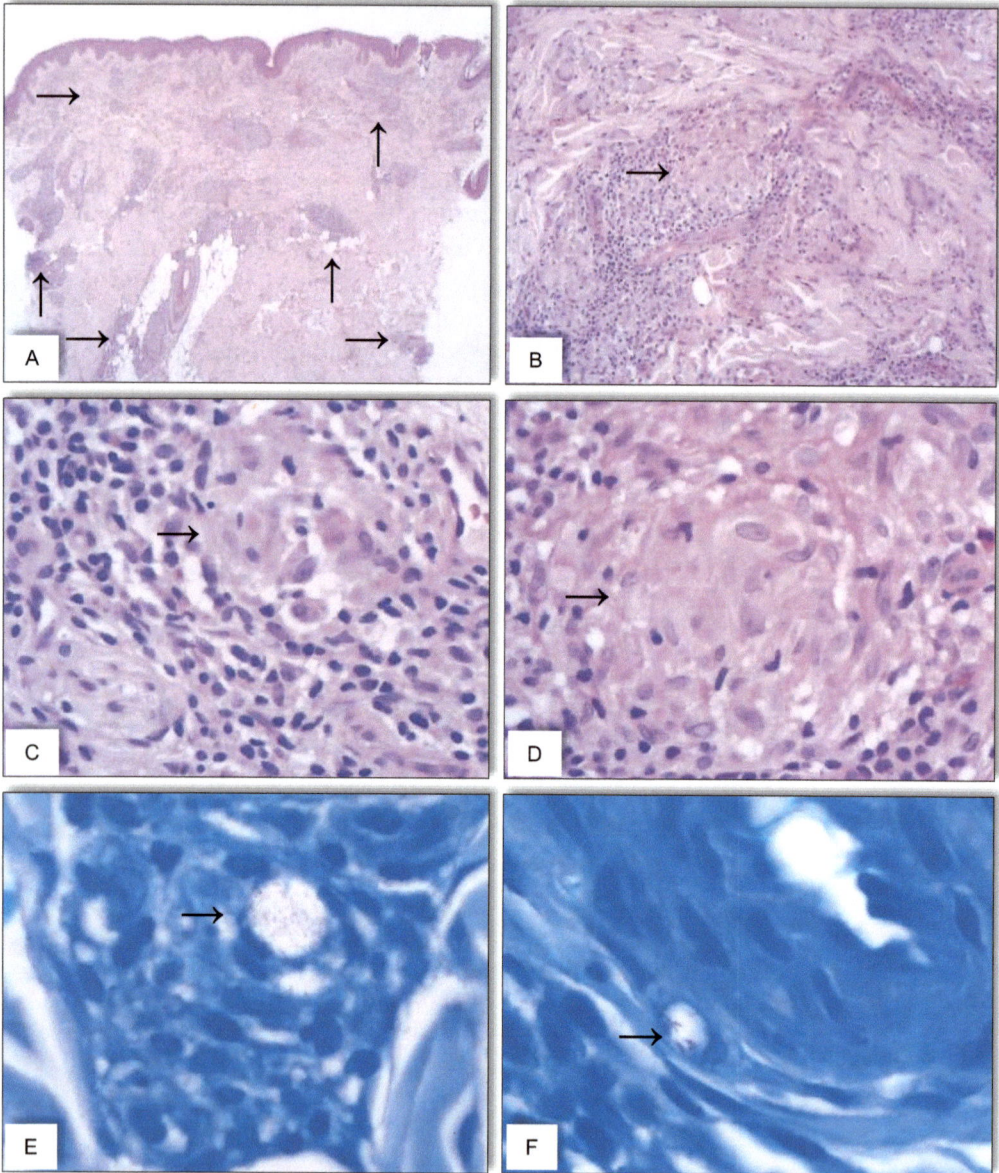

Fig. (16). Example of borderline leprosy with T1R associated post-treatment with non-specific antibiotics for leprosy. Patient underwent cesarean delivery using prophylactic antibiotic therapy. Six months after delivery, she developed erythematous plaques all over her body and clinical suspicion of a drug reaction. Histopathological examination showed a BB/BL leprosy lesion with associated T1R, characterized by an inflammatory infiltrate with tuberculoid pattern granulomas involving the entire dermis (→) (A, B, C and D). Bacilloscopic examination showing slightly colored, multifragmented bacilli within granulomas (→) **(E)** and solid bacilli on the vessel wall (→) (BI ≥ 4+) **(F)**. HE staining (A-D) and FF staining (E and F).

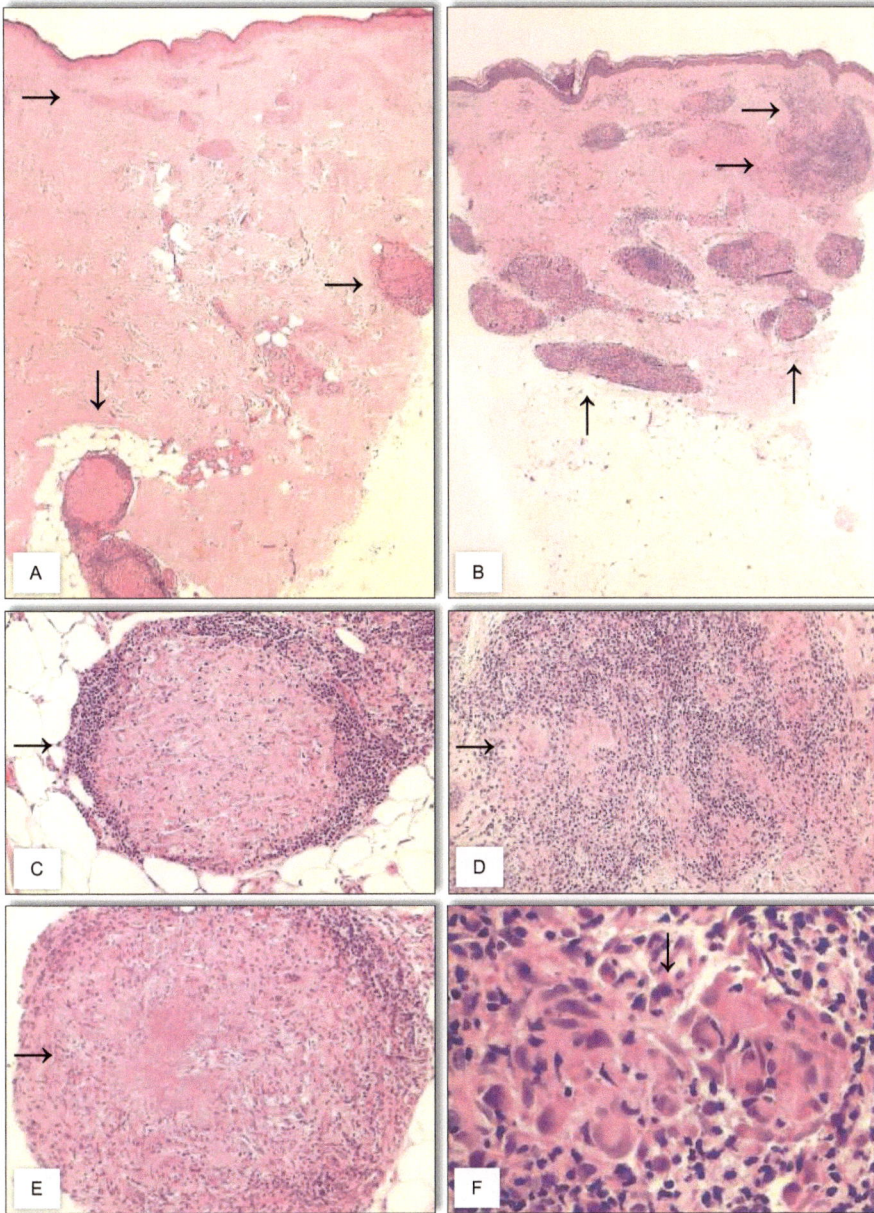

Fig. (17). Histopathological characteristics of a T1R over TT (A, C and E) and over BT (B, D and F). In both cases, T1R is restricted to neural branches, pili muscle and parasitized papillary derma areas (→). Other skin areas and components do not have T1R. HE staining.

The histopathological and bacilloscopic characteristics of a T1R over a lesion in the tuberculoid band (TT/BT) are different from that over BB/BL. The reactions occur on tissues or clusters of parasitized cells. Therefore, the T1Rs that affect TT/BT are more restricted and generally involve neural branches, pili muscle, and mononucleated cells or neural threads in the papillary dermis. BI is commonly 0 or 1+. Interstitium, vessels, endothelium, sweat glands, pilosebaceous follicle and other skin components, where *M. leprae* is not observed, do not usually have T1R (Fig. **17**). On the other hand, T1Rs on BB and BL lesions are more comprehensive and diffuse as there are a greater number of parasitized cells and tissues. The BI can vary from 0 to 5+, but it is usually ≥2+. Histopathological features that show a T1R with more extensive and confluent granulomas present in the interstitium, wall of vessels, glands, and pilosebaceous follicle are indicative of a T1R over a BB/BL lesion (Fig. **18**). In this context, the extent of the reaction process may reflect the patient's classification according to the R&J spectrum, especially if they are divided into two groups: TT/BT and BB/BL.

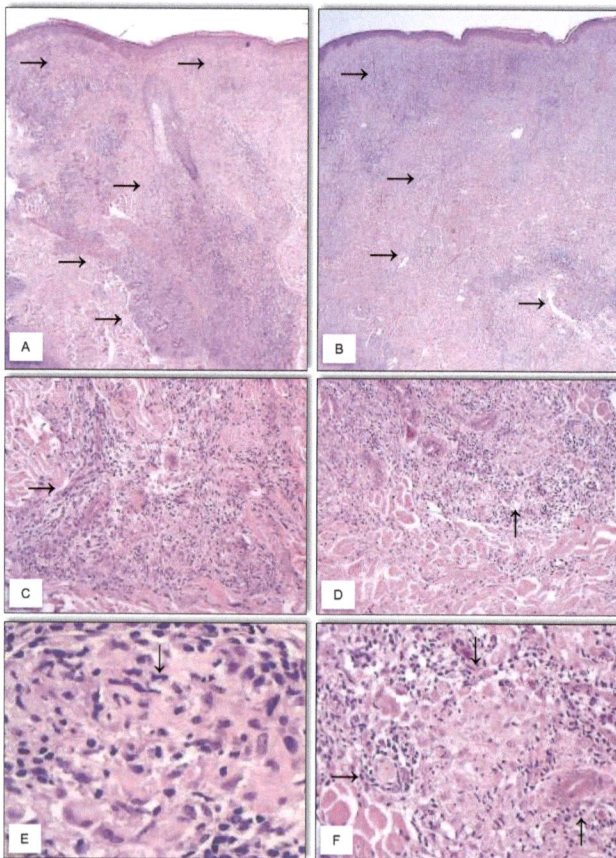

Fig. (18). Histopathological characteristics of a T1R over BB (A, C and E) and BL (B, D and F) lesions. T1R affecting BB and BL lesions are more comprehensive and diffuse, with T1R granulomas present in different skin tissues (→). HE staining.

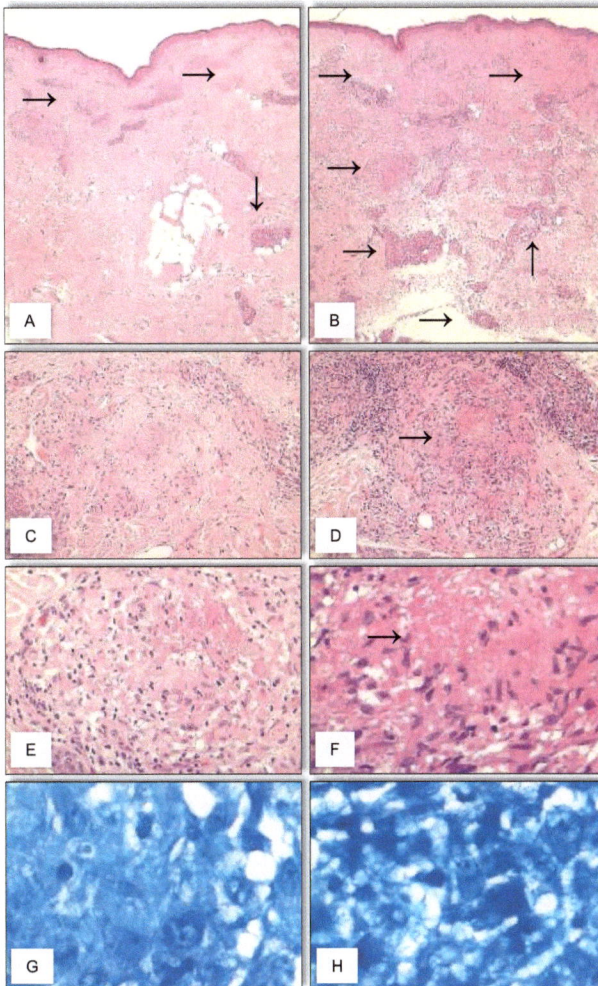

Fig. (19). Differences in T1R extension and intensity in the same patient. Abdominal lesion (→) (A, C, E and G) is less extensive and intense when compared to the elbow lesion (→) (B, D, F and H). Note that the reaction process in the elbow lesion compromises different skin tissues and there are well-defined areas of necrosis (→) (D and E). In both, the BI is 0 (G and H). HE staining (A-F) and FF staining (G and H).

The conditions for the onset of T1R differ among leprosy lesions found on various parts of the body. Clinically, the patient may have a single lesion with T1R and consequently develop T1R in several other lesions on different parts after a few days or weeks. In the case of T1R over TT, it is common for the reaction process to be restricted to a few injuries (≤5 injuries). It is not uncommon for a BB/BL patient with development of T1R in one or a few lesions to be mistakenly classified as TT or paucibacillary (Fig. **10 - 11**). In these cases, the development of T1R over several other skin lesions during disease progression or after initiation of treatment indicates that it is actually borderline or multibacillary leprosy. Histopathological examination of these lesions confirms characteristics of T1R with a BI greater than 2+. Additionally, skin lesions with T1R that appear at the beginning of reaction episodes may have histopathological and bacilloscopic characteristics with some differences from the more recent ones, both in the extension of the reaction process and in the intensity and bacilloscopic characteristics (Figs. **19 - 20**).

Biopsies of skin with T1R also show that the reaction process is not homogeneous in all skin components. In some samples, the reaction process can be extensive and involve almost all skin components. It is common for the reaction process to be observed in a specific component with no observable histopathological signs of T1R in other skin components (Fig. **21**). In other words, T1R can occur selectively over any parasitized skin tissues: interstitium, papillary dermis, subcutaneous adipose tissue, neural branches, vessels, glands of the skin appendages and epidermis. T1R is common in the papillary dermis over all borderline lesions and in TT. T1R granulomas are observed adjacent to the basal layer of the epidermis and associated with lymphocyte epidermotropism and hyperplasia with hyperkeratosis of the epidermis (Fig. **22**). A histopathological picture of aggression to the epidermis can also be seen in TT and BT forms (chapters 3 and 4) without histopathological signs of associated T1R, but it is usually less intense than in cases with associated T1R. T1R affecting the interstitium is characterized by granulomas containing multinucleated giant cells, sometimes with phagocytosis of collagen fibers, interstitial edema, and stellate fibroblasts (Fig. **23**). T1R can occur over small- and medium-sized vessels with involvement of the different layers, as well as characterizing granulomatous vasculitis (Fig. **24 - 25**). When it occurs over the neural branches, their involvement can vary from discrete perineural inflammatory infiltrates to the complete replacement of neural components by T1R granulomas (Fig. **26**). The reaction process occurring in BB and BL commonly involves glands and the pilosebaceous follicle, partly due to parasitism of neural branches, macrophages, and perianexial tissues by *M. leprae* (Fig. **27**). If there is parasitism of the glandular epithelial and myoepithelial cells or epithelial cells of the pilosebaceous follicle, T1R can also occur directly on these structures with the possibility of their destruction. The intensity of the reaction process varies among different lesions on the body and also within the same skin biopsy sample. The reaction picture ranges from low intensity with outline of reactive granulomas in few lesions or in focal areas of the biopsy to high intensity with caseous necrosis present in the granuloma centers or involving other areas of the skin and parasitized tissues (Fig. **28**). Bacilloscopic examination in areas of necrosis within T1R granulomas does not usually exhibit bacilli.

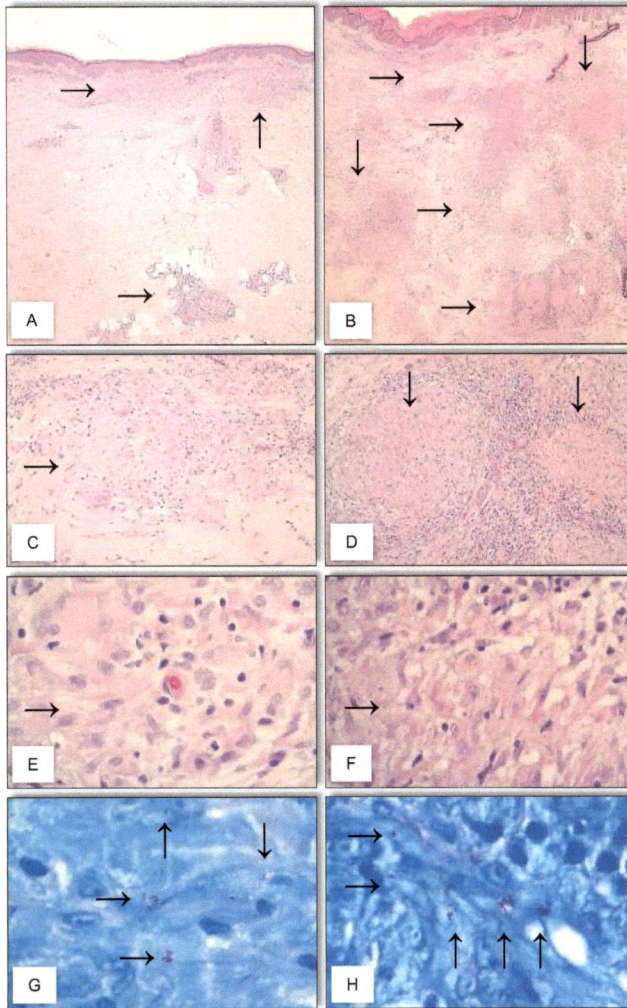

Fig. (20). T1R example showing differences in the extent and intensity of the reaction process. Patient with erythematous and scaly lesions in the knee (A, C, E and G) and elbow (B, D, F and H), with clinical suspicion of syphilis. Histopathological examination shows characteristics of BB/BL leprosy with associated T1R. Note that the knee injury (→) is less extensive than that of the elbow (→). Bacilloscopic index of both is similar (→) (BI ≥ 4+). HE staining (A-F) and FF staining (G and H).

The same histopathological characteristics of a T1R occurring in cutaneous lesions are also observed in neural trunks and viscera (Fig. **29**) [2]. T1R affecting viscera occurs in BB or BL patients, where parasitism is more extensive and diffuse and can affect different viscera. Autopsies of leprosy patients with T1R, mainly in those with subpolar lepromatous leprosy (LLsp), revealed T1R granulomas in lymph nodes, liver, spleen, bone marrow, synovial membranes, mucous membranes of the upper respiratory tract (nasal, buccal, pharyngeal, laryngeal and vocal folds), salivary gland, testis, epididymis, adrenal gland, and eyeballs [2]. Parasitism is infrequent or absent in kidneys, central nervous system, lungs, heart, large vessels, digestive system, pancreas, urinary system and organs of the female reproductive system [2].

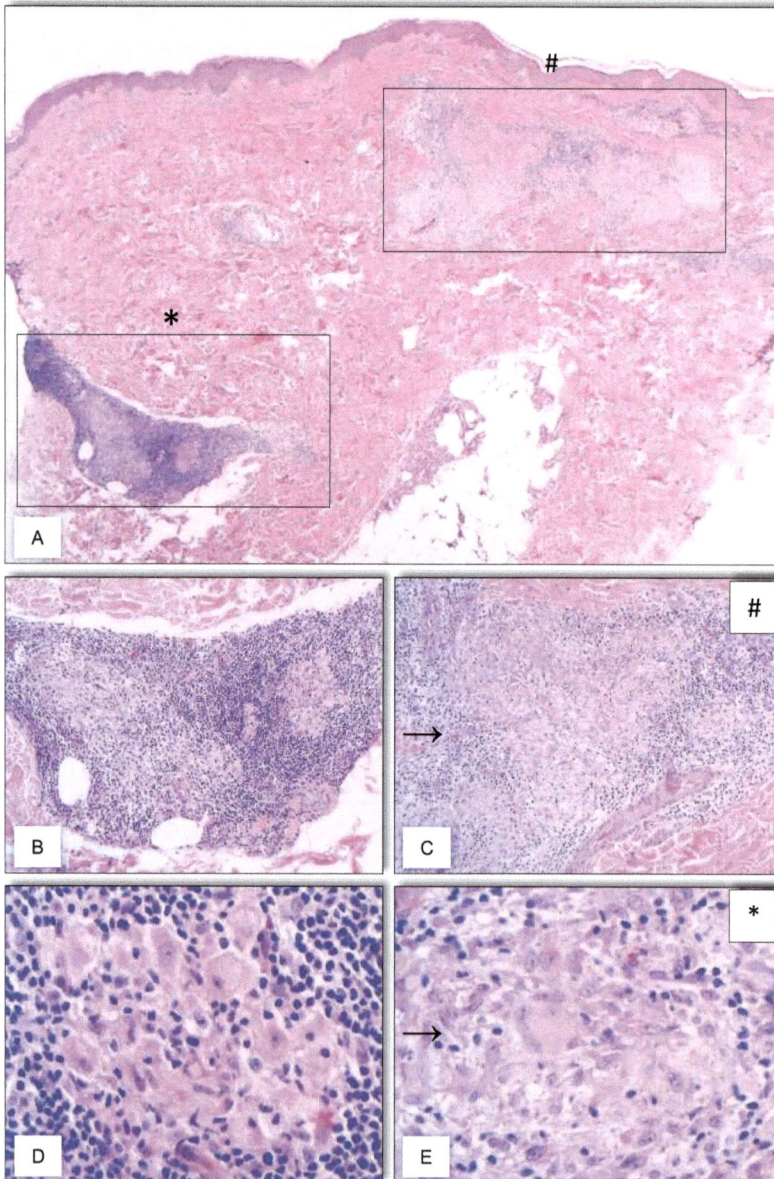

Fig. (21). Example of BT with T1R occurring selectively in part of the sample. The reaction process is present in the papillary/reticular dermis (→) (#; A, C and E) while other skin components, including the deep neural branches involved by tuberculoid granuloma (*; A, B and D) show no signs of T1R. HE staining.

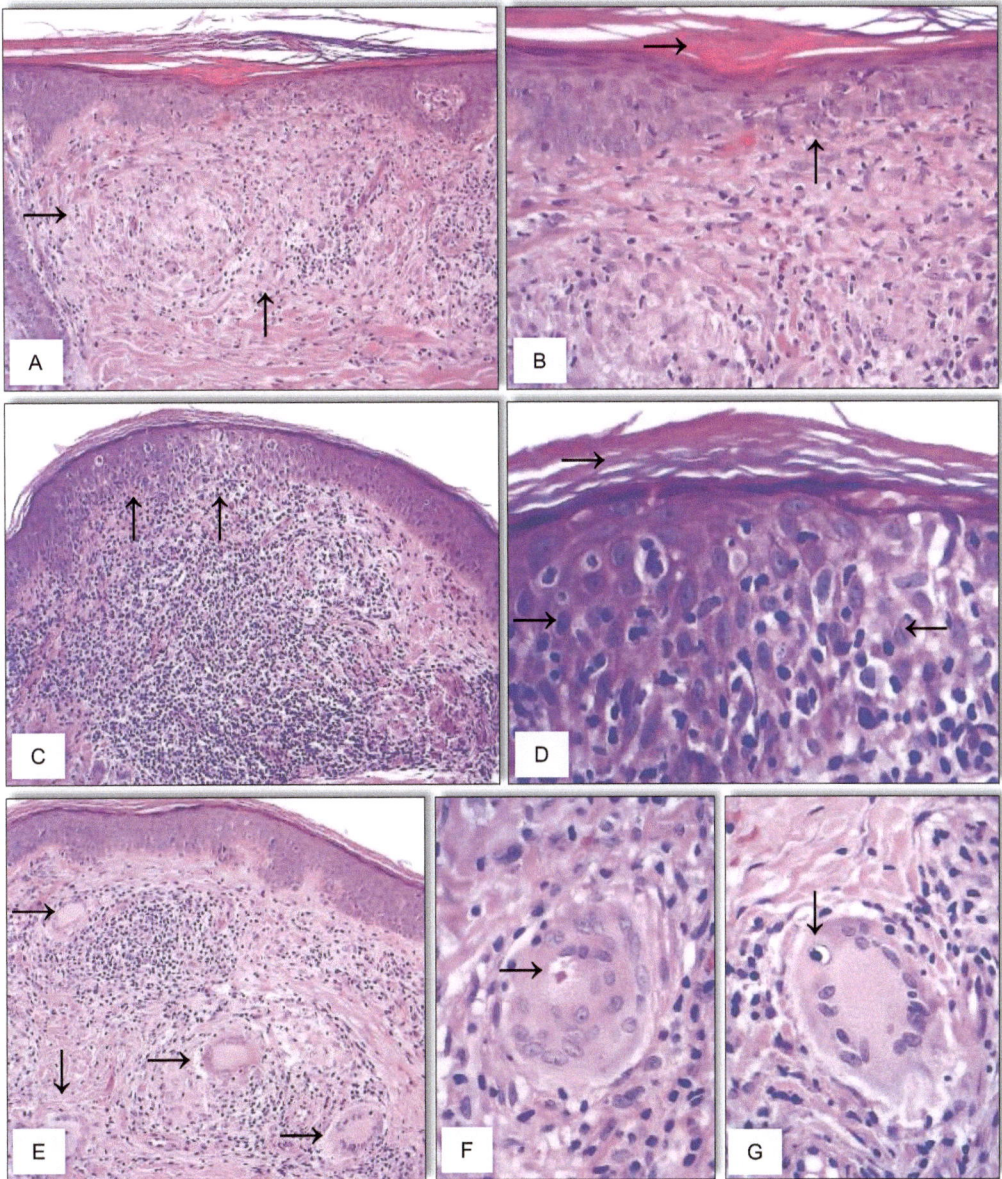

Fig. (22). T1R present in the papillary dermis. Tuberculoid granulomas of T1R with multinucleated giant cells (A and E). Lymphocytes on the periphery of granulomas also permeate the keratinocytes of the epidermis, giving a pagetoid aspect (→) (B, C and D), and associated with hyperkeratosis and parakeratosis (→) (B and D). Some multinucleated giant cells may contain an asteroid body (→) **(F)** or calcifications (→) **(G)**. HE staining.

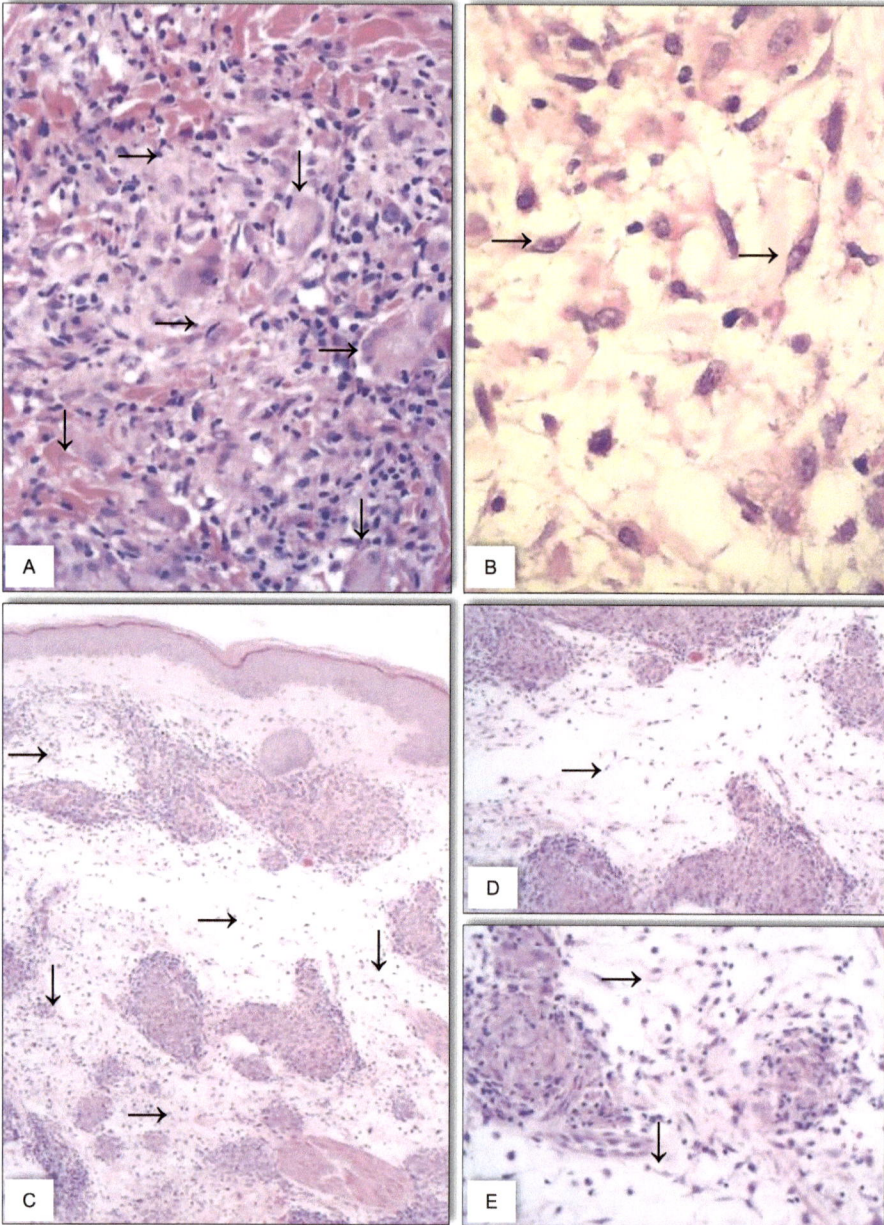

Fig. (23). T1R in the interstitium. Granulomas involve collagen bands, sometimes with multinucleated giant cells containing collagen fibers (→) **(A)**. Fibroblasts inside or adjacent to granulomas are stellate, with an evident nucleolus (→) (B and E). The T1R reaction process can present intense edema affecting all skin segments (→) (C, D and E). HE staining.

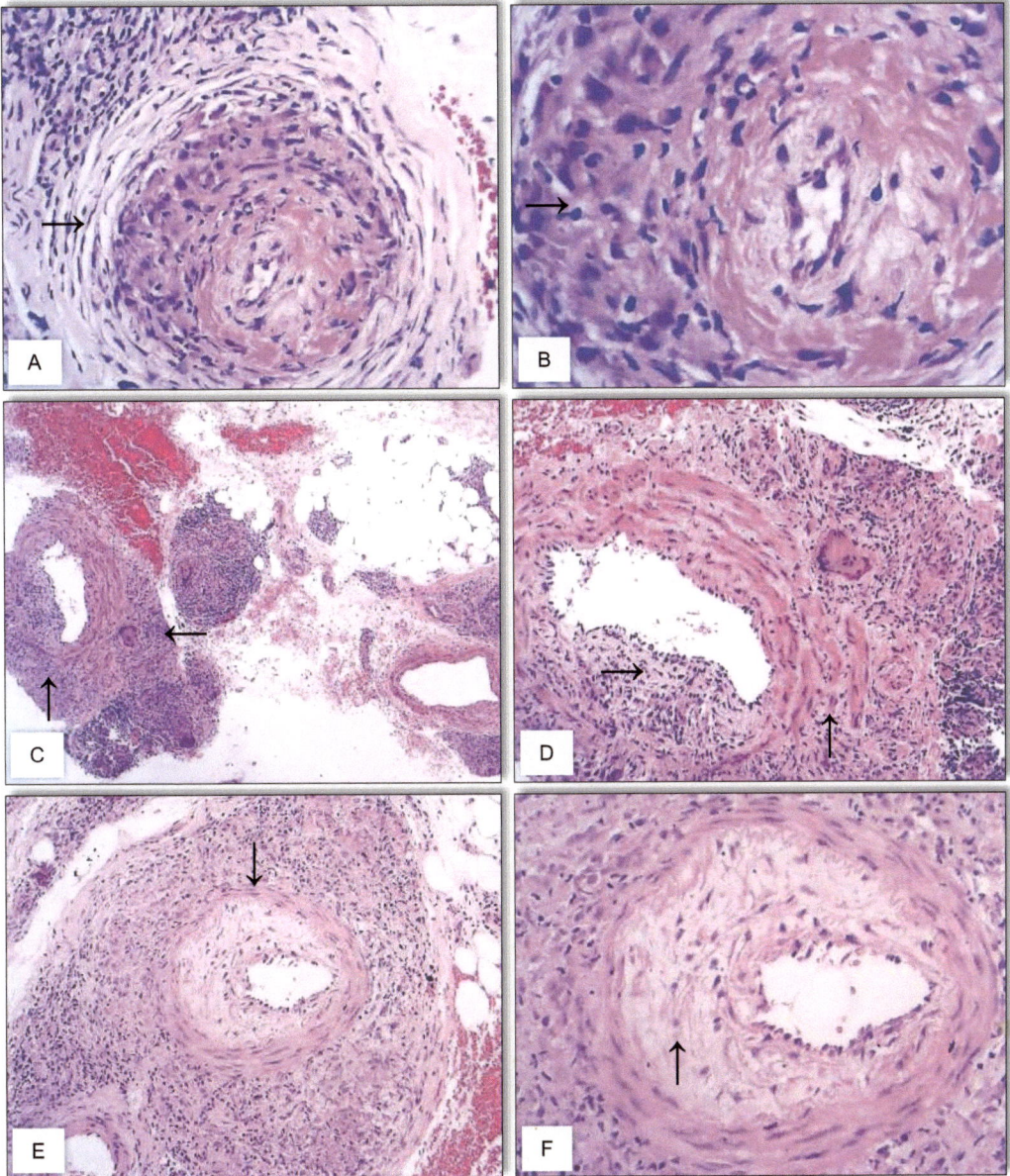

Fig. (24). T1R in the vessel. Reaction process involving veins (A, B, C and D) and artery (E and F). Note that the reaction process of T1R compromises from the perivascular tissues to the endothelium (→) (A, B C and D). In **(E)** and **(F)** T1R completely encompasses the artery associated with the arterial wall and intense sub-endothelial edema (→). HE staining.

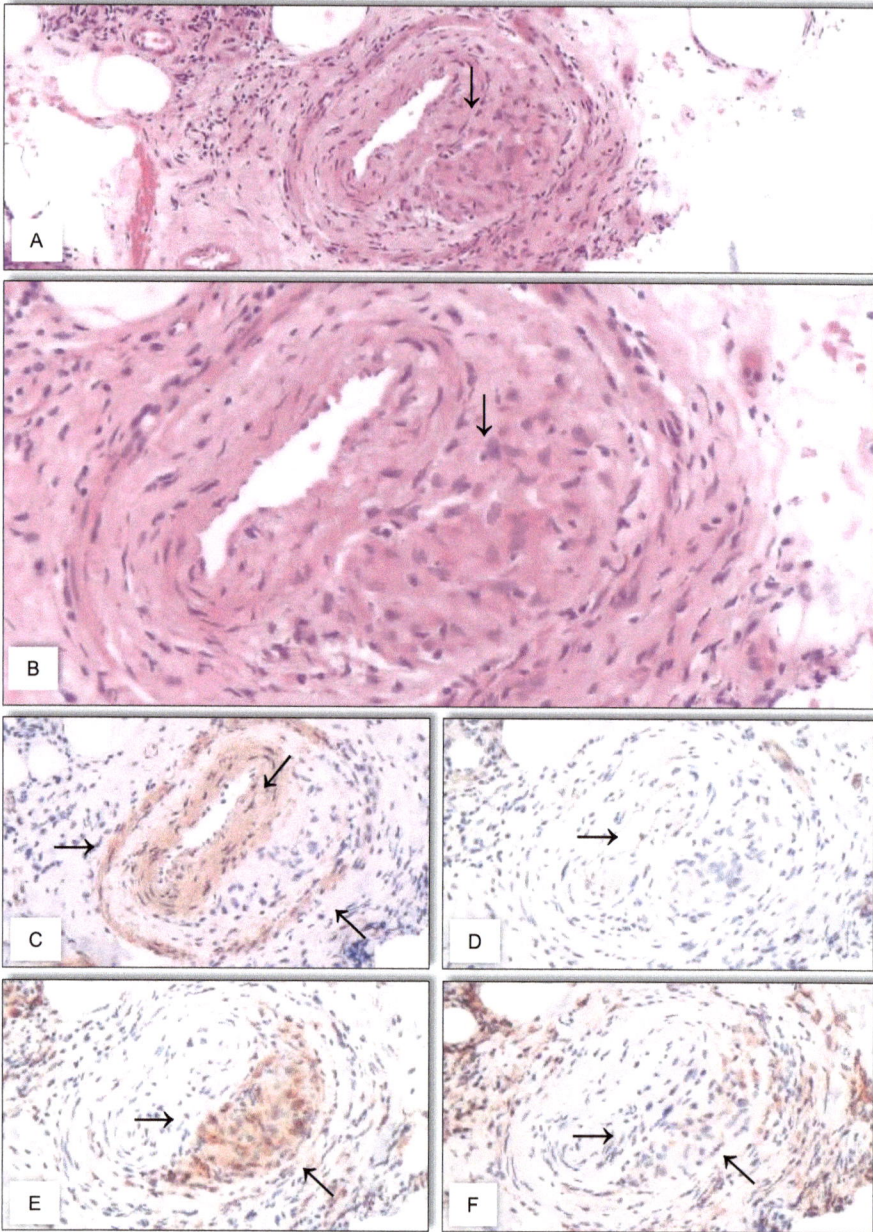

Fig. (25). T1R in the vessel. Reaction process showing T1R granuloma on the vessel wall (→) (A and B). Immunohistochemistry staining demonstrates the reaction process inside the muscle layer **(C)** (smooth muscle actin 1A4), center endothelium **(D)** (CD31) and granuloma consisting of epithelioid macrophages of M1 pattern (CD68 positive in **(E)** and CD163 negative in **(F)**). HE staining (A and B).

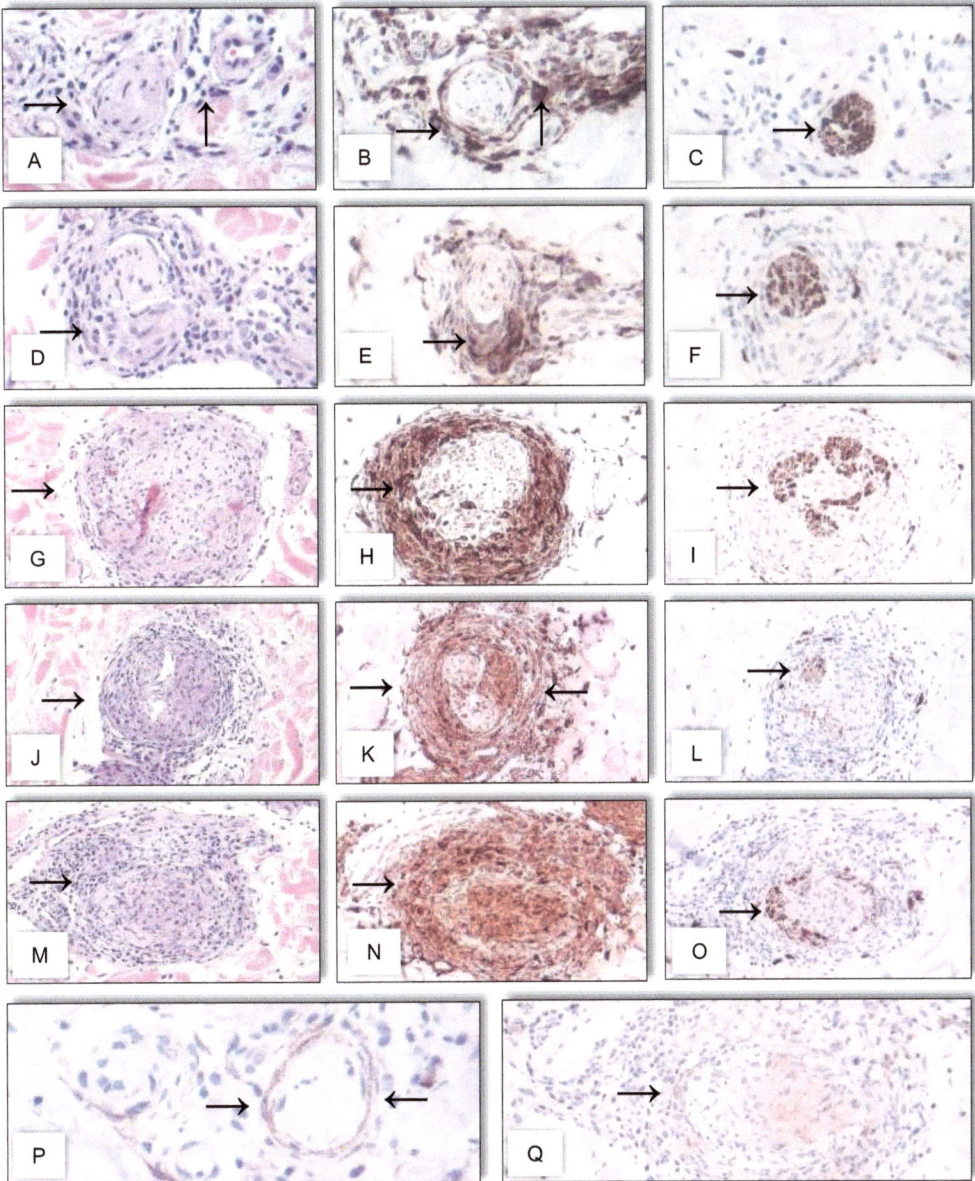

Fig. (26). T1R in the nerve. Different levels of neural involvement by T1R in the same sample. From **(A)** to **(F)**, T1R granulomas (→) are in formation and on the periphery of the neural branches (→). From **(G)** to **(I)**, the involvement is complete with partial destruction of the nerve (→). From **(J)** to **(O)**, a fragment of neural branches is left inside the granulomas (→). In **(A)** and **(P)**, there is little aggression to the neural branch, evidenced by immunohistochemical staining showing the intact perineurium (→) (positive EMA) **(P)**. In **(M)** and **(Q)**, the disappearance of the perineurium by the action of the T1R granuloma is noted (→) (negative EMA) **(Q)**. HE staining (A, D, G, J and M). Immunohistochemistry staining showing CD68 epithelioid macrophages in T1R granulomas (B, E, H, K and N) and Schwann cells from neural branches S-100 (C, F, I, L and O).

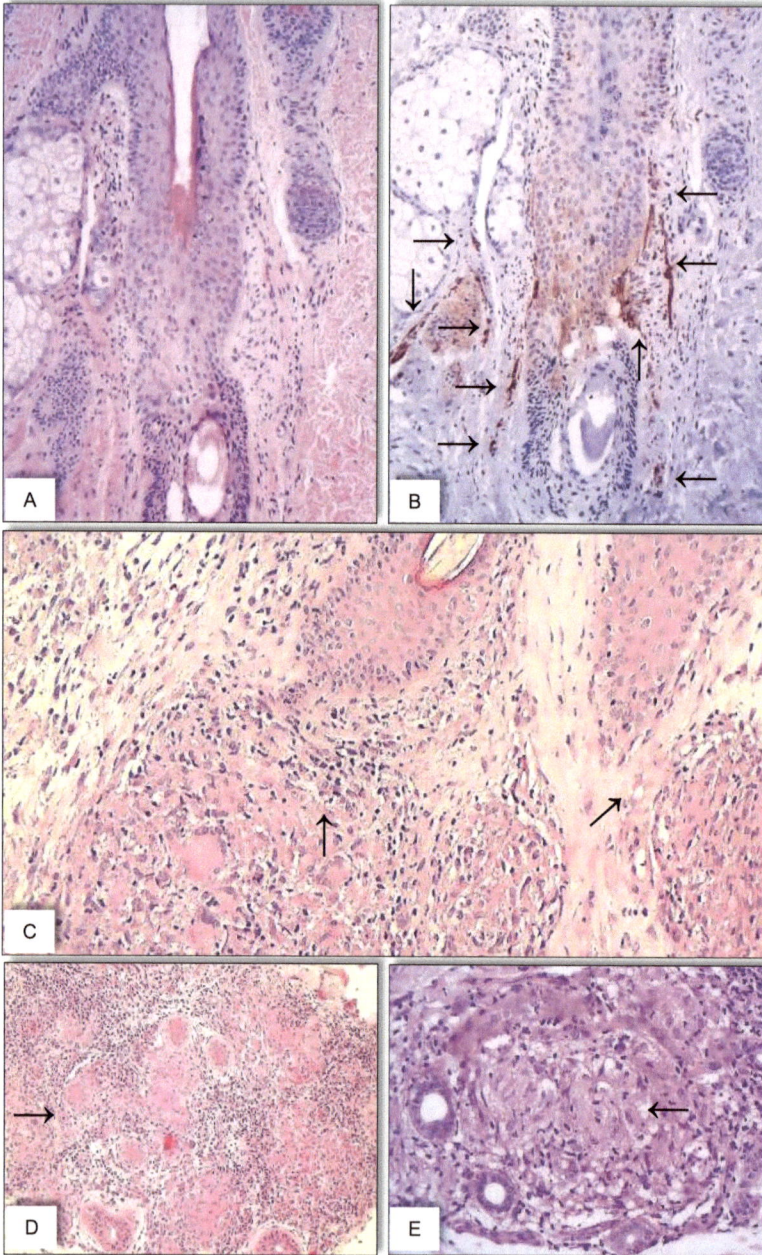

Fig. (27). T1R involving pilosebaceous follicle and sweat glands. Longitudinal histological section of a pilosebaceous follicle **(A)** with numerous neural threads surrounding them (→) (S-100 +) **(B)**. In **(C)** T1R granulomas involve the pilosebaceous follicle (→) and in **(D)** and **(E)** the sweat glands (→). HE staining (A, C-E) and S-100 immunohistochemistry **(B)**.

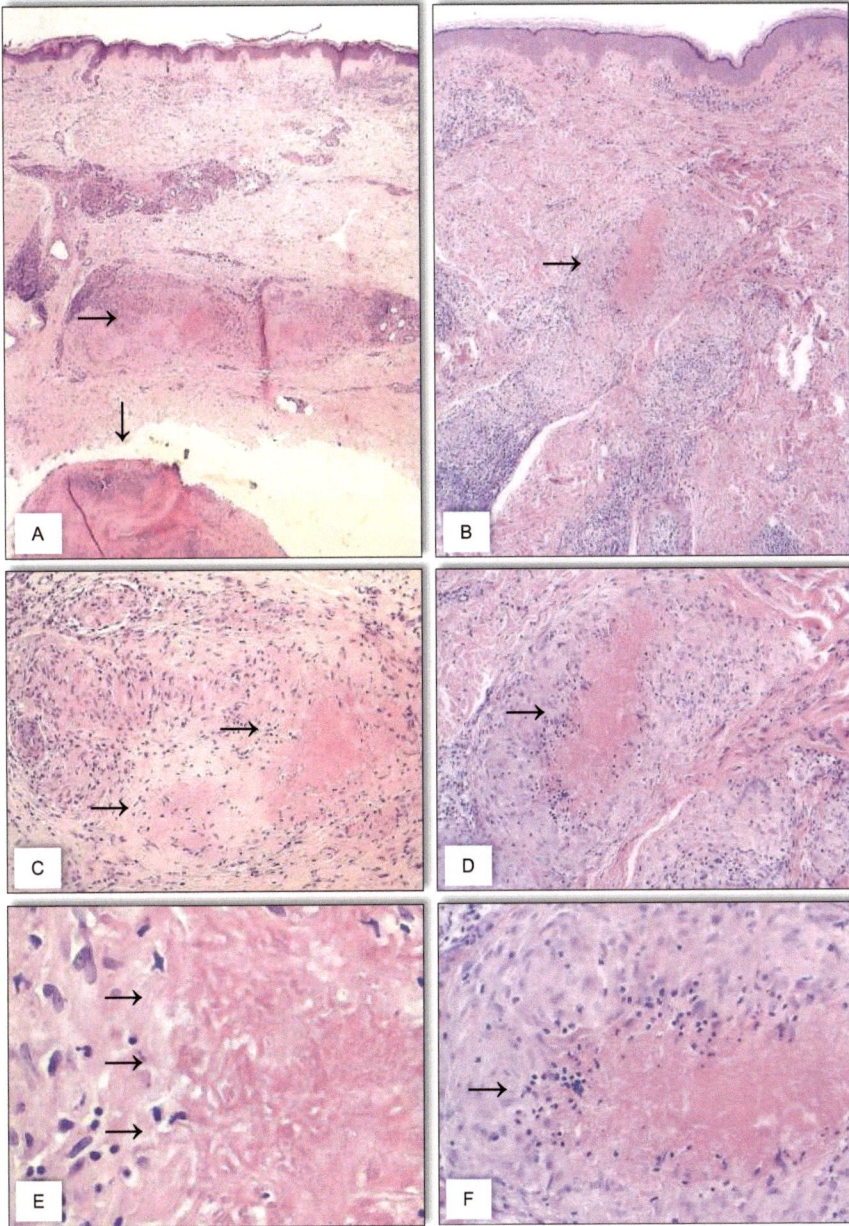

Fig. (28). Two examples of T1R with intense reaction ((A, C and E) and (B, D and F)). Various T1R granulomas at different levels with associated central necrosis (→). HE staining (A-F).

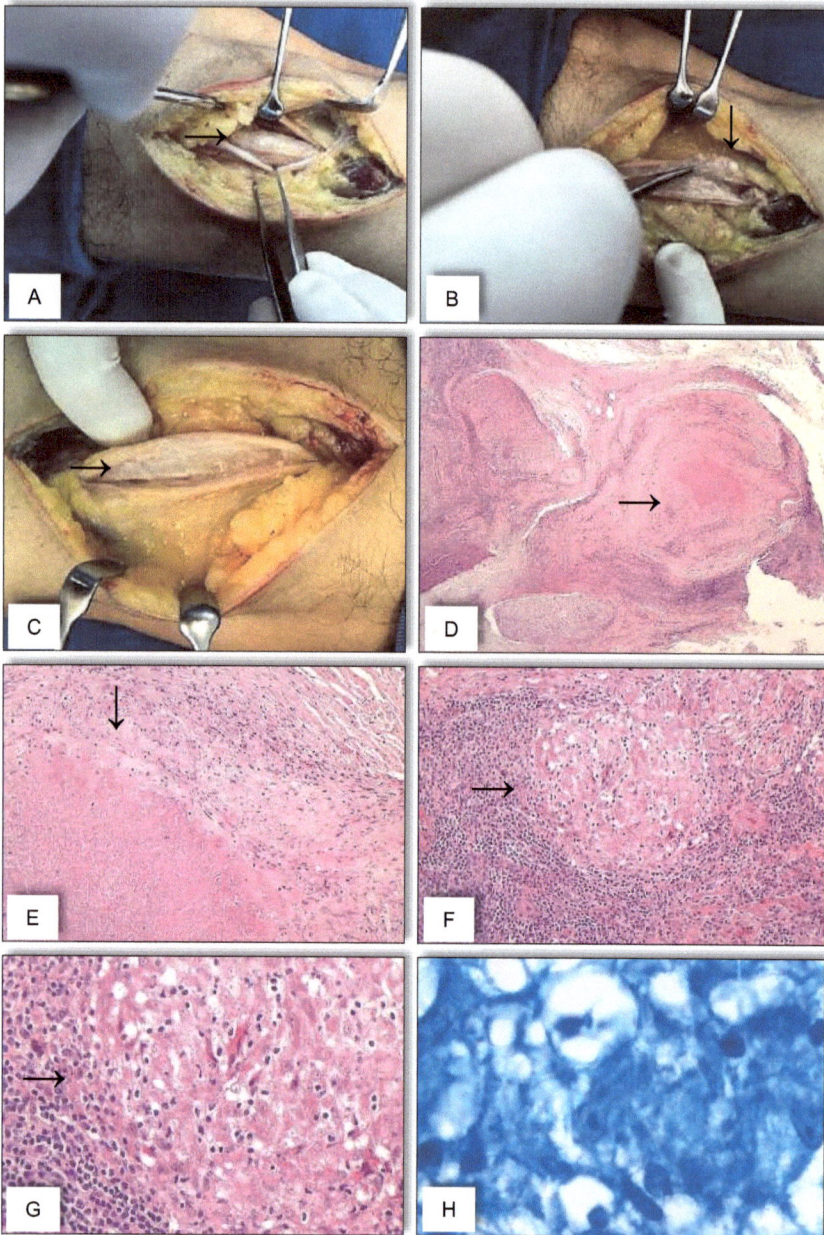

Fig. (29). T1R in the tibial nerve. Patient with expansive lesion of the tibial nerve, at the level of the popliteal fossa, associated with neural thickening in its most distal portions, as well as imaging studies with suspected expansive lesion for neurilemoma or neurofibroma. Intraoperative examination shows a thickened nerve with caseous necrosis (A, B and C). Clinical-pathological characteristics of borderline leprosy with T1R granulomas and extensive caseous necrosis ($\rightarrow$). (D-G) Absence of bacilli (BI = 0) in T1R granulomas and necrotic areas. HE staining (D-G) and FF staining **(H)**. Photos (A-C) courtesy of Dr. Milton Cury Filho.

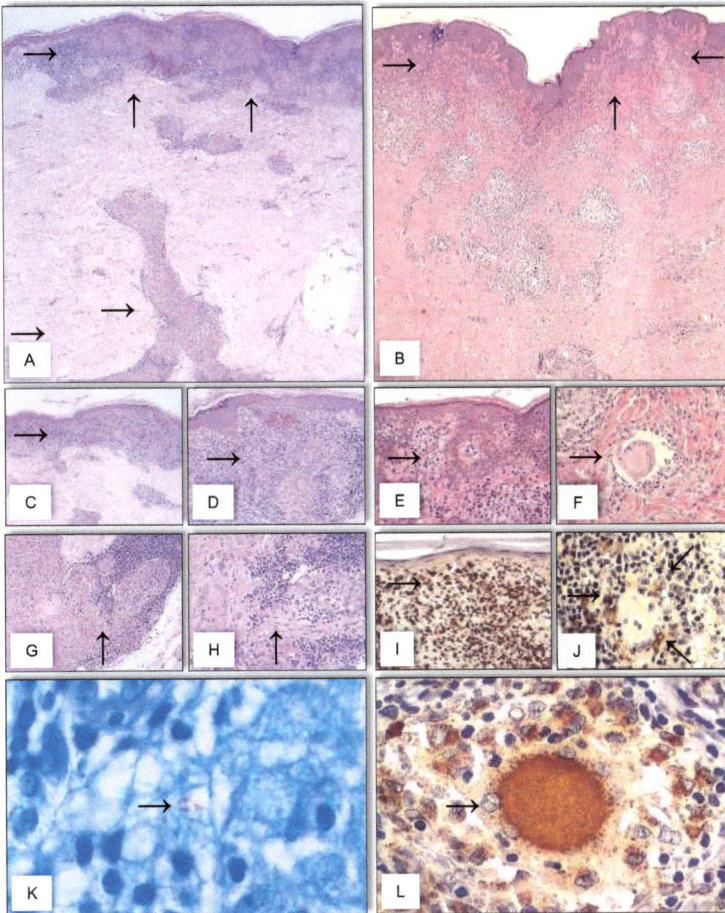

Fig. (30). Leprosy lesion with T1R simulating mycosis fungoides in the papillary dermis, and case of mycosis fungoides. T1R on BT lesion (A, C, D, G, H and K) with intense reaction process in the papillary dermis, coupled with the presence of multinucleated giant cells and aggression to the epidermis (→) and involvement of neural branches in the deep dermis. Granulomatous slack skin (B, E, F, I, J and L), a rare and indolent subtype of mycosis fungoides, with lymphocytic infiltrate in the papillary dermis, CD4+ T lymphocyte epidermotropism and presence of multinucleated giant cells (→) (B, E, F, I, J and L). HE staining (A, B, C, D, E F, G and H). Immunohistochemistry for CD4 (→) **(I)** T lymphocytes, CD1a antigen presenting cells (→) **(J)** and CD68 (→) **(L)** macrophages. FF staining **(K)** showing bacilli fragmented in macrophages (→).

Differential Diagnoses of T1R

Skin lesions of erysipelas, Sweet's syndrome, drug reaction, mycosis fungoides, granuloma annulare, different types of necrobiosis, actinic granuloma, and vasculitis can be clinically similar to leprosy lesions with associated T1R [8, 12]. From the histopathological point of view, several diseases, infectious and non-infectious granulomatous lesions, especially localized annular granuloma, are part of the differential diagnosis (Fig. **30** - **32**) [13, 14]. The presence of granulomatous vasculitis should not be confused with several diseases that cause granulomatous vasculitis of small and medium vessels [15]. In all these cases, it is important to observe the presence of granulomas involving neural branches in adjacent tissues, indicating that it is a leprosy lesion with T1R. It is noteworthy that leprosy patients can develop different types of diseases or skin lesions during the progression of leprosy or in regression after treatment (chapter 7) [16, 17]. In these cases, skin lesions of different types of disease can coexist with leprosy lesions and both can be identified in the same skin biopsy (Fig. **33**). Among the leprosy lesions on the R&J spectrum, the histopathological features that differentiate a T1R from TT and BT lesions were discussed in this chapter.

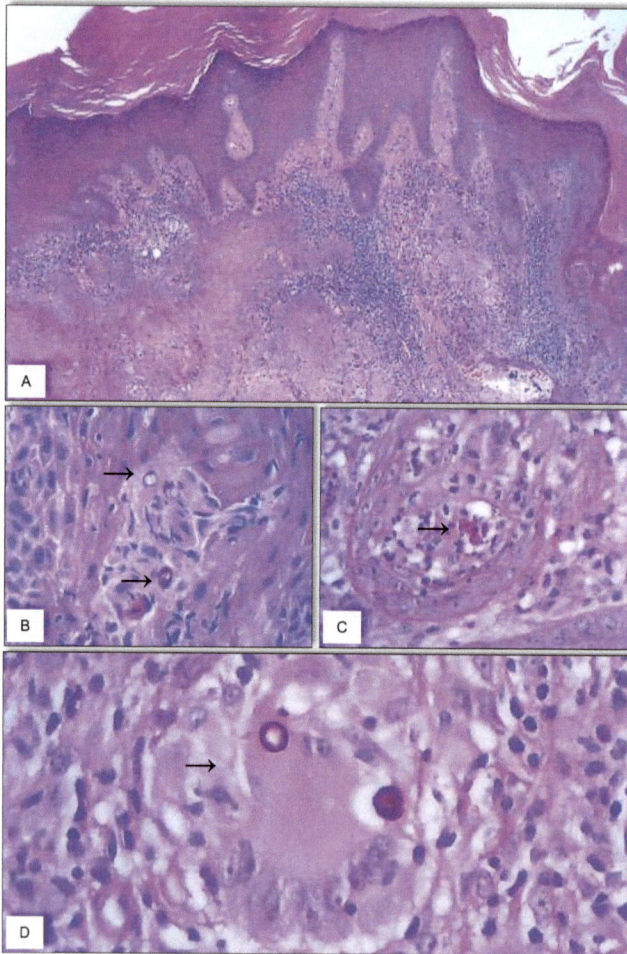

Fig. (31). Chromoblastomycosis clinically simulating TT/BT leprosy with T1R. Epidermis with intense epithelial hyperplasia (A and B) and microabscesses within the epidermis (→) **(C)**. Pigmented cells (sometimes septated) in macrophages in the papillary dermis, within microabscesses and in multinucleated giant cells (→). (B, C and D). HE staining.

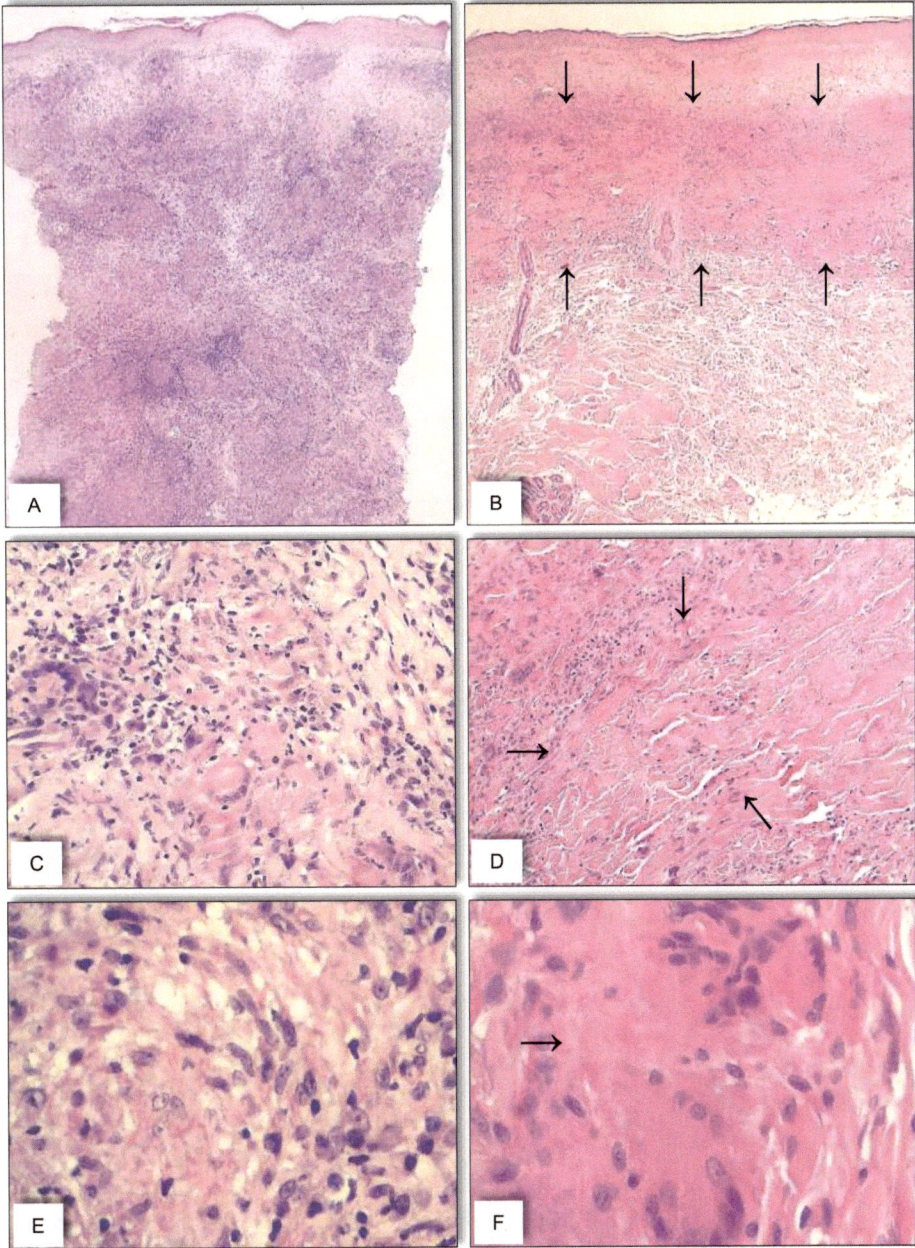

Fig. (32). Common histopathological characteristics of the T1R reaction and localized annular granuloma. T1R interstitial granuloma is diffuse and affects neural branches (A, C, and D). In annular granuloma, interstitial necrobiosis with epithelioid macrophages and giant cells in the periphery is common, forming a palisade granuloma, and absence of neural branch involvement (→) (B, D and F). HE staining.

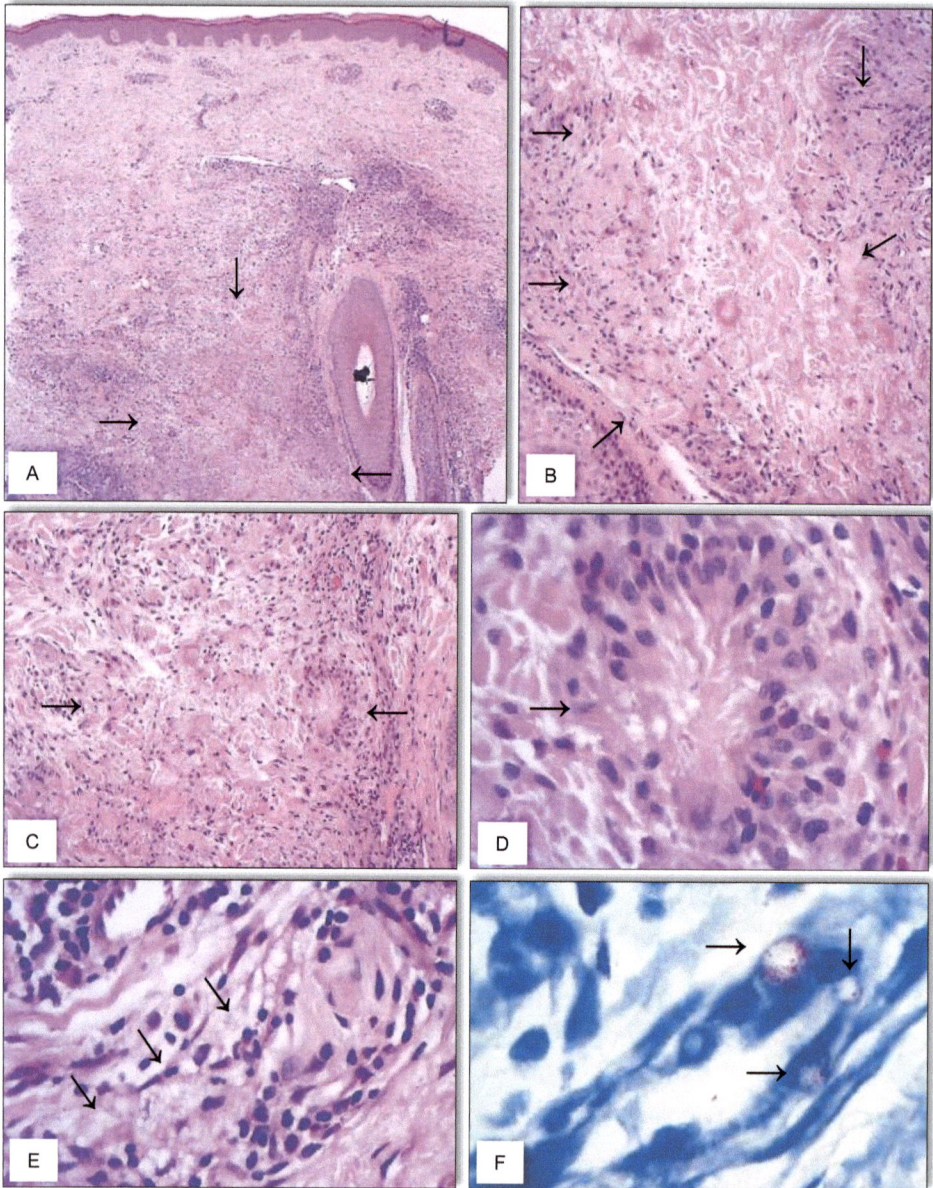

Fig. (33). Annular granuloma coexisting with leprosy injury. BL patient undergoing treatment had a cutaneous lesion on the elbow with a clinical hypothesis of annular granuloma. Histological sections demonstrated an interstitial granulomatous reaction in a palisade involving an area of necrobiosis compatible with annular granuloma (→) (A, B, C, and D). Other areas showed leprosy lesions in regression (→) (**E**). Bacilloscopic examination showing multi fragmented bacilli in the vessel wall (→) (**F**). HE staining (A-E) and FF staining (**F**).

CONCLUSION

T1R is a reaction phenomenon that occurs in patients with tuberculoid (TT) and borderline (BT, BB, and BL) leprosy. Its intensity and extent are variable, and it can cause permanent sequelae. Early recognition of the histopathologic characteristics of T1R is essential for determining appropriate treatment and reducing its possible sequelae.

REFERENCES

[1]   Opromolla DVA. Manifestações Clínicas e Reações.Noções de Hansenologia. 2nd ed. Bauru, Brazil: Centro de Estudo Dr. Reynaldo Quagliato, Instituto Lauro de Souza Lima 2000; pp. 51-8.

[2]   Fleury RN. Patologia e Manifestações Viscerais.Noções de Hansenologia. 2nd ed. Bauru, Brazil: Centro de Estudo Dr. Reynaldo Quagliato, Instituto Lauro de Souza Lima 2000; pp. 63-71.

[3]   Maymone MBC, Venkatesh S, Laughter M, *et al*. Leprosy: Treatment and management of complications. J Am Acad Dermatol 2020; 83(1): 17-30.
[http://dx.doi.org/10.1016/j.jaad.2019.10.138] [PMID: 32244016]

[4]   Ridley DS, Jopling WH. Classification of leprosy according to immunity. A five-group system. Int J Lepr Other Mycobact Dis 1966; 34(3): 255-73.
[PMID: 5950347]

[5]   Fachin LR, Soares CT, Belone AF, *et al*. Immunohistochemical assessment of cell populations in leprosy-spectrum lesions and reactional forms. Histol Histopathol 2017; 32(4): 385-96.
[PMID: 27444702]

[6]   Lazo-Porras M, Prutsky GJ, Barrionuevo P, *et al*. World Health Organization (WHO) antibiotic regimen against other regimens for the treatment of leprosy: a systematic review and meta-analysis. BMC Infect Dis 2020; 20(1): 62.
[http://dx.doi.org/10.1186/s12879-019-4665-0] [PMID: 31959113]

[7]   Lockwood DNJ, Lambert S, Srikantam A, *et al*. Three drugs are unnecessary for treating paucibacillary leprosy-A critique of the WHO guidelines. PLoS Negl Trop Dis 2019; 13(10)e0007671
[http://dx.doi.org/10.1371/journal.pntd.0007671] [PMID: 31671087]

[8]   Talhari C, Talhari S, Penna GO. Clinical aspects of leprosy. Clin Dermatol 2015; 33(1): 26-37.
[http://dx.doi.org/10.1016/j.clindermatol.2014.07.002] [PMID: 25432808]

[9]   Girão RJS, Opromolla DVA, Soares CT, Stump MV. Tuberculoid leprosy in AIDS patient. Hansenol Int 2004; 29(2): 137-40.

[10]   Sanghi S, Grewal RS, Vasudevan B, Lodha N. Immune reconstitution inflammatory syndrome in leprosy. Indian J Lepr 2011; 83(2): 61-70.
[PMID: 21972657]

[11]   Lockwood DN, Sinha HH. Pregnancy and leprosy: a comprehensive literature review. Int J Lepr Other Mycobact Dis 1999; 67(1): 6-12.
[PMID: 10407623]

[12]   Kundakci N, Erdem C. Leprosy: A great imitator. Clin Dermatol 2019; 37(3): 200-12.
[http://dx.doi.org/10.1016/j.clindermatol.2019.01.002] [PMID: 31178103]

[13]   Motta LMD, Soares CT, Nakandakari S, Silva GVD, Nigro MHMF, Brandão LSG. Granulomatous slack skin: a rare subtype of mycosis fungoides. An Bras Dermatol 2017; 92(5): 694-7.
[http://dx.doi.org/10.1590/abd1806-4841.20175099] [PMID: 29166509]

[14]   Queiroz-Telles F, de Hoog S, Santos DW, *et al*. Chromoblastomycosis. Clin Microbiol Rev 2017; 30(1): 233-76.

[http://dx.doi.org/10.1128/CMR.00032-16] [PMID: 27856522]

[15]   Sharma A, Dogra S, Sharma K. Granulomatous Vasculitis. Dermatol Clin 2015; 33(3): 475-87.
        [http://dx.doi.org/10.1016/j.det.2015.03.012] [PMID: 26143427]

[16]   Fleury RN, Opromolla DVA, Taborda PR, Nakandakari MTCBR, Soares CT, de Campos Bonfim A.
        Mycosis fungoides succeeding long-term borderline leprosy with multiple episodes of type 1 reaction.
        Hansenol Int 1999; 24(2): 137-43.

[17]   Singh SK, Manchanda K, Bhayana AA, Verma A. Allopurinol induced granuloma annulare in a
        patient of lepromatous leprosy. J Pharmacol Pharmacother 2013; 4(2): 152-4.
        [http://dx.doi.org/10.4103/0976-500X.110915] [PMID: 23761716]

CHAPTER 6

Type 2 Reaction (T2R)

Abstract: Type 2 reaction (T2R), also called erythema nodosum leprosum (ENL), is a reactional phenomenon that occurs in response to *Mycobacterium leprae* antigens in patients with borderline lepromatous or lepromatous forms of leprosy. T2R usually occurs after starting treatment and can affect any parasitic tissue in the body, causing neuritis, arthritis, painful lymphadenitis, buccopharyngeal lesions, laryngitis, hepatomegaly, splenomegaly, bone injuries, iridocyclitis, uveitis, orchitis, glomerulitis with proteinuria, and hematuria. Recognition of the histopathological characteristics of T2R is important for guiding early treatment of the reaction process, decreasing the likelihood of developing serious sequelae, especially when T2R affects the nerves, and to exclude different diseases that can simulate T2R over leprosy lesions during the course of the disease. In this chapter, the histopathological characteristics that allow T2R diagnosis are described, and some of its differential clinicopathological diagnoses and their possible pathophysiological mechanisms are discussed.

Keywords: Differential diagnosis, Erythema nodosum leprosum, Hansen′s disease, Leprosy, *Mycobacterium leprae*, T2R, Type 2 reaction.

INTRODUCTION

Type 2 reaction (T2R), or erythema nodosum leprosum, is a type of inflammatory response that affects patients with low levels of cellular immunity or anergy and occurs in tissues parasitized by *Mycobacterium leprae*. Patients that develop T2R are those located on the lepromatous side of the Ridley & Jopling classification spectrum, which corresponds to borderline lepromatous (BL) and lepromatous leprosy (LL) [1 - 3] (Fig. **1**).

T2R rarely occurs before treatment begins but commonly occurs after the first 6 months of leprosy-specific multidrug therapy [1, 2]. T2R is commonly characterized by erythematous nodules or plaques on leprosy lesions in regression (Figs. **2 - 6**). Intense forms of T2R present nodules or plaques that might undergo suppuration, necrosis, and/or ulceration (Fig. **2** and **3**). Additionally, T2R on skin lesions is accompanied by general systemic manifestations, such as fever, myalgia, asthenia, and inappetence and inflammatory manifestations that can occur all over the body containing bacillary antigens. Moreover, neuritis, arthritis, painful lymphadenitis, bucco-pharyngeal lesions, laryngitis, hepatomegaly, splenomegaly, bone lesions, iridocyclitis, uveitis, orchitis, and, rarely, glomerulitis with proteinuria and hematuria can be observed [2].

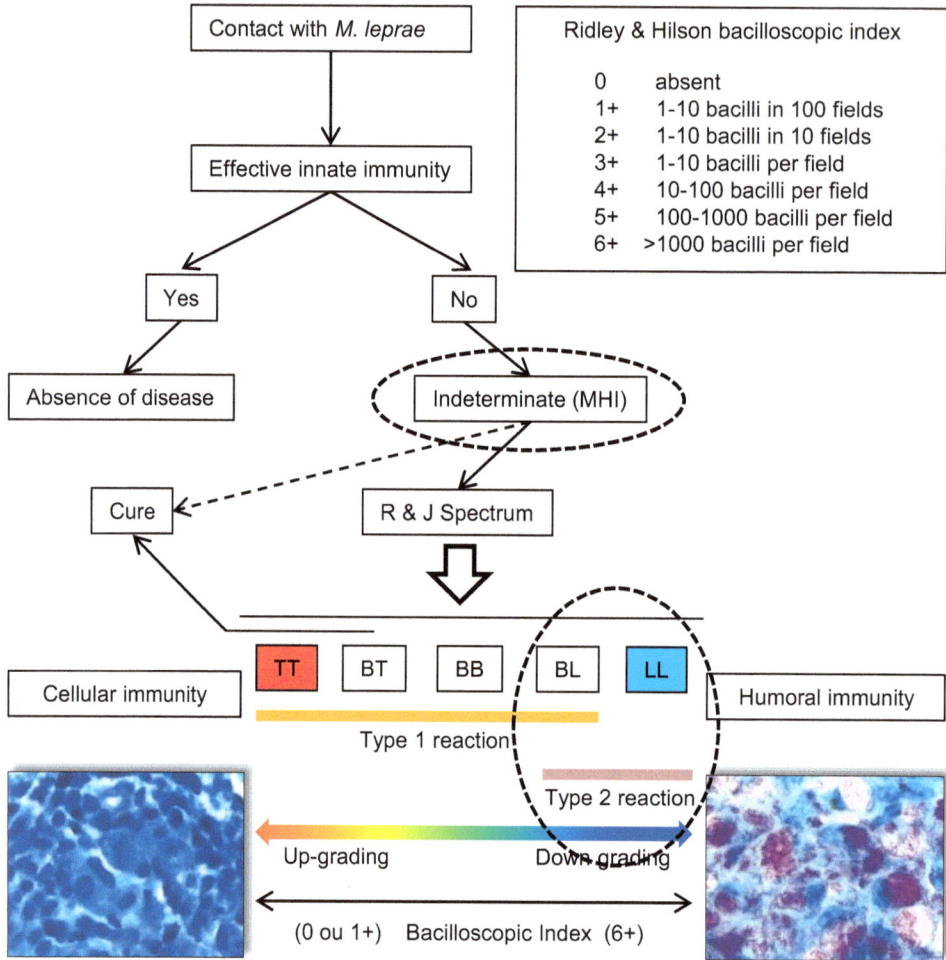

Fig. (1). Clinical spectrum and bacilloscopic index of leprosy forms and reactions. Patients exposed to *M. leprae* can eliminate the bacilli *via* mechanisms of the primary immune response and do not develop the disease. If the primary immune defense cannot refrain bacilli proliferation, the patient develops indeterminate leprosy (I), the early stage of the disease preceding the polarized forms of the Ridley and Jopling (R&J) classification: tuberculoid (TT), borderline-tuberculoid (BT), borderline-borderline (BB), borderline-lepromatous (BL), and lepromatous or virchowian (LL). Late recognition of bacillary antigens by the individual could result in an intense and effective immune response (TT and BT pattern) which might lead to the destruction of the bacilli and spontaneous cure. TT individuals are those with effective cellular immunity. Ineffective cellular immunity results in persistent proliferation and dissemination of the bacilli and disease progression toward the lepromatous pole. LL individuals are anergic and react to the bacilli through humoral immunity. Type 1 reaction (T1R) affects patients in the range from TT to BL. Type 2 reaction (T2R) affects patients on the lepromatous side (BL and LL). The bacilloscopic index ranges from 0 to 6+.

Neural impairment is particularly important when T2R affects the peripheral nervous system, causing severe neuritis triggered by the acute inflammatory reaction in a poorly expanding neural structure [2]. Unlike type 1 reaction (TIR; Chapter 5), T2R has a shorter duration and a higher recurrence rate during and after treatment, with each reactional episode lasting ~15 days.

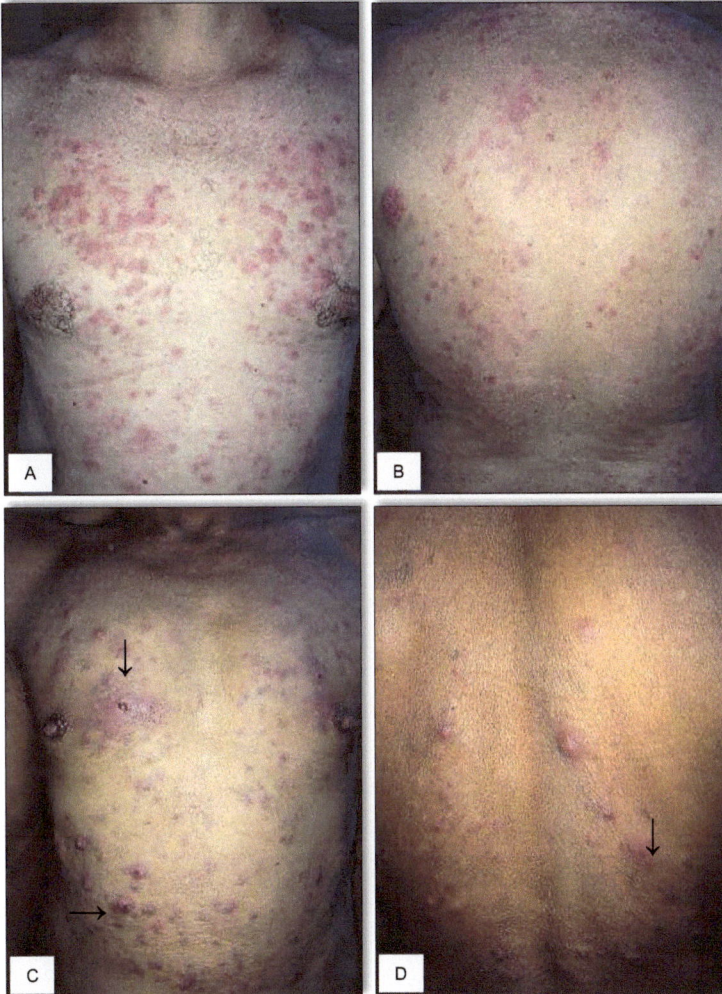

Fig. (2). Clinical characteristics of the type 2 reaction (T2R). LL patient with sudden onset of painful nodules and plaques throughout the body (A and B), some with ulceration (→) (C and D). Courtesy of Dr. Cássio C. Ghidella.

The intensity and frequency of reaction episodes vary according to the patient [1, 2], and to date, no medication has been identified capable of preventing T2R development. Generally, treatment of reactional episodes is insufficient to repair damage caused to neural structures and other tissues affected by T2R [4]. Previous molecular studies suggest several genes as important targets for understanding T2R pathophysiology and its potential prevention [5 - 8].

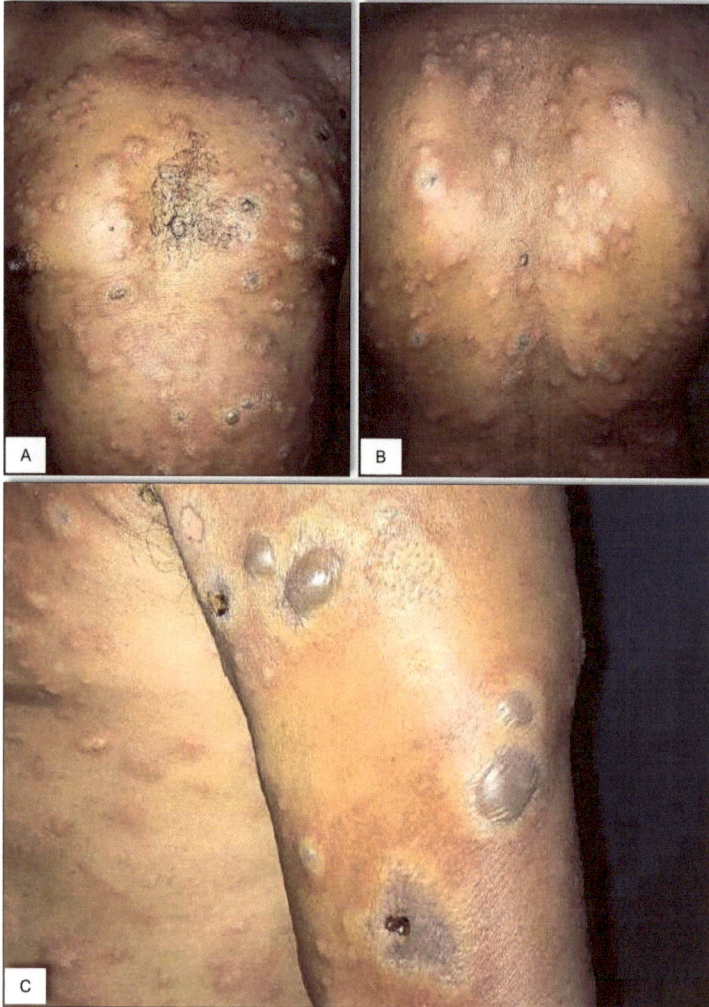

Fig. (3). Clinical characteristics of the type 2 reaction (T2R). LL patient with T2R lesions in different parts of the body along with the formation of pustules, vesicles, necrosis, and ulceration (also called necrotizing erythema nodosum leprosum) (A–C). Courtesy of Dr. Cássio C. Ghidella.

Histopathological and Bacilloscopic Characteristics of T2R

Whenever T2R occurs, histopathological changes are caused by an acute or subacute inflammatory reaction (non-granulomatous) on a regression-like granuloma (BL/LL) or, rarely, on an active lesion (Figs. **4** and **5**). Generally, vascular dilatation, endothelial swelling, and sero-fibrinous and neutrophil exudation are observed that disorganize pre-existing granulomas [2] (Fig. **4**). Venocapillary thrombosis and microabscesses can be observed in the most intense T2R (Figs. **4** - **6**); therefore, T2R present in a skin lesion can have different degrees of intensity and extension. A hypothetical T2R grading system would be: 1) "GRADE 1 or mild", describing a mononuclear inflammatory reaction with few neutrophils and slight vascular dilation with endothelial swelling; 2) "GRADE 2 or moderate", corresponding to changes in GRADE 1 along with a generalized histiocytic reaction, intense neutrophilic exudate, and vascular thrombosis; and (3) "GRADE 3 or intense", representing the sum of GRADES 1 and 2 and associated with abscesses, necrosis, generalized thrombosis, and ulcerations (Fig. **6**).

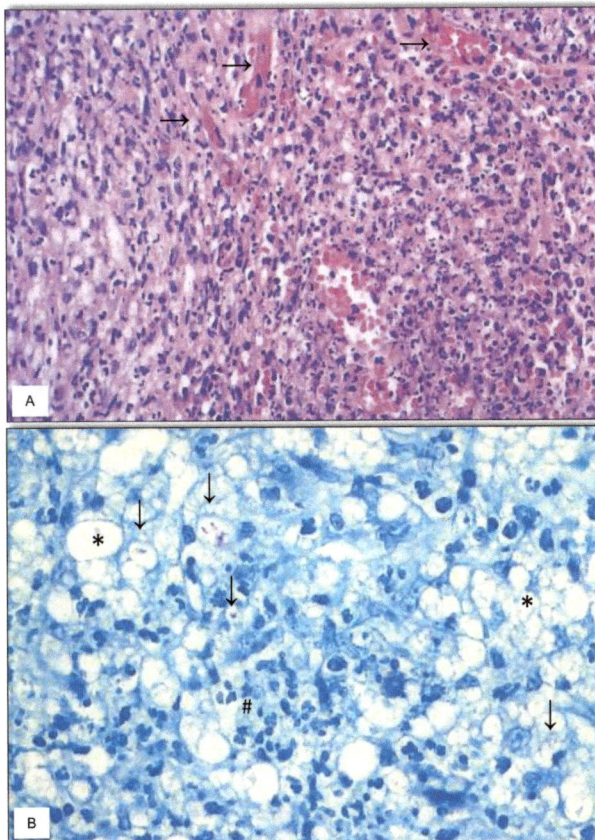

Fig. (4). Histopathological characteristics of the type 2 reaction (T2R). Presence of neutrophils disorganizing the pre-existing BL/LL lesion **(A)**. In the central areas, there is an accumulation of neutrophils outlining the formation of neutrophilic microabscesses and congested capillary vessels with fibrin deposits (→) **(A)**. Bacilloscopic examination showing a regressive lesion on the periphery, with multivacuolated macrophages containing weakly stained or discolored fragmented bacilli (→) (*) and a neutrophil cluster in the center (#). Hematoxylin and eosin **(A)** and Fite–Faraco **(B)** staining.

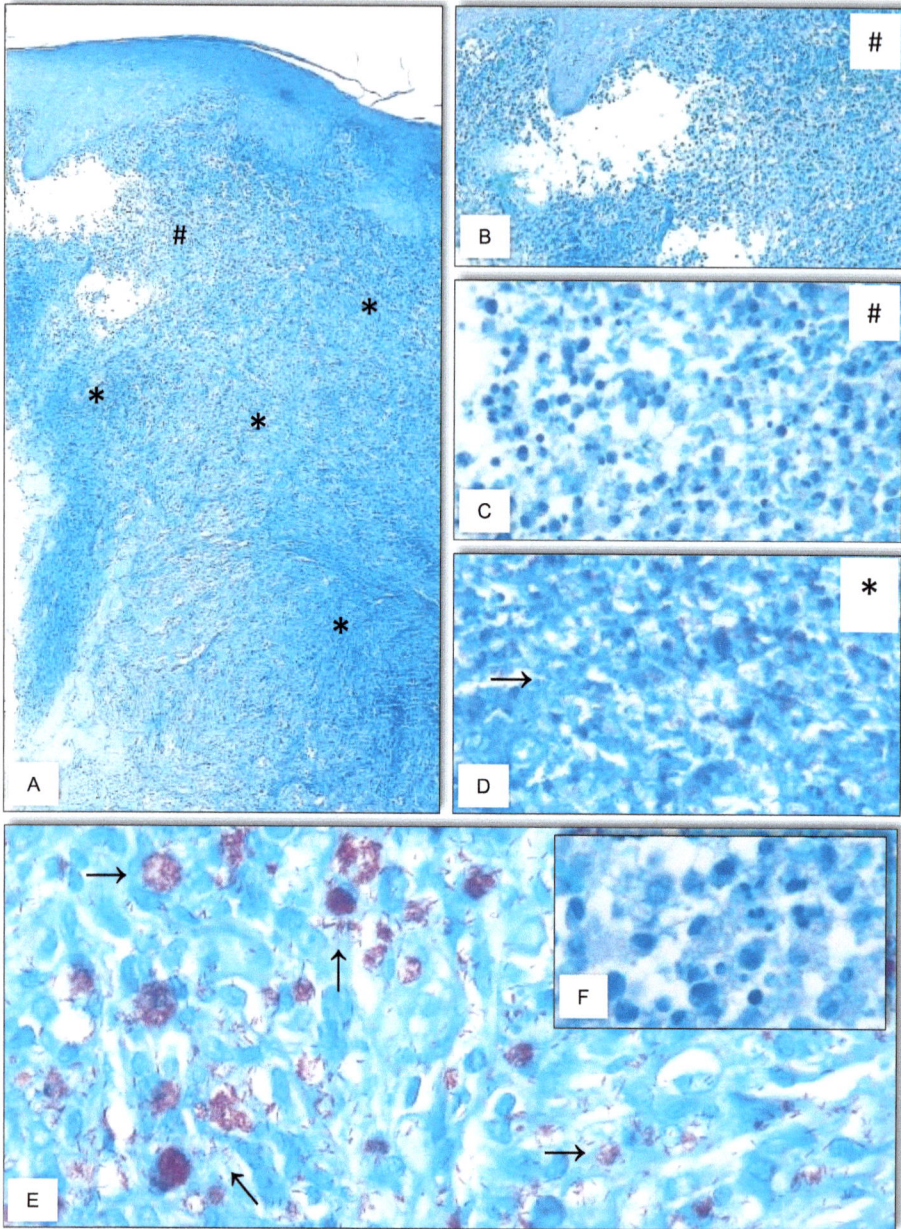

Fig. (5). T2R on an active LL lesion. The reaction process affects the papillary dermis (#), and adjacent areas present an active lesion (*) **(A)**. Bacilloscopic examination showing intense bacillary fragmentation and disappearance of bacilli in the center of microabscesses (B, C, and F), whereas adjacent active areas show intense parasitism by *M. leprae* along with solid bacilli inside some globi (→) (D and E). Fite–Faraco staining.

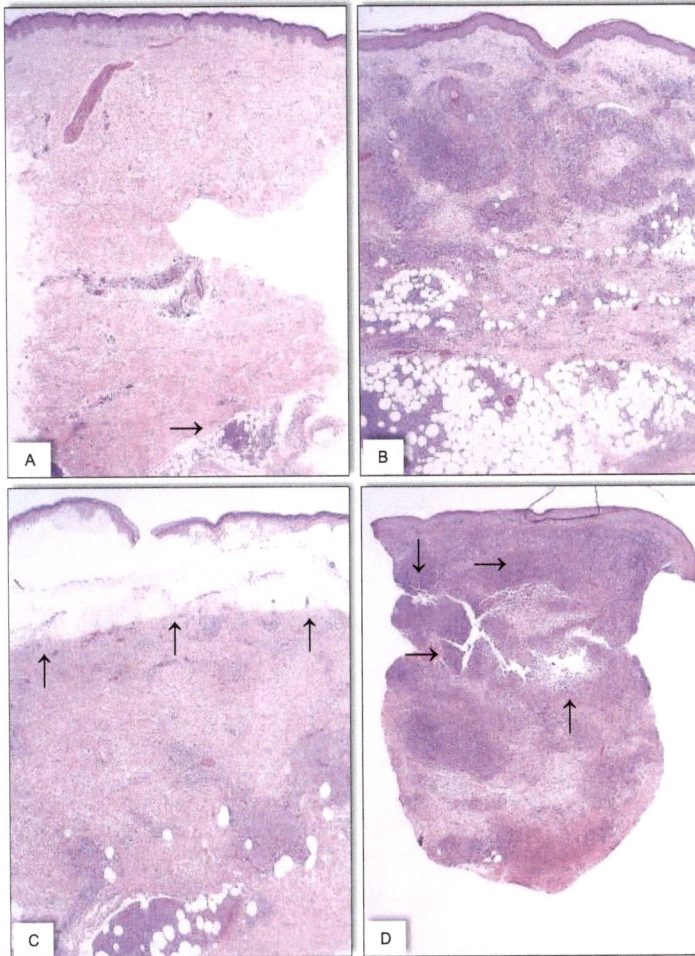

Fig. (6). T2R with different lengths and intensities. Example of focal T2R affecting adipose tissue (→) **(A)** and absence of involvement of all other skin components (GRADE 1). T2R compromises different tissues in the dermis and adipose tissue (GRADE 2) **(B)**. Intense edema in the papillary dermis along with the formation of a subepidermal blister (GRADE 3) **(C)**. Extensive T2R along with the formation of neutrophilic abscesses and necrosis (→) (GRADE 3) **(D)**. Hematoxylin and eosin staining.

The presence of neutrophils is the hallmark of T2R, as they are absent or insignificant in all forms of leprosy and T1R. In T2R, the number of neutrophils varies, although they are always present, with their levels depending on the stage at which the lesion has been biopsied (beginning, middle, or end) and the intensity of the reaction process [9]. At any stage, there is an influx of neutrophils into specific parasitic tissue, or BL/LL granulomatous infiltrates, and neutrophilic clusters can subsequently form microabscesses. At a later stage, neutrophil fragmentation occurs along with leakage of enzymes into parasitized tissues and the appearance of necrotic foci. On the periphery of neutrophilic microabscesses or areas of necrosis, there is a pre-existing BL/LL lesion characterized by multivacuolated macrophages containing fragmented bacilli and permeated by a small number of lymphocytes, plasma cells, and neutrophils. Around the foci of microabscesses, M1 macrophages can be observed containing cellular debris in the cytoplasm but in the absence of granuloma formations [9]. Therefore, the histopathological characteristics of a T2R sample are the sum of the pre-existing histopathological characteristics before the establishment of the reaction process and usually a BL or LL lesion in regression, with characteristics typical of T2R (Figs. **7** and **8**).

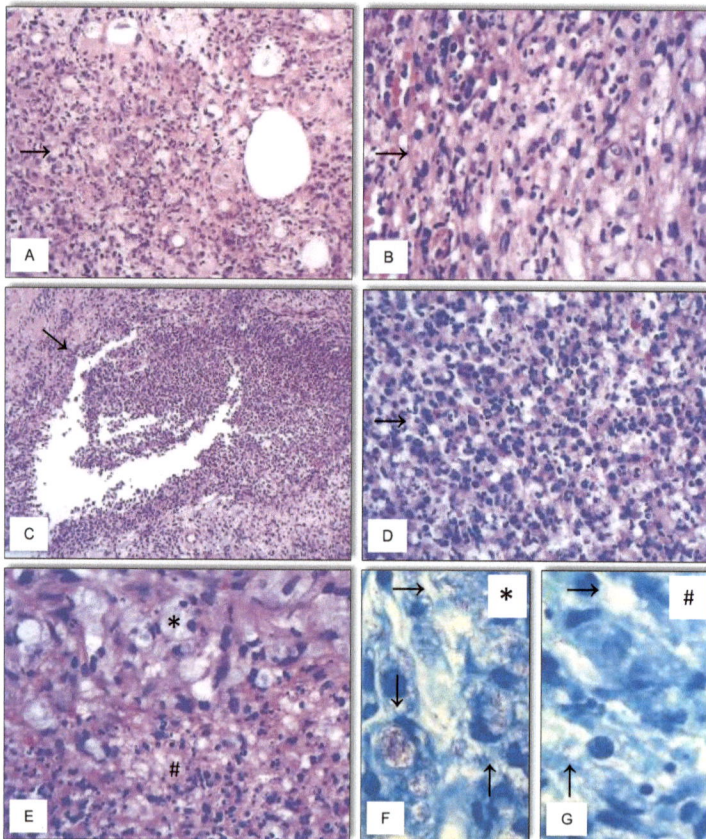

Fig. (7). Histopathological characteristics of T2R in the interstitium. Neutrophils involved with BL/LL-related macrophage clusters in regression (→) **(A)**. Neutrophils permeate macrophages (→) **(B)**, sometimes forming neutrophilic microabscesses (→) **(C)**. The center of microabscesses predominantly comprise neutrophils and cellular debris (→) **(D)**. At the periphery of the reaction process, there is a transition between the pre-existing regressive lesion (*) and the microabcess (#) **(E)**. In the peripheral areas of regressive lesions (→) **(F)**, bacilloscopic examination shows numerous fragmented bacilli, and in the center of the microabscesses, a marked decrease in the number of bacilli, as well as their intense fragmentation (→) **(G)**. Hematoxylin and eosin (A–E) and Fite–Faraco (F and G) staining.

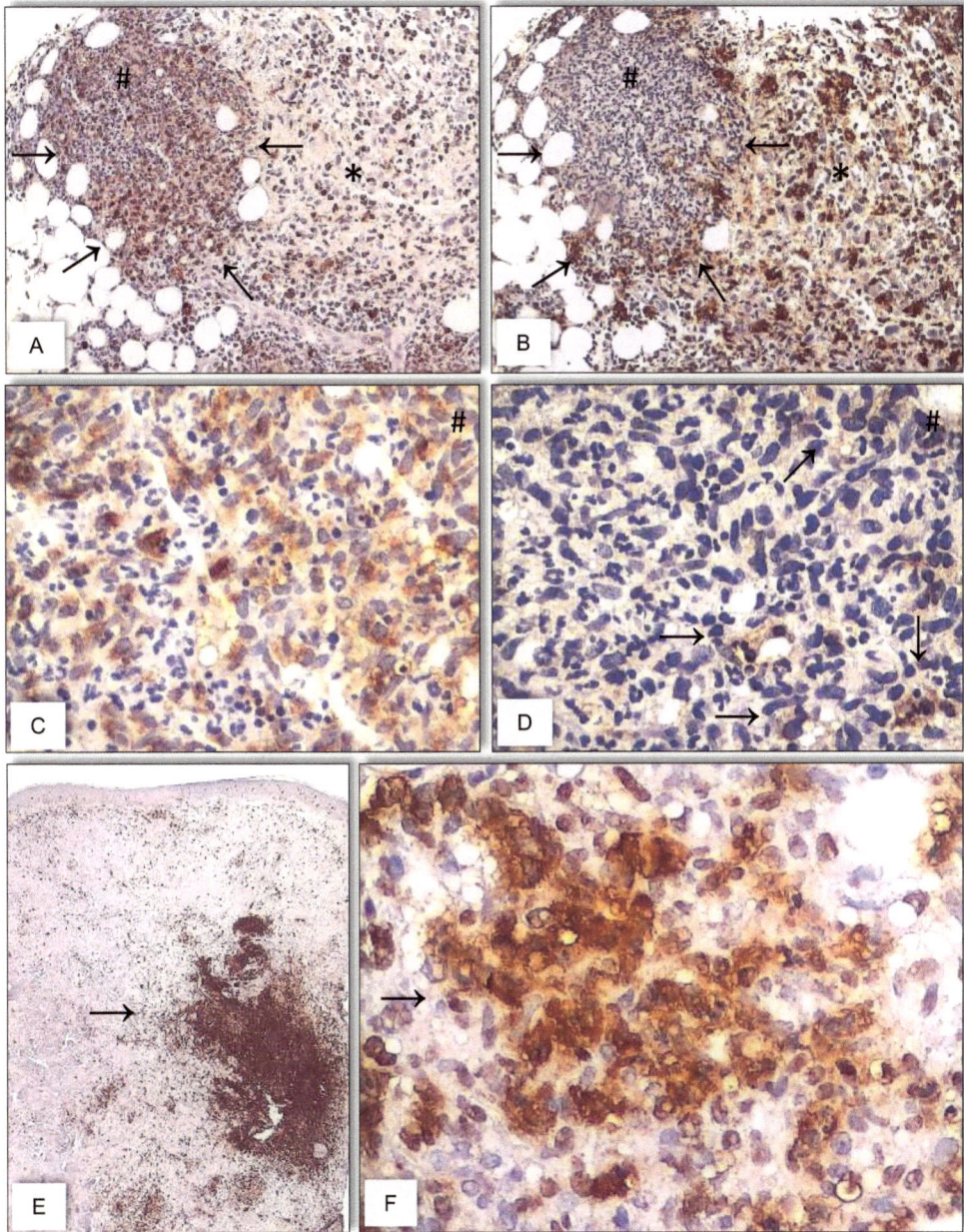

Fig. (8). Histopathological and immunohistochemical characteristics of T2R. Macrophages parasitized by *M. leprae* from pre-existing lesions (#) are permeated by neutrophils and new macrophages (*). Note that in the neutrophilic microabscess areas (#) there is a predominance of CD68+/CD163− (→) macrophages, whereas in peripheral areas of BL/LL lesions in regression (*), the macrophages are CD68+/CD163+ (→) (A and B). At the center of neutrophilic microabscesses, there are numerous CD68+ **(C)** macrophages, with few CD163+ macrophages (→) **(D)**. CD15+ neutrophils form neutrophilic microabscesses (→) (E and F). Immunohistochemistry for CD68 (A and C), CD163 (B and D), and CD15 (E and F).

As in T1R, the conditions that trigger T2R differ between leprosy lesions distributed in different parts of the body (Figs. **2** and **3**). Histopathological characteristics suggest that in the same skin biopsy fragment, the T2R process can selectively affect one or more skin components. BL and LL patients (especially LL) present parasitism of different skin tissues by *M. leprae*, with any of these parasitized tissues capable of presenting T2R. In rare cases, T2R mainly affects the pili muscle (Fig. **9**). The involvement of sweat glands in the T2R can be from the reaction process affecting vessels, nerves, and parasitized periglandular tissues, causing secondary changes in the glands, as well as directly affecting the glandular cells. The glandular components are permeated by neutrophils that cause epithelial and myoepithelial changes characterized by hypercomasia, pycnosis, nuclear fragmentation, and even necrosis of all glandular components (Fig. **10**).

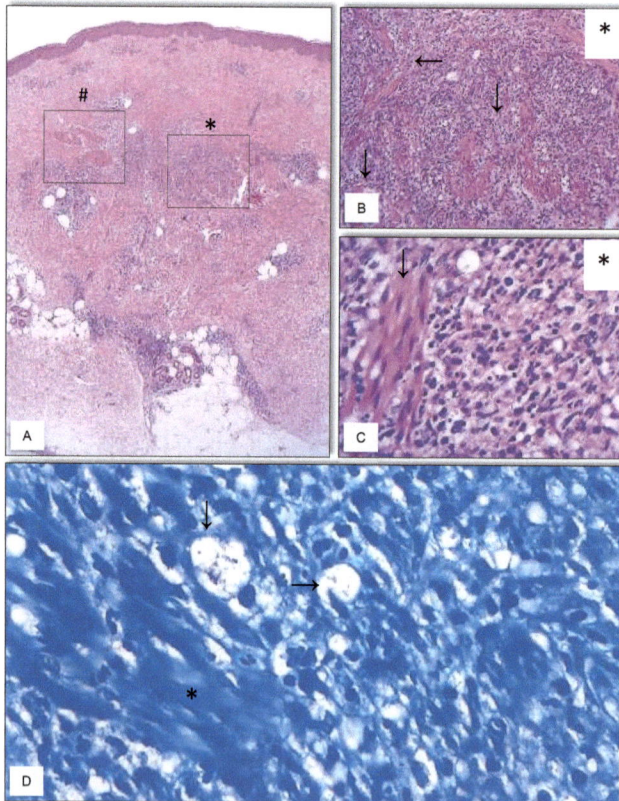

Fig. (9). T2R sample showing predominant effect on the pili muscle. Focal T2R involving only part of the pili muscle (*) **(A)**. In other areas, the pili muscle is unaffected by the reaction process (#). T2R involves and fragments part of the pili muscle, with some muscle bundles remaining inside the reaction process (→) (B and C). Bacilloscopic examination showing a BL/LL lesion in regression with multivacuolated macrophages containing discolored or weakly stained multifragmented bacilli (→) and T2R neutrophils involving the pili muscle segment (*) **(D)**. Hematoxylin and eosin (A–C) and Fite–Faraco **(D)** staining.

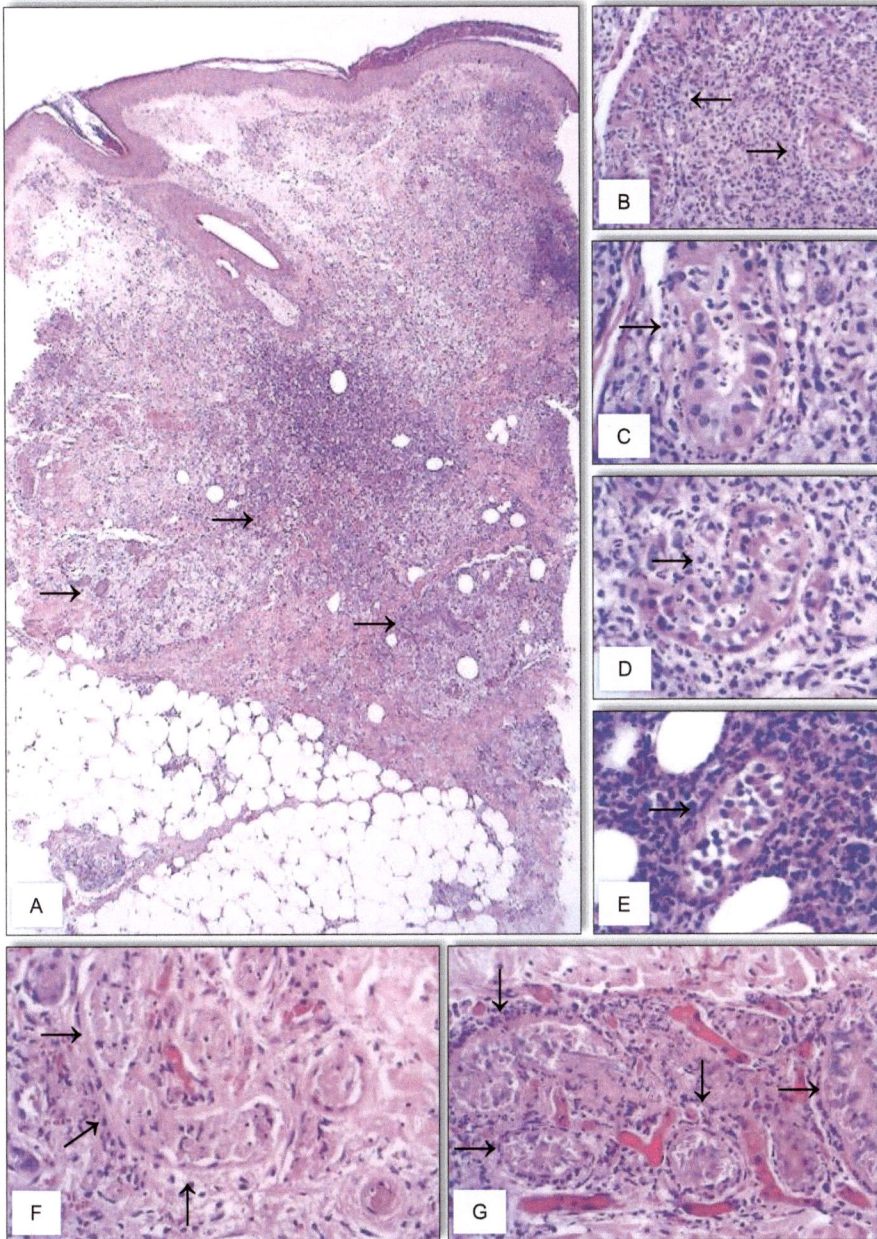

Fig. (10). T2R affecting sweat glands. Presence of interstitial T2R with involvement of sweat glands (→) **(A)**. Reaction process involving parasitized periglandular tissues and the sweat glands themselves (→) **(B)**. Neutrophils directly infiltrate the glandular epithelium, which presents hypercomasia, degenerative changes, and pycnotic nuclei (→) (C–E). All glandular components are necrotic (→) (F and G). Hematoxylin and eosin staining.

The pilosebaceous follicle is frequently parasitized by *M. leprae* in BL and LL forms, and T2R can affect any segment of the pilosebaceous follicle, including the sebaceous glands (Fig. **11**). T2R affecting tissues of the papillary dermis and the epidermis can cause edema accompanied by formations of subepithelial bubbles and epidermal necrosis. T2R-related changes in the dermis and epidermis might be due to the reaction process directly affecting parasitic tissues and dermal vessels, with some vessels showing thromboembolic phenomena, as well as direct aggression of the reaction process to the epidermis by subepithelial neutrophilic clusters and neutrophil exocytosis in all epidermal layers (Figs. **12** and **13**).

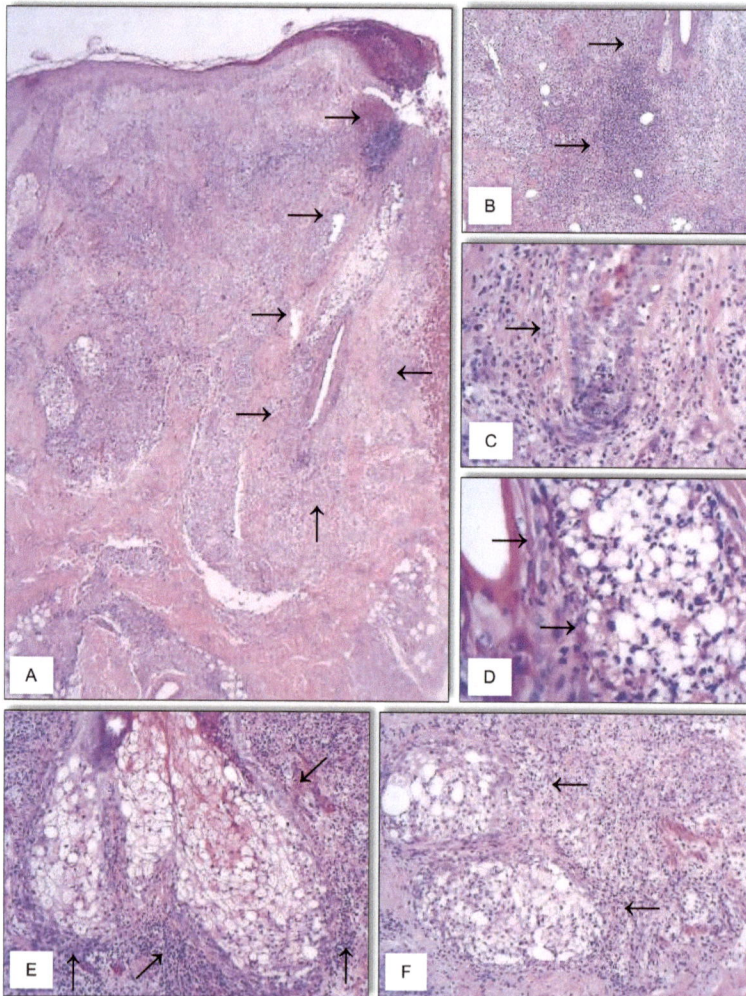

Fig. (11). T2R compromising the pilosebaceous follicle. T2R affects the entire pilosebaceous follicle (→) **(A)**. T2R with formation of neutrophilic microabscesses involving the pilosebaceous follicle (→) **(B)**. Neutrophils permeate the hair sheath and the sebaceous gland (→) (C–F). Hematoxylin and eosin staining.

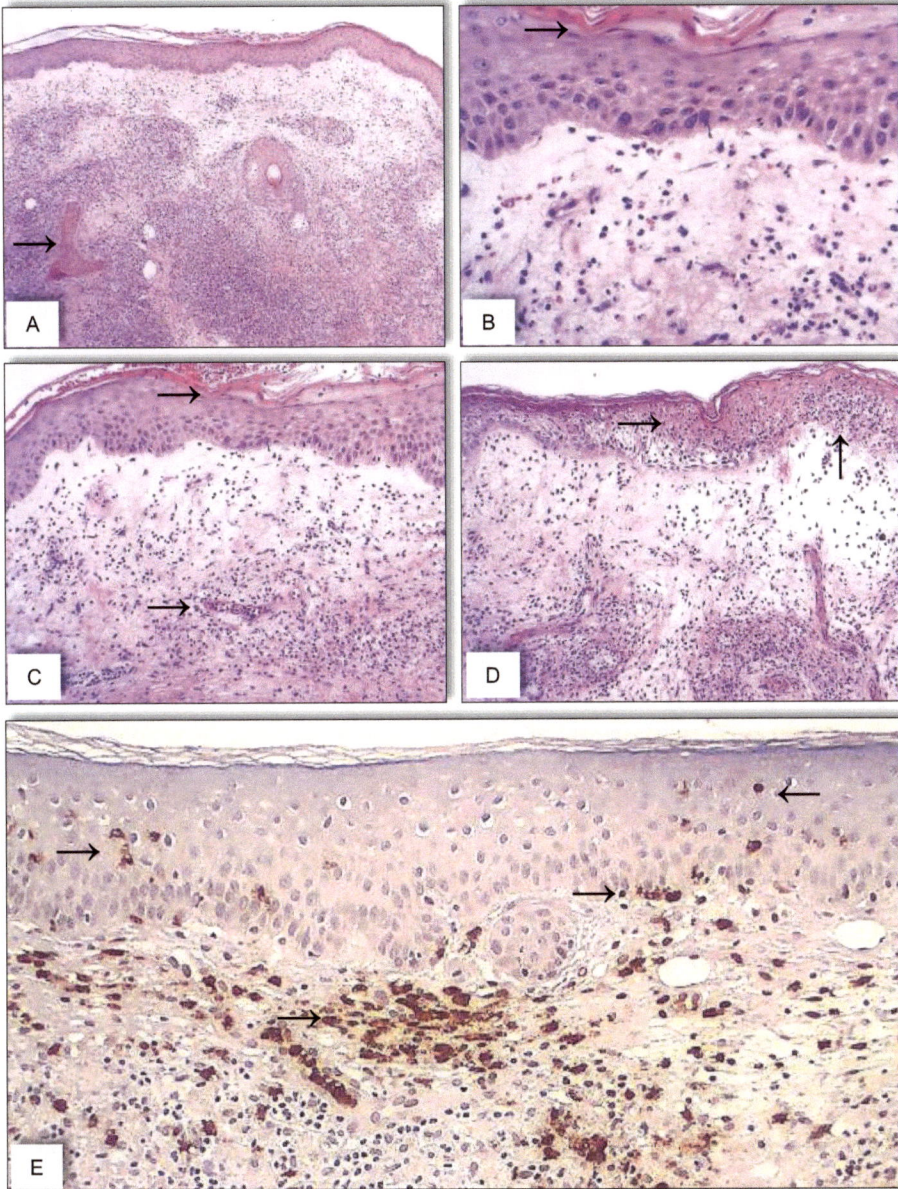

Fig. (12). Histopathological characteristics of T2R affecting the papillary dermis and epidermis. T2R compromising the papillary dermis, with vessels showing congestion, fibrinoid necrosis (→), and interstitial edema **(A)**. Neutrophils permeating the vessels and tissues of the papillary dermis and epidermis associated with epithelial hyperplasia, hyperkeratosis, and parakeratosis (→) **(B and C)**. More extensive neutrophilic infiltrate, intense edema in the papillary dermis, and aggression to the epidermis with keratinocyte necrosis (→) **(D)**. Presence of CD15+ neutrophils (→) in the papillary dermis and the formation of neutrophilic clusters and neutrophil exocytosis at different levels in the epidermis **(E)**. Hematoxylin and eosin staining (A–D) and immunohistochemistry **(E)**.

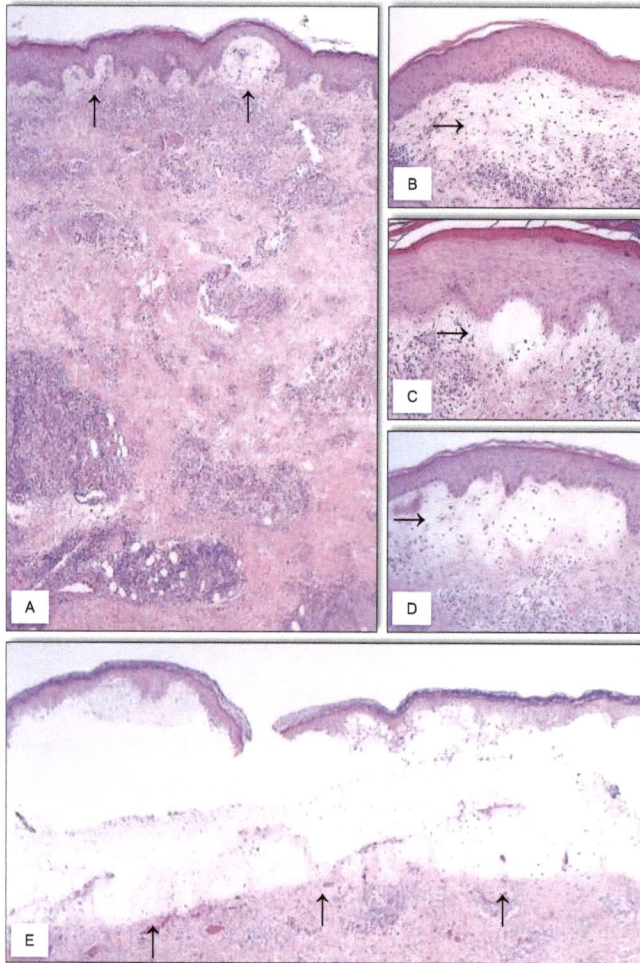

Fig. (13). Histopathological characteristics of T2R affecting the papillary dermis. T2R causing mild interstitial edema in the papillary dermis (→) (A–C) to intense edema (→) **(D)** and subepithelial bubble formation (→) **(E)**. Hematoxylin and eosin staining.

In many cases, only deep tissues associated with transition between the dermis and subcutaneous adipose tissue present evidence of the reaction process (Fig. **14**). Adipose tissue is frequently compromised in BL/LL lesions, with intense parasitism of macrophages, vessels, and adipocytes occurring in the adipose septa and lobes (described in Chapters 1, 3, and 4). Treatment generates an intense fragmentation of the bacilli in the different parasitized cells in adipose tissue, which creates a favorable environment for triggering T2R (Fig. **15**). Therefore, the mechanisms that trigger T2R in adipose tissue and cause panniculitis are the same as those observed in other components of parasitic skin or internal organs. In all cases of T2R in subcutaneous adipose tissue, there is a BL/LL lesion in associated regression, which compromises the lobes and septa. Bacilloscopic examination usually identifies weakly stained or discolored fragmented bacilli within macrophages and other cells on the periphery of subcutaneous neutrophilic microabscesses (Fig. **14**). The histopathological and bacilloscopic changes in regression of leprosy lesions affecting the parasitized adipose tissue are detailed in Chapter 7.

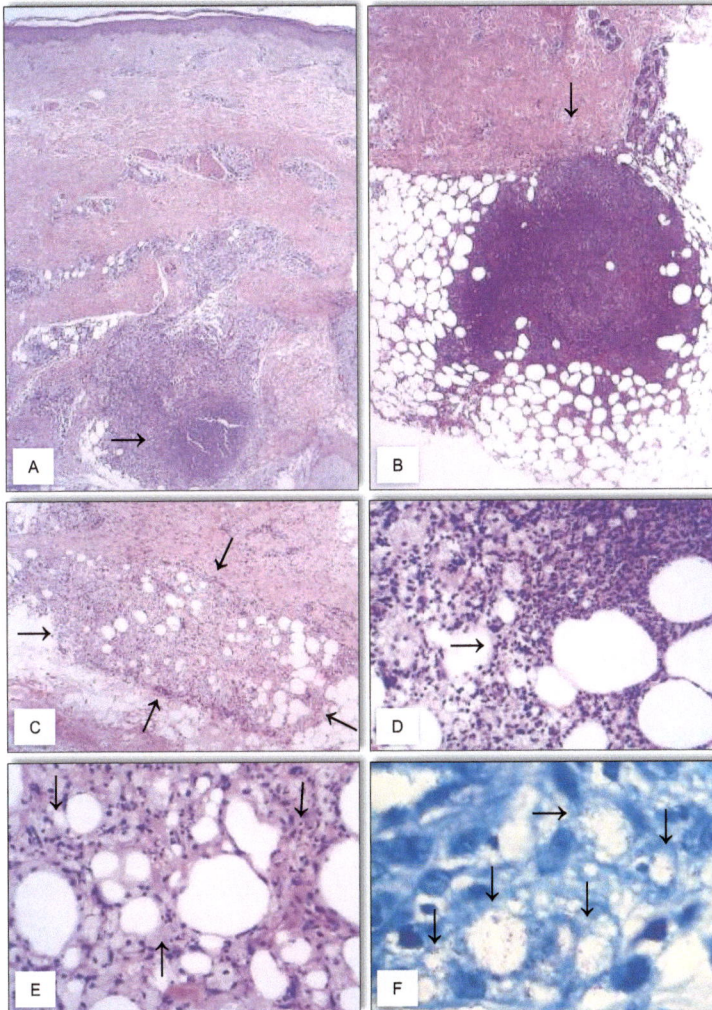

Fig. (14). T2R on subcutaneous adipose tissue. Exclusive compromise of adipose tissue, which causes panniculitis (→) (A and B). The entire lobe and the adipose septum present inflammatory infiltrate from the T2R (→) **(C)**. Neutrophils among adipocytes, macrophages, and other cells in the adipose lobes (→) (D and E). Bacilloscopic examination showing numerous fragmented bacilli that are poorly stained or discolored in the parasitized cells (→) **(F)**. Hematoxylin and eosin (A–E) and Fite–Faraco **(F)** staining.

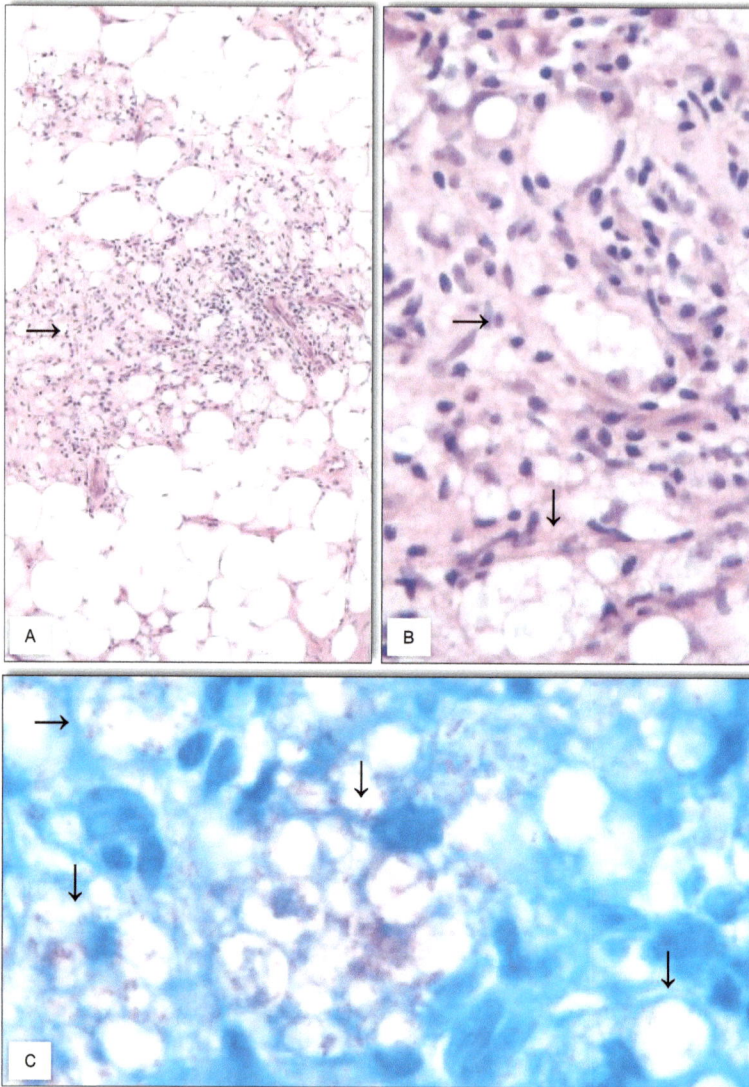

Fig. (15). Subcutaneous adipose tissue with BL/LL infiltrate in regression. Multivacuolated macrophages, vessels, fibroblasts, and adipose cells are commonly parasitized in these lesions (→) (A and B). Bacilloscopic examination showing numerous multifragmented and poorly stained or discolored bacilli mainly inside vacuoles in the macrophage cytoplasm (→) **(C)**. Hematoxylin and eosin (A and B) and Fite–Faraco **(C)** staining.

T2R affecting the neural branches is a common event observed in skin biopsies with leprosy lesions. Nerves are frequently intensely parasitized and susceptible to development of the reaction process at different points in the neural pathway. Moreover, it is possible to observe T2R at different stages or intensity in cutaneous neural branches (Fig. **16**). Similar to other tissues, bacilloscopic examination of T2R-affected neural branches shows multifragmented bacilli in different endoneural and perineural cells. When T2R affects deep nerves where the perineurium is thicker, thereby hindering neural expansion during the reaction process, it is possible to observe areas of ischemic necrosis (Fig. **17**).

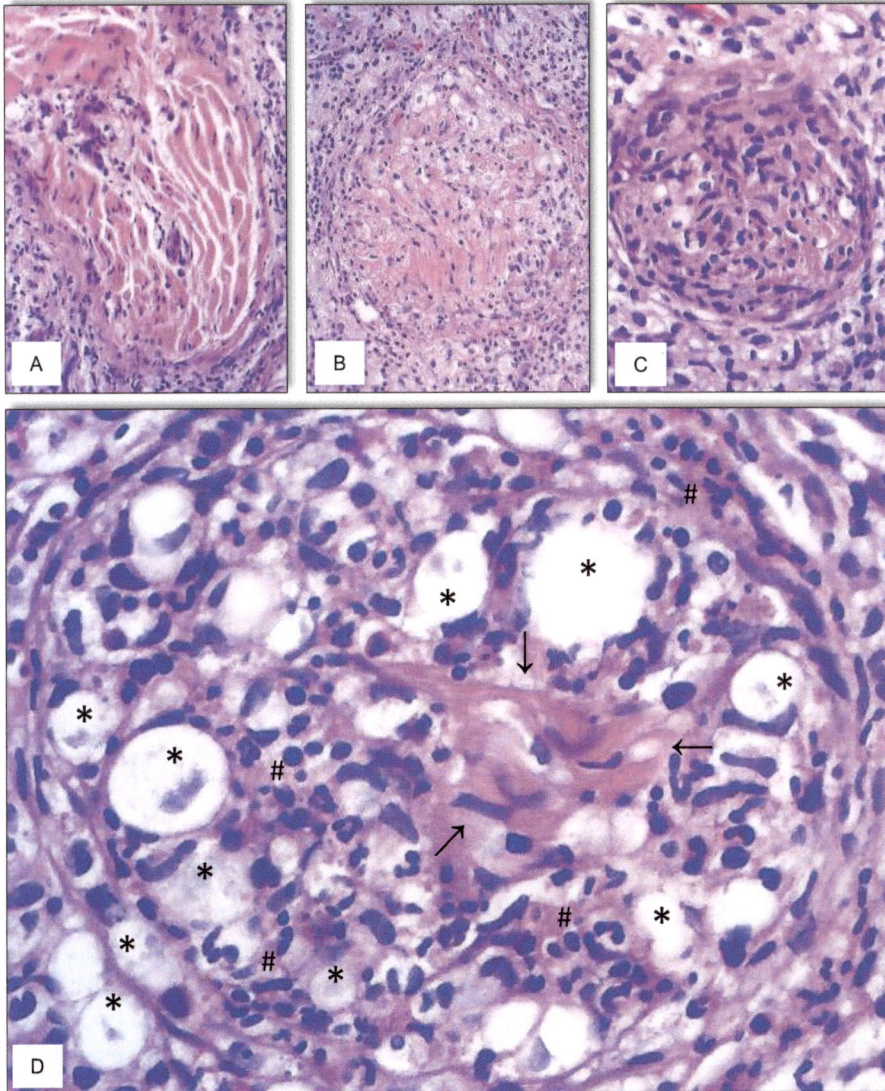

Fig. (16). T2R affecting nerves. Cutaneous neural branches can present T2R predominantly perineurally but with mild endoneural involvement **(A)**, whereas others present a gradually more intense reaction process, sometimes with significant endoneural involvement (B–D). An intensely parasitized neural branch showing numerous multivacuolated macrophages containing fragmented bacilli from the BL/LL lesion in regression (*) and, in the center, neutrophils forming endoneural neutrophilic clusters (#) involving neural fragments (→) **(D)**. Hematoxylin and eosin staining.

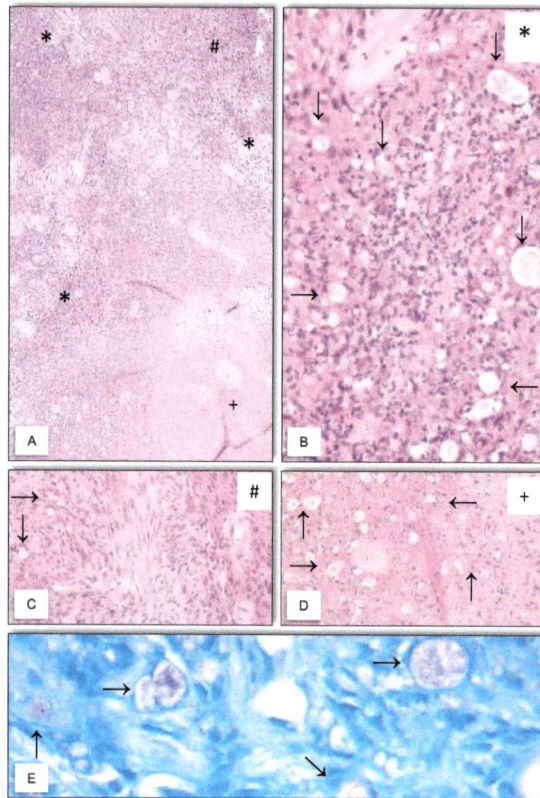

Fig. (17). Sural nerve with T2R. Nerve portion without the reaction process (#) (A and C). Areas displaying T2R characteristics along with formation of neutrophilic microabscesses (*) (A and B). Central areas of ischemic necrosis (+) (A and D). In all areas, multivacuolated macrophages are noted as containing multifragmented bacilli (→) (B–D). Poorly stained or discolored multifragmented bacilli are inside intracytoplasmic vacuoles (→) **(E)**. Hematoxylin and eosin (A–D) and Fite–Faraco **(E)** staining.

T2R effects on the vessels are important phenomena in leprosy. Early studies suggested T2R as a classic example of immune-complex disease, similar to the Arthus phenomenon, which displays a histopathological basis as an acute vasculitis [10, 11]. Subsequent studies have not demonstrated these complexes containing mycobacterial antigens, immunoglobulin, or their complement in vessels [12]. Our experience at Instituto Lauro de Souza Lima shows that vessels affected by T2R are present in <30% of cases in skin biopsies. When the vessels present reactive phenomena, multifragmented bacilli are also observed in the endothelium, the vessel wall, or perivascular tissues (Figs. **18** and **19**). We have not observed the presence of thromboembolic phenomena or leukocytoclastic vasculitis associated with the deposition of immune-circulating complexes in vessels occurring on tissues not parasitized by *M. leprae* in skin or nerve biopsies from patients with leprosy. The histopathological characteristics of T2R in most skin biopsies show an acute inflammatory process, which in evolution might become subacute due to reductions in exudative phenomena and later association of mononuclear inflammatory infiltrate. Changes in the more peripheral vessels (arterioles, capillaries, and venules) reflect the participation of these vascular segments in the acute or subacute inflammatory reaction, with the most intense alteration being thrombosis inside or in the vicinity of microabscesses and fibrinoid necrosis of the vessel wall (Fig. **20**). Vasculitis with destructive inflammation of vascular walls in vessels not parasitized by *M. leprae* are not observed, and small-caliber arteries and veins of the deep dermis and subcutaneous cellular tissue are less affected. Commonly, all components of the vessels, regardless of caliber, are parasitized by *M. leprae* in BL and LL forms (described in Chapters 1, 3, and 4). The pathophysiological mechanisms of T2R are poorly understood [12]; however, molecular studies report exclusive hyperexpression of several genes and microRNAs in T2R [5 - 8].

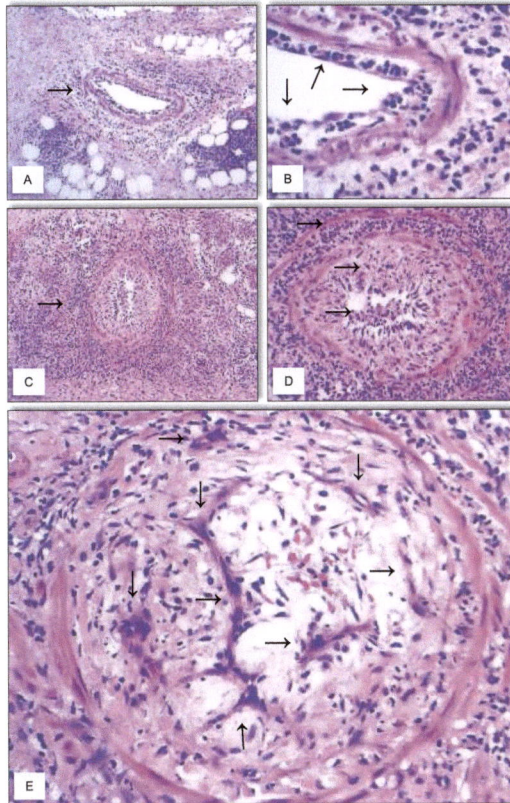

Fig. (18). T2R in different stages affecting vessels. T2R affecting mainly the endothelium and subendothelial tissues (→) (A and B). T2R compromises all vascular layers and perivascular tissues (→) (C and D). In a later stage, the vessel presents thrombi in organization and recanalization (→) **(E)**. Hematoxylin and eosin staining.

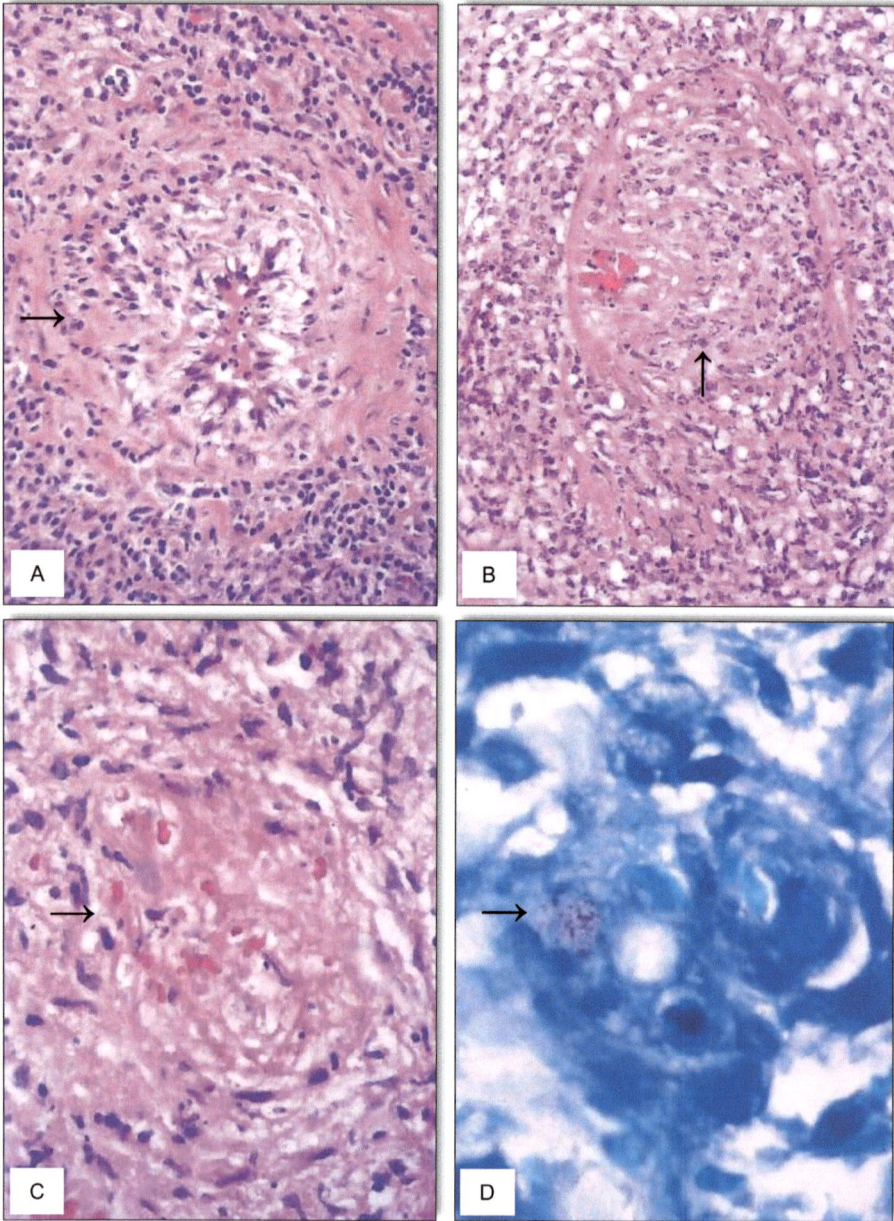

Fig. (19). T2R with different intensities affecting vessels. T2R compromises all vascular layers, but the vascular architecture is preserved (→) **(A)**. Intense and destructive reaction process in the vessel wall accompanied by endothelial and subendothelial extension, causing complete obstruction of the vascular lumen (→) **(B)**. Necrosis of all layers of the vessel (→) **(C)**. Bacilloscopic examination showing the presence of fragmented bacilli (→) in vessels affected by T2R **(D)**. Hematoxylin and eosin staining (A–C) and Fite–Faraco **(D)** staining.

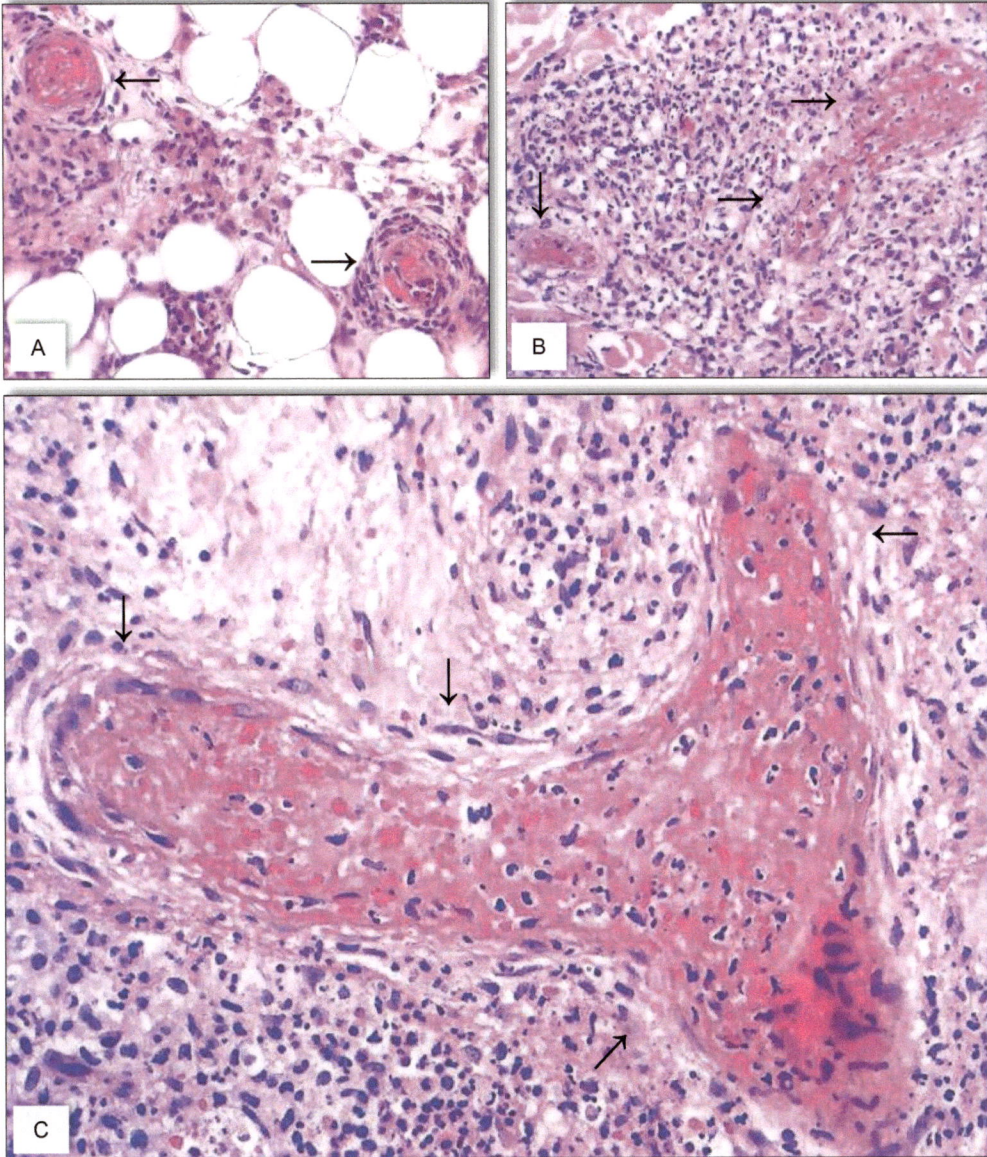

Fig. (20). T2R affecting vessels. T2R-affected vessels on the periphery or inside tissues and showing fibrinoid necrosis (→) (A and B) and thrombi (→) **(C)**. Hematoxylin and eosin staining.

Vascular proliferation and endothelial changes in capillaries are also important. Capillary endothelial cells have a broad, eosinophilic, and vacuolar cytoplasm associated with a vesicular nucleus and prominent nucleoli. It is possible to observe mitosis of endothelial cells. Capillary vascular proliferation characterizes the angiogenesis that occurs in T2R and mainly around neutrophilic microabscesses, with this proliferation better identified by the expression of endothelial markers [13] (Fig. **21**).

Some LL patients with long disease progression present intense parasitism of the wall and endothelium of the superficial vessels and might display a peculiar clinical presentation of T2R as a panflebitis characterized clinically by hyperemic areas following the path of the vessels in the papillary dermis (Fig. **20**). The histopathology of these cases shows T2R permeating all layers of parasitized vessels in the papillary dermis and with the same characteristics previously described as T2R affecting any other parasitized tissue (Fig. **22**).

Differential Clinical and Histopathologic Diagnoses of T2R

Clinical features, such as erysipelas, Sweet's syndrome, drug reaction, mycosis fungoides, annular granuloma, necrobiosis lipoidica, actinic granuloma, diseases that cause vasculitis, erythema nodosum, bullous diseases, and various autoimmune diseases, especially lupus erythematosus, polyarteritis nodosa, and rheumatoid arthritis can present skin lesions clinically similar to leprosy lesions with associated T2R [14 - 17]. In all of these conditions, histopathologic examination is important to exclude these diseases. Leprosy diagnoses can be made according to the presence of BL or LL leprosy lesion, either active or in regression, according to bacilloscopic examination and showing nerve parasitism and T2R-associated changes. Some patients might present T2R clinically similar to erythema multiforme; however, observation of histological and bacilloscopic characteristics of a BL/LL lesion with T2R affecting vessels and tissues of the papillary dermis and the absence of classic features of erythema multiforme (hyperkeratosis and/or hydropic degeneration of the basal layer and cytoid bodies) rule out this hypothesis [18, 19] (Fig. **23**).

Leprosy can simulate, in both the clinic and laboratory, different autoimmune diseases, especially lupus erythematosus. Some cases of leprosy mistakenly diagnosed as lupus erythematosus might display T2R episodes during disease progression. Biopsy of these lesions shows a BL/LL pattern of leprosy associated with T2R changes, resulting in diagnosis of leprosy usually at an advanced stage. It is important to note that leprosy, as a long-term spectral disease, can occur in patients with different types of chronic diseases, including autoimmune diseases (Figs. **24** and **25**). Late T2R vasculitis can reproduce subcutaneous polyarteritis nodosa. Additionally, Lucio's phenomenon, another important differential diagnosis of T2R, presents important changes in blood coagulation and tissue necrosis due to the specific inflammatory involvement of cutaneous vessels. The histopathological characteristics that differentiate T2R (necrotizing ENL) from the Lucio phenomenon are described in Chapter 8.

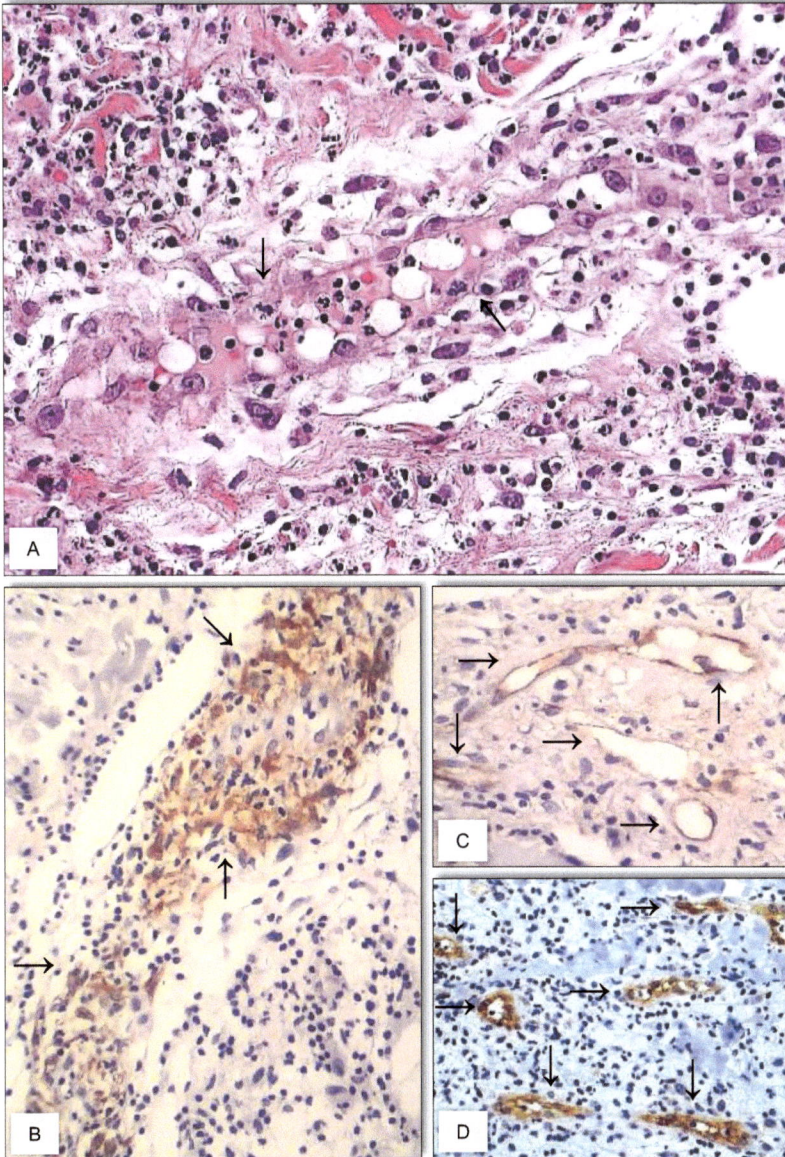

Fig. (21). T2R affecting capillary vessels. Capillary vessel showing endothelial cells with eosinophilic and vacuolar cytoplasm associated with prominent nucleoli and mitosis (→) **(A)**. Smooth muscle cells of the venule wall (→) (calponin+) permeated by numerous neutrophils **(B)**. Angiogenesis characterized by the proliferation of capillary vessels identified by endothelial expression of CD31 (→) **(C)** and CD105 (→) **(D)**. Hematoxylin and eosin **(A)** and immunohistochemistry [calponin **(B)**, CD31 **(C)**, and CD105 **(D)**] staining.

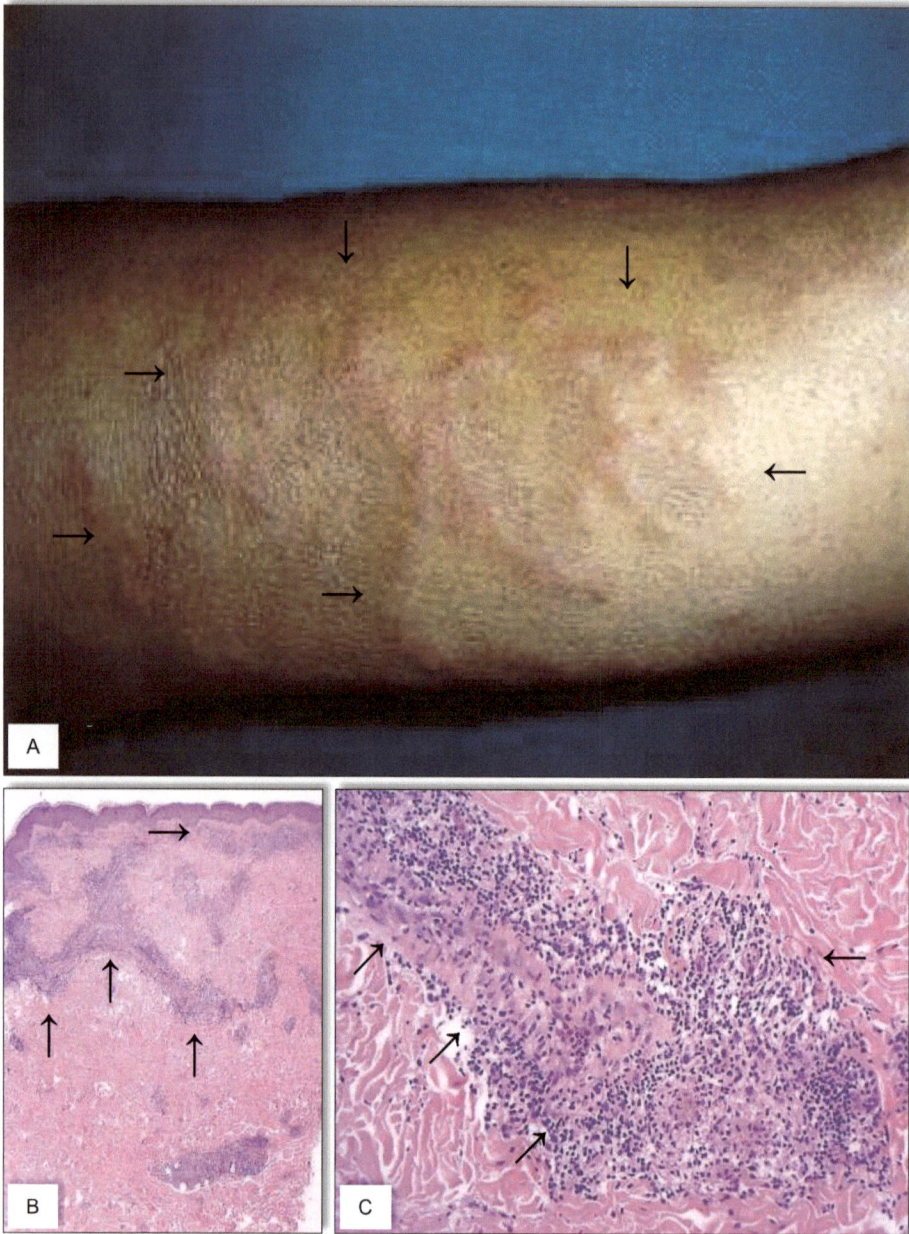

Fig. (22). T2R affecting superficial vessels. Peculiar clinical presentation of T2R over superficial vessels characterized by panphlebitis following the path of the vessels (→) **(A)**. Histopathology showing T2R predominantly affecting the venules and capillaries in the dermis (→) (B and C). Courtesy of Dr. Cássio C. Ghidella **(A)**. Hematoxylin and eosin staining (B and C).

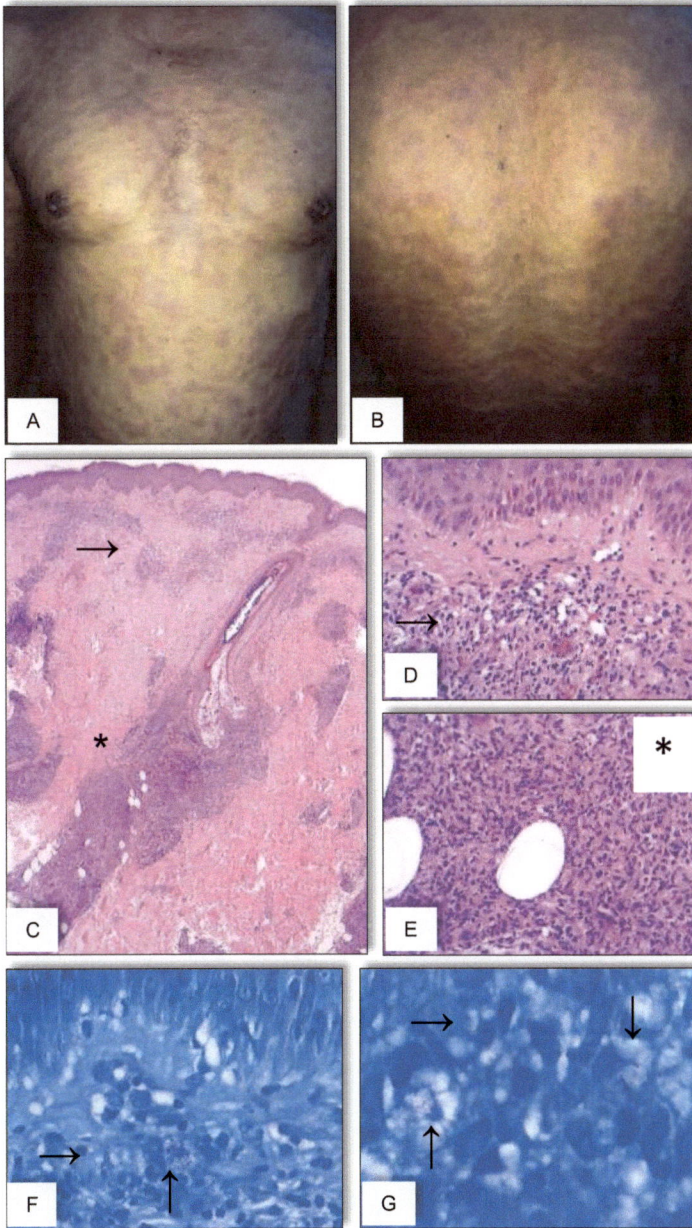

Fig. (23). T2R presenting as plaques. T2R presenting clinically as flat erythematous-violaceous plaques ("target" lesions) similar to erythema multiforme (A and B). Histopathological features are similar to T2R affecting vessels and tissues in the papillary dermis (→) (C and D) and deep tissues (*) (C and E). Bacilloscopic examination showing intense parasitism of tissues at the dermoepidermal interface, with numerous fragmented bacilli (F and G). Courtesy of Dr. Cássio C. Ghidella (A and B). Hematoxylin and eosin (C–E) and Fite–Faraco (F and G) staining.

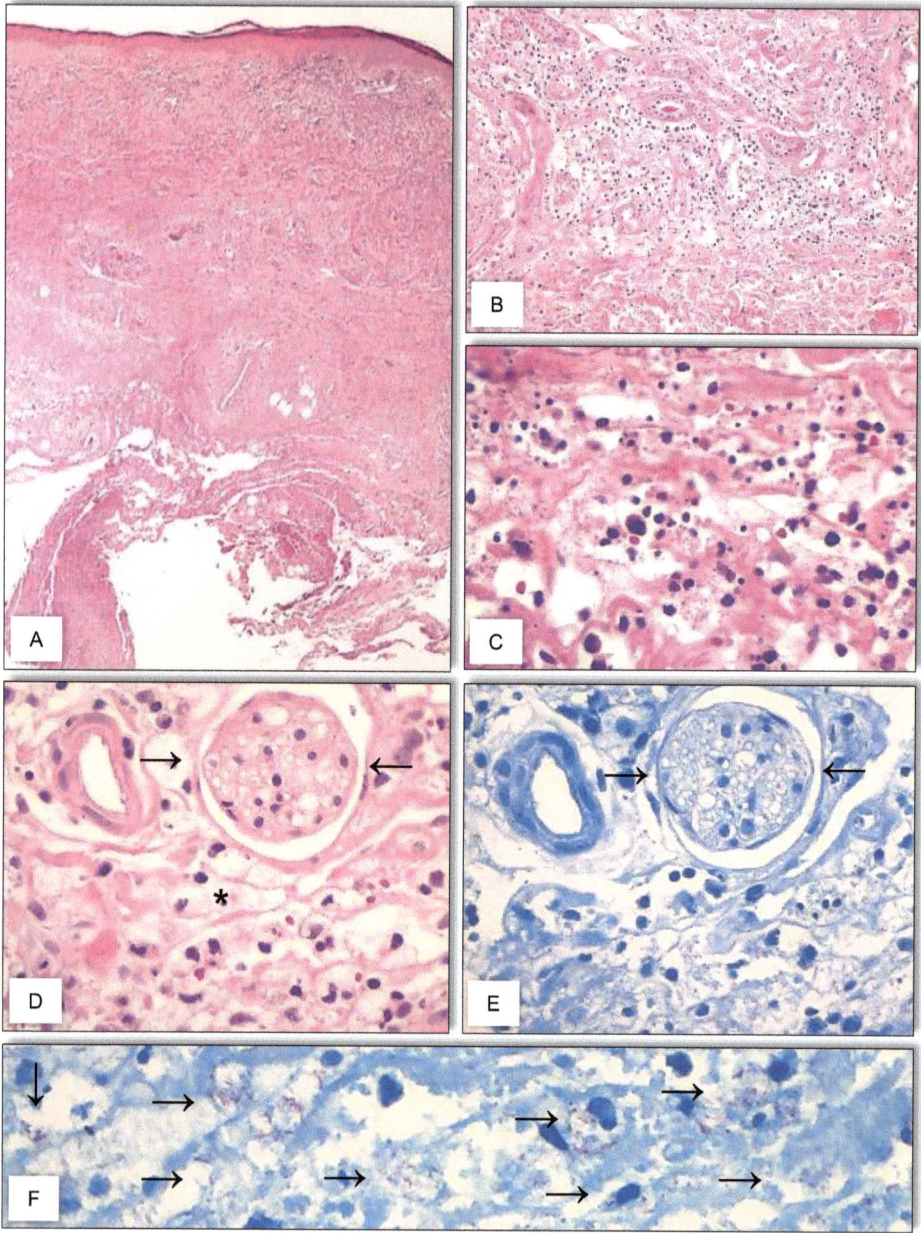

Fig. (24). T2R on LL lesions simulating lupus erythematosus. A patient mistakenly diagnosed for lupus erythematosus presented erythematous and some necrotic skin lesions with suspected lupus vasculitis. Histopathological features show an LL lesion with T2R (necrotizing erythema nodosum leprosum) (→) (A–C). Evidence of an intensely parasitized neural branch surrounded by multivacuolated macrophages (*) **(D)**. The neural branch (→) **(E)** and macrophages (→) **(F)** contain numerous multifragmented bacilli and show a bacilloscopic index (BI) of 6+. Hematoxylin and eosin (A–D) and Fite–Faraco (E and F) staining.

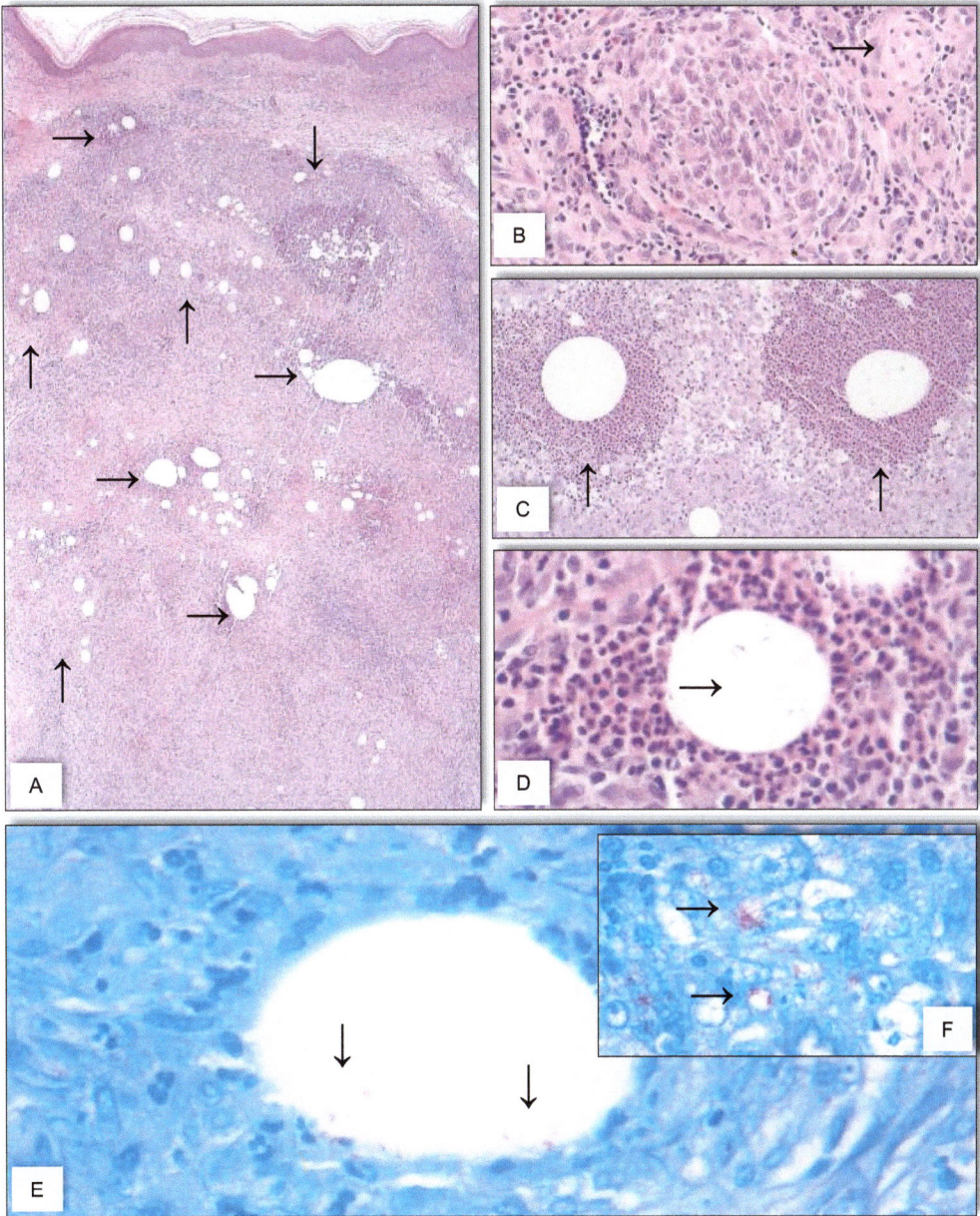

Fig. (25). *Mycobacterium fortuitum chelonae* infection simulating leprosy with T2R. Patient with numerous abscesses in the lower limbs. Granulomatous and suppurative inflammatory process affecting the entire dermis and subcutaneous tissue (→) **(A)**. Granulomas include epithelioid macrophages without neural aggression (→) **(B)**. Numerous vacuoles (→) **(A)** surrounded by neutrophils (→) (C and D) and filled with clusters of bacilli visible by hematoxylin and eosin **(D)** and Fite–Faraco (→) **(E)** staining. Identification of bacilli in granulomatous areas adjacent to the neutrophilic clusters (→) **(F)**. Hematoxylin and eosin (A–D) and Fite–Faraco (E and F) staining.

CONCLUSION

In summary, T2R mainly affects patients with BL and LL forms and focuses on parasitized skin or viscera. Parasitism of different types of tissue in skin lesions is a favorable environment for triggering T2R in any parasitized tissue, and T2R can be observed in the form of neuritis, vasculitis, panniculitis, folliculitis, and adenitis, among others. In all presentations, there is an influx of neutrophils, sometimes forming neutrophilic microabscesses, and in the most intense cases, it is possible to observe tissue necrosis at different levels and intensities.

REFERENCES

[1]   Opromolla DVA. Manifestações clínicas e reações.Noções de Hansenologia. 2nd ed. Bauru, Brazil: Centro de Estudo Dr Reynaldo Quagliato, Instituto Lauro de Souza Lima 2000; pp. 51-8.

[2]   Fleury RN. Patologia e manifestações viscerais.Noções de Hansenologia. 2nd ed. Bauru, Brazil: Centro de Estudo Dr Reynaldo Quagliato, Instituto Lauro de Souza Lima 2000; pp. 63-71.

[3]   Ridley DS, Jopling WH. Classification of leprosy according to immunity. A five-group system. Int J Lepr Other Mycobact Dis 1966; 34(3): 255-73.
[PMID: 5950347]

[4]   Maymone MBC, Venkatesh S, Laughter M, *et al.* Leprosy: treatment and management of complications. J Am Acad Dermatol 2020; S0190-9622: 30473-4.

[5]   Belone A de F, Rosa PS, Trombone AP, *et al.* Genome-wide screening of mRNA expression in leprosy patients. Front Genet 2015; 6: 334.
[http://dx.doi.org/10.3389/fgene.2015.00334] [PMID: 26635870]

[6]   Soares CT, Trombone APF, Fachin LRV, *et al.* Differential expression of microRNAs in leprosy skin lesions. Front Immunol 2017; 8: 1035.
[http://dx.doi.org/10.3389/fimmu.2017.01035] [PMID: 28970833]

[7]   Soares CT, Fachin LRV, Trombone APF, Rosa PS, Ghidella CC, Belone AFF. Potential of AKR1B10 as a biomarker and therapeutic target in type 2 leprosy reaction. Front Med (Lausanne) 2018; 5: 263.
[http://dx.doi.org/10.3389/fmed.2018.00263] [PMID: 30320113]

[8]   Mi Z, Liu H, Zhang F. Advances in the immunology and genetics of leprosy. Front Immunol 2020; 11: 567.
[http://dx.doi.org/10.3389/fimmu.2020.00567] [PMID: 32373110]

[9]   Fachin LR, Soares CT, Belone AF, *et al.* Immunohistochemical assessment of cell populations in leprosy-spectrum lesions and reactional forms. Histol Histopathol 2017; 32(4): 385-96.
[PMID: 27444702]

[10]   Wemambu SN, Turk JL, Waters MFR, Rees RJW. Erythema nodosum leprosum: a clinical manifestation of the arthus phenomenon. Lancet 1969; 2(7627): 933-5.
[http://dx.doi.org/10.1016/S0140-6736(69)90592-3] [PMID: 4186599]

[11]   Waters MFR, Ridley DS. Necrotizing reactions in lepromatous leprosy. Int J Lepr 1963; 31: 418-36.
[PMID: 14166267]

[12]   Polycarpou A, Walker SL, Lockwood DN. A systematic review of immunological studies of erythema nodosum leprosum. Front Immunol 2017; 8: 233.
[http://dx.doi.org/10.3389/fimmu.2017.00233] [PMID: 28348555]

[13]   Soares CT, Rosa PS, Trombone AP, *et al.* Angiogenesis and lymphangiogenesis in the spectrum of leprosy and its reactional forms. PLoS One 2013; 8(9)e74651
[http://dx.doi.org/10.1371/journal.pone.0074651] [PMID: 24040306]

[14]   Gunawan H, Yogya Y, Hafinah R, Marsella R, Ermawaty D, Suwarsa O. Reactive perforating leprosy, erythema multiforme-like reactions, sweet's syndrome-like reactions as atypical clinical manifestations of Type 2 leprosy reaction. Int J Mycobacteriol 2018; 7(1): 97-100.
[http://dx.doi.org/10.4103/ijmy.ijmy_186_17] [PMID: 29516895]

[15]   Cuevas J, Rodríguez-Peralto JL, Carrillo R, Contreras F. Erythema nodosum leprosum: reactional leprosy. Semin Cutan Med Surg 2007; 26(2): 126-30.
[http://dx.doi.org/10.1016/j.sder.2007.02.010] [PMID: 17544965]

[16]   Gao LN, Zhong B, Wang Y. Rheumatoid arthritis-like features in Hansen disease: A case report. Medicine (Baltimore) 2018; 97(29)e11590
[http://dx.doi.org/10.1097/MD.0000000000011590] [PMID: 30024562]

[17]   Andrade TCPC, Martins TY, Vieira BC, Santiago TM, Soares CT, Barreto JA. Lepromatous leprosy simulating rheumatoid arthritis - Report of a neglected disease. An Bras Dermatol 2017; 92(3): 389-91.
[http://dx.doi.org/10.1590/abd1806-4841.20175423] [PMID: 29186255]

[18]   Chiaratti FC, Daxbacher EL, Neumann AB, Jeunon T. Type 2 leprosy reaction with Sweet's syndrome-like presentation. An Bras Dermatol 2016; 91(3): 345-9.
[http://dx.doi.org/10.1590/abd1806-4841.20164111] [PMID: 27438203]

[19]   Chavez-Alvarez S, Herz-Ruelas M, Ocampo-Candiani J, Gomez-Flores M. Type 2 leprosy reaction resembling Sweet syndrome: Review of new and published cases. Australas J Dermatol 2020; 61(2): e234-7.
[http://dx.doi.org/10.1111/ajd.13224] [PMID: 31984474]

CHAPTER 7

Regression and Relapse

Abstract: Immediately after leprosy treatment initiation, changes in leprosy lesions also commence. The histopathological and bacilloscopic characteristics of the regressing lesions undergo continuous changes over years or decades. It is important to recognize these changes as they allow for the assessment of whether a particular lesion is in regression or if there are signs of disease reactivation. Interpretation of the findings will depend on a close correlation among histopathological patterns, bacilloscopic characteristics, and clinical data. This chapter discusses the main factors that allow the recognition of the histopathological characteristics of regressive phenomena from initial phases to late or residual phases, the changes typical in regressive leprosy granulomas and their importance for assessing treatment effectiveness, the reaction phenomena triggered after treatment initiation on regressing lesions, and the evaluation of leprosy recurrence. Further, this chapter includes a discussion on the main differential diagnoses of leprosy regression and relapse.

Keywords: Hansen's disease, Leprosy, *M. leprae*, Regression, Relapse.

INTRODUCTION

Regression changes in leprosy lesions begin as soon as the first treatment dose is administered. Leprosy in its active phase is a long-term spectral disease in which tissues are progressively parasitized. In its regression phase, especially in BL and LL patients, changes occur continuously for many years or decades. These regression changes predispose to various phenomena in leprosy lesions. The most important are the leprosy reaction type 1 (T1R) and type 2 (T2R) described in chapters 5 and 6. Other phenomena are interstitial fibroblastic proliferations simulating a scar reaction, the development of neoplastic lesions, and the healing and tissue repair processes of the various parasitized tissues, mainly in those affected by T1R or T2R.

Regression changes are also visible in the bacilloscopic examination. Treatment leads to bacillary fragmentation with the bacilloscopic index (BI) continuously decreasing, according to the ability to eliminate fragmented bacilli until a minimum index (BI-zero) is reached. Bacillary fragmentation and antigen removal are not homogeneous in different parasitized tissues. Consequently, bacilli identification and BI are different among the tissues in a sample.

Furthermore, it is important to be aware of the histopathological and bacilloscopic characteristics that indicate disease reactivation by looking for signs of bacillary proliferation in previously parasitized tissues.

Therefore, recognition of the histopathological characteristics of regressive phenomena is important in the assessment of treatment effectiveness, in the recognition of associated reaction phenomena and overlapping lesions in regression, in the detection of neoplastic and non-neoplastic stromal changes that are liable to occur by regressive changes in parasitized tissues, and in the assessment of disease recurrence.

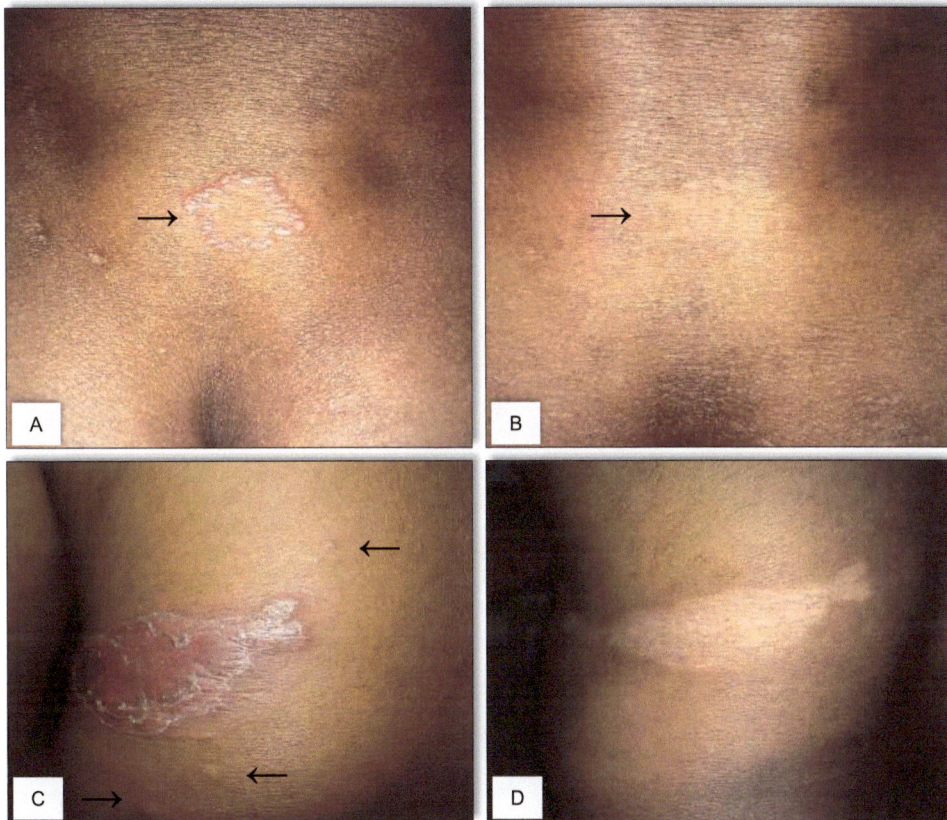

Fig. (1). Active and regressing lesions in the tuberculoid side (TT and BT). **(A)** TT active lesion characterized by a small erythematous-hypochromic plaque in the sacral region, with edges formed by tiny papules (→). **(B)** Six months after MDT-PB treatment, atrophy and residual hypochromia of the same TT lesion were noted (→). **(C)** Active BT lesion characterized by erythematous and scaling plaque of imprecise limits associated with tiny satellite lesions close to a larger lesion (→). **(D)** Five years after MDT-MB treatment (12 doses), the same lesion appears as an atrophic plaque with residual hypochromia (→) and disappearance of satellite lesions. Courtesy of Dr. Cássio C. Ghidella.

CLINICO PATHOLOGICAL AND BACILLOSCOPIC CHARACTERISTICS OF LEPROSY REGRESSION

The treatment for leprosy involves multidrug therapy (MDT) and employs different drug combinations for a duration ranging from six months (paucibacillary, MDT/PB) to up to two years (multibacillary, MDT/MB) [1 - 3]. After the first dose, intense bacilli fragmentation begins. In the tuberculoid side forms (TT and BT), with few lesions and a low BI (0-2), these lesions disappear in a few months or years, and, in general, new biopsies are not collected for evaluation of cure (Fig. **1**). In contrast, lesions on the lepromatous side (BL and LL) are extensive, involve a large part of the integument, and have a high BI (5 or 6), and their disappearance or the formation of residual lesions is a very late phenomena (Figs. **2 - 3**). Just as the disease progresses slowly and over a long period, the regression of lesions in BL and LL patients can take years or decades from the diagnosis of an active lesion to the regression being almost completed in the form of residual lesions (Figs. **4 - 5**).

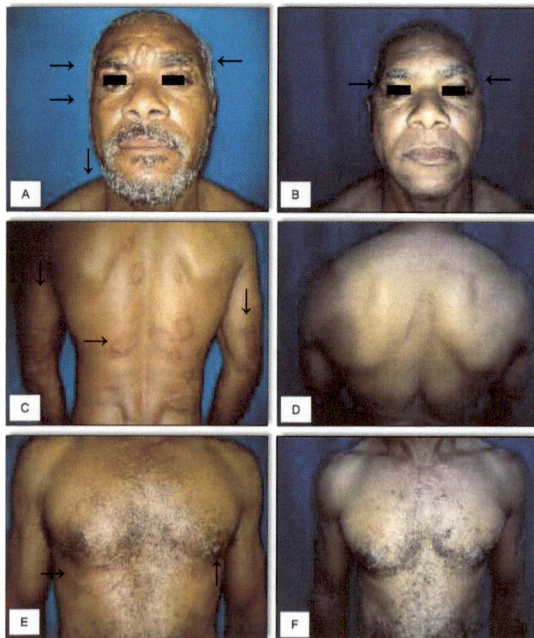

Fig. (2). Active lesions and in regression of a borderline-borderline (BB) patient. Sequential photographs of active (A, C, and E) and regression lesions (B, D, and F) five years after the end of MDT-MB treatment. (**A**) Erythematous pigmented infiltrative plaques on the face, affecting the eyelids, forehead, and right clavicular region (→). (**B**) After treatment, bilateral supraciliary residual pigmentation and atrophy was noted (→). (**C**) Trunk and limbs showing ring lesions with imprecise limits like "Swiss cheese" (→). (**D**) After treatment, lesions disappeared. (**E**) Right inframammary infiltrative annular plaque and nodule in the left nipple (→). (**F**) After treatment, lesions disappeared completely. Courtesy of Dr. Cássio C. Ghidella.

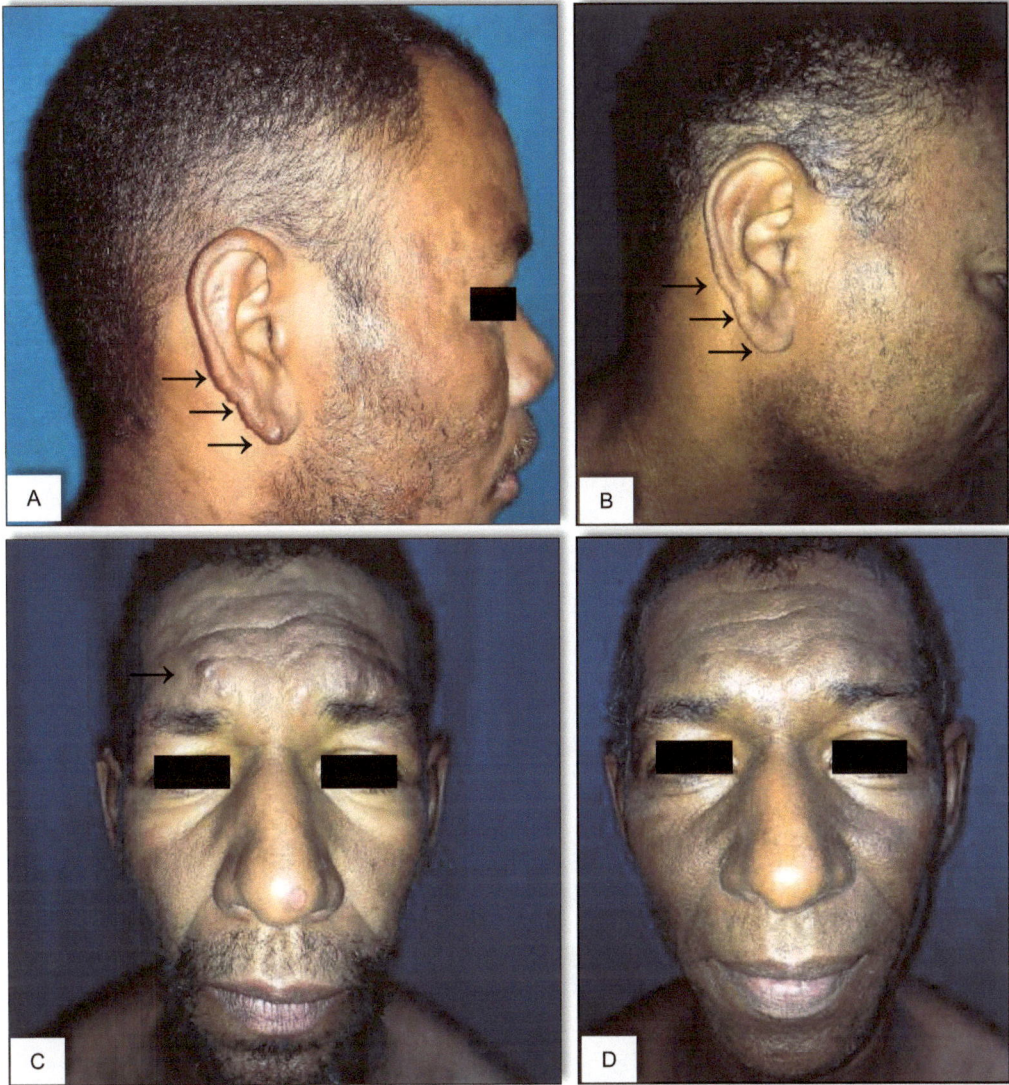

Fig. (3). Active and regression lesions in two lepromatous borderlines (BL) patients. Active lesions (A and C) and in regression (B and D). **(A)** Erythematous-brown plaques with imprecise limits on infiltrated skin and small nodules or tubers (lepromas) (→) in the ear. **(B)** Ten years after specific treatment (MDT/MB - 24 doses), there was a complete disappearance of the specific lesions and the presence of anetodermal lesions in the auricle (→) caused by regression of pre-existing lepromas. **(C)** Diffuse involvement of the entire face with areas of greater infiltration, forming small nodules (lepromas) (→). **(D)** Marked regression of all lesions after treatment (MDT/MB - 24 doses). Courtesy of Dr. Cássio C. Ghidella.

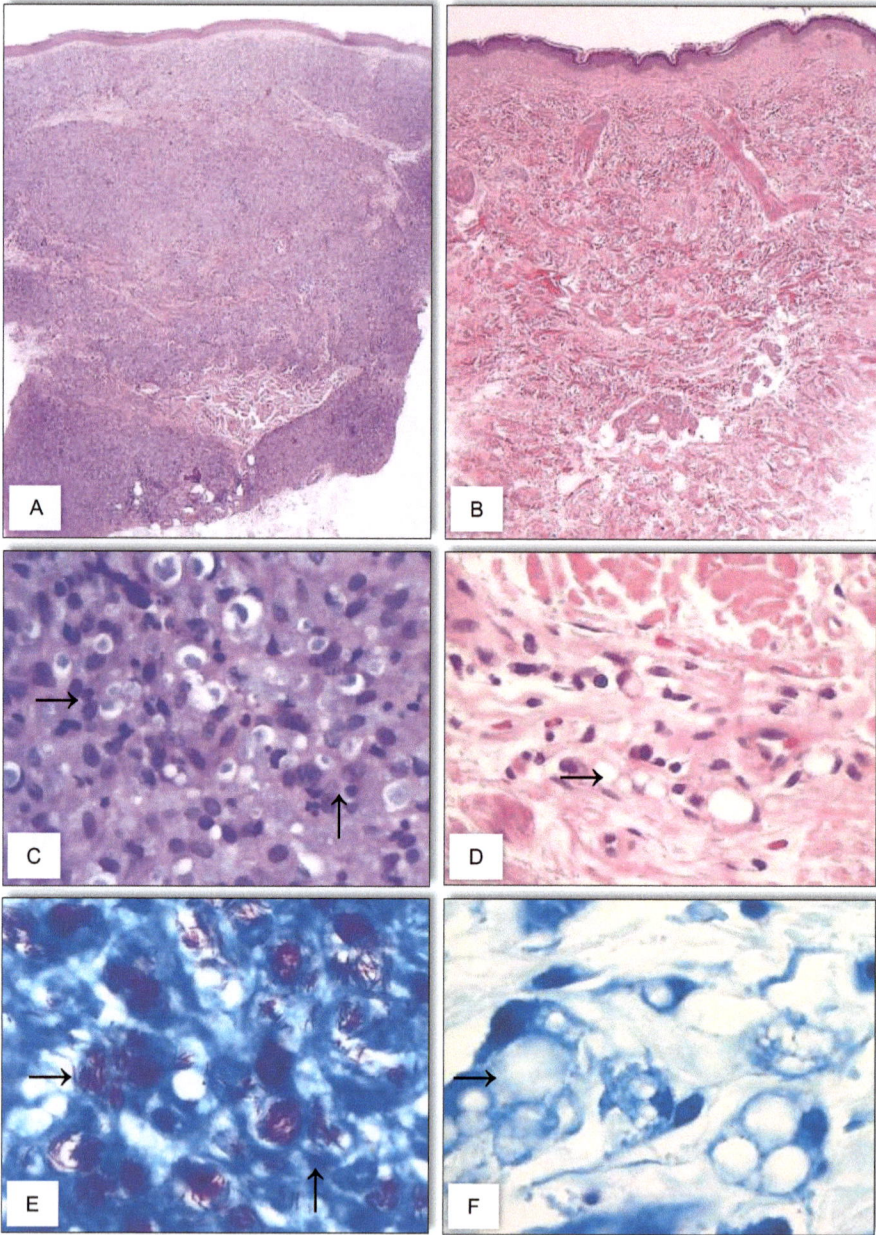

Fig. (4). Example of active and residual injury. Lesion in the lepromatous band (BL-LL) active and in progression (A, C, and E). Residual lesion in the lepromatous band (BL-LL) ten years after treatment - MDT/MB (B, D, and F). The active lesion shows extensive inflammatory infiltrate **(A)** and vacuolated macrophages **(C)** containing a large number of bacilli **(E)** (→). In the residual lesion, the inflammatory infiltrate practically disappears **(B)**, leaving small foci of vacuolated macrophages **(D)** and absence of bacilli **(F)** (→). Hematoxylin and eosin (A-D) and Fite–Faraco (E and F) stainings.

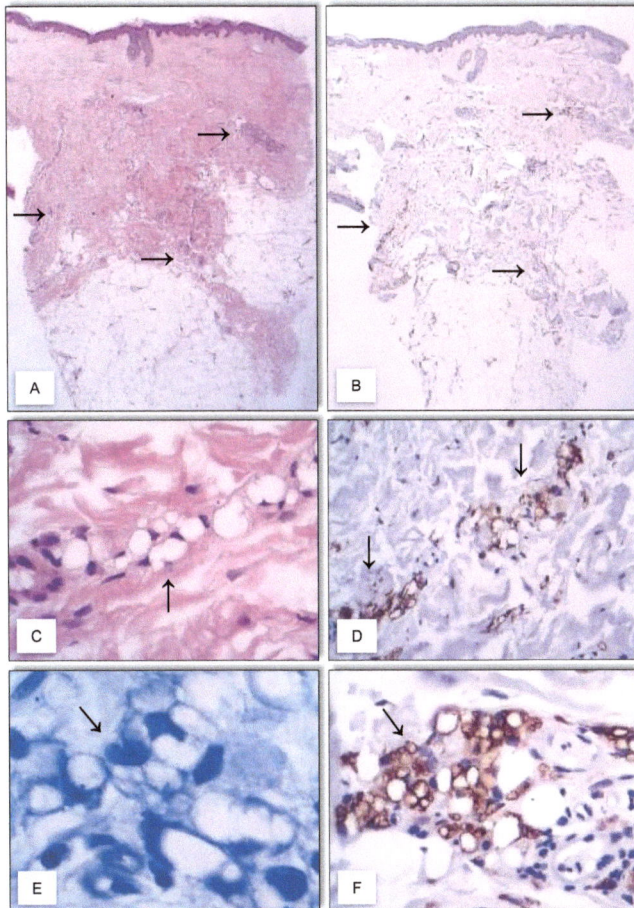

Fig. (5). Residual lesion of lepromatous leprosy 16 years after the end of treatment MDT/MB - 24 doses. The epidermis, dermis, and subcutaneous adipose tissue present usual histological characteristics except for the presence of a residual LL lesion characterized by multivacuolated macrophages following the vasculo-neural pathways (→) (A and C) and negative bacilloscopic examination (→) **(E)**. Macrophages are best observed by immunohistochemistry (IHC) for macrophage markers (→) (B, D, and F). HE (A and C), Fite–Faraco **(E)**, and IHC (anti-CD163 in B, D, and F) staining.

The clinical characteristics of regressing lesions vary constantly and the histopathological and bacilloscopic characteristics found in the biopsies depend on the treatment and its duration, namely, the chosen drugs and the interval between treatment initiation and time of biopsy. Modifications of regression lesions also have different dynamics in the various parasitized tissues. The regression in histiocytic granulomas of borderline-borderline (BB), BL, and LL lesions is caused by progressive intracytoplasmic vacuolization of macrophages due to bacilli fragmentation and by formation of multinucleated giant cells containing large clusters of fragmented bacilli. Macrophages become continuously multivacuolated with vacuoles occupying the entire cytoplasm. After a long time, the vacuoles become larger and compress the nuclei, giving residual macrophages a similar appearance to lipoblasts (Fig. **6**). Macrophage vacuolization is accompanied by intense bacilli fragmentation and progressive color loss until they are no longer stained by Fite–Faraco (Fig. **7**). In the center of the histiocytic granulomas, it is common to find multinucleated giant cells containing a large vacuole filled with multi-fragmented bacilli discolored or poorly stained by Fite–Faraco (Fig. **8**). Some of these large vacuoles may eventually be surrounded by neutrophils (Fig. **9**). Both situations are common as changes in the regression of histiocytic granulomas of the forms BB, BL, and LL usually present in the first 12 months after treatment initiation. Such findings should, however, not be interpreted as T1R or T2R.

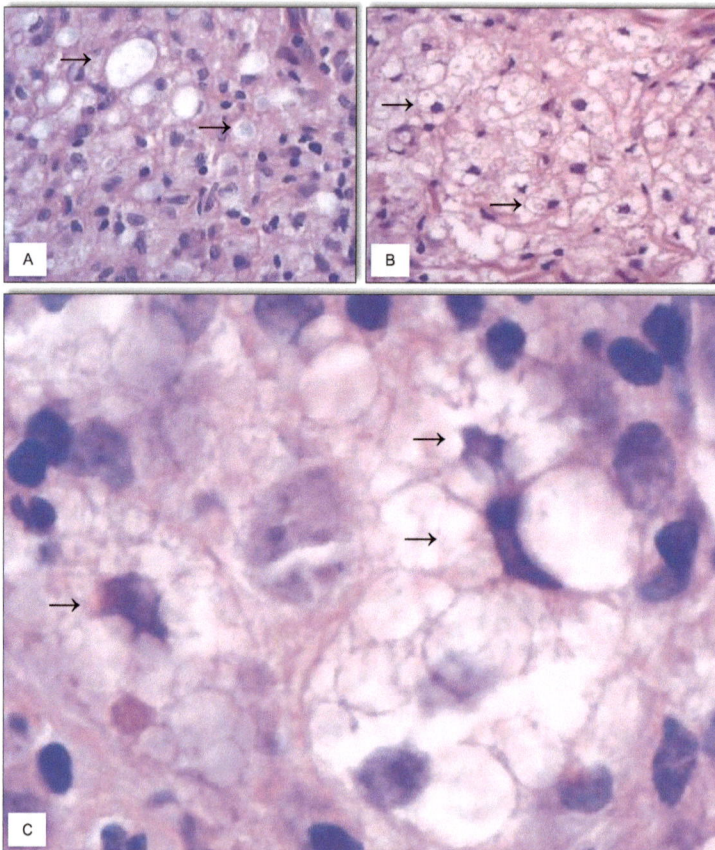

Fig. (6). Regression changes in macrophages of leprosy lesions. **(A)** An active LL lesion presents macrophages with few and large intracytoplasmic vacuoles containing large amounts of bacilli characterized by gray amorphous material (→). **(B)** LL lesion after six months of MDT/MB treatment showing multivacuolated macrophages of different sizes and filled with fragmented bacilli. **(C)** The intense intracytoplasmic vacuolization causes indentations to macrophage's nucleus resembling a lipoblast (→). HE staining.

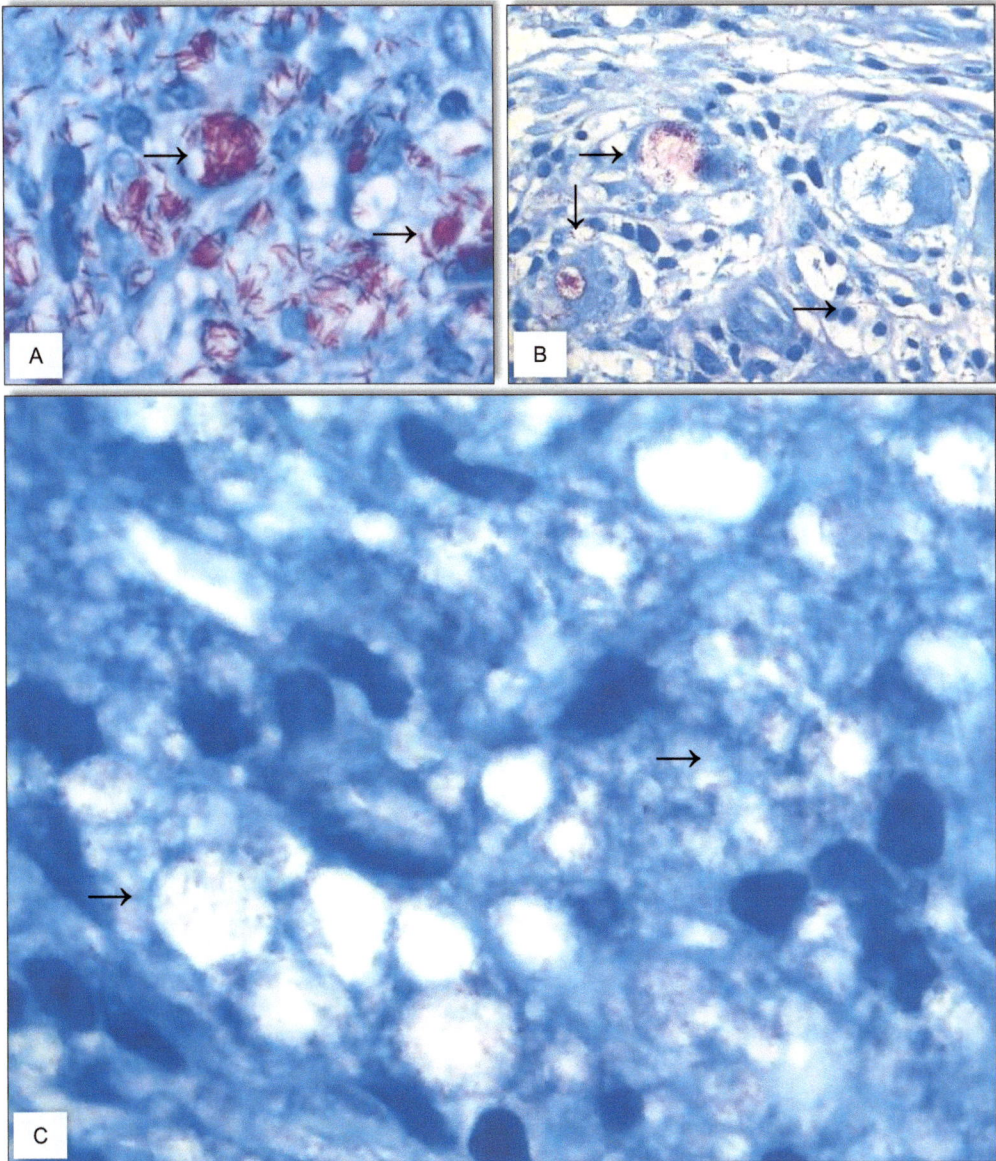

Fig. (7). Regression changes in bacilloscopic examination of macrophages in leprosy lesions. **(A)** Active LL lesion with macrophages showing large intracytoplasmic vacuoles containing a large quantity of intact bacilli (globi) (→). **(B)** LL lesion after 12 months of MDT/MB treatment showing macrophages with vacuoles filled with well-stained fragmented bacilli (→). **(C)** LL lesion at the end of MDT/MB - 24 doses treatment with intensely fragmented and discolored bacilli (→). Fite–Faraco staining.

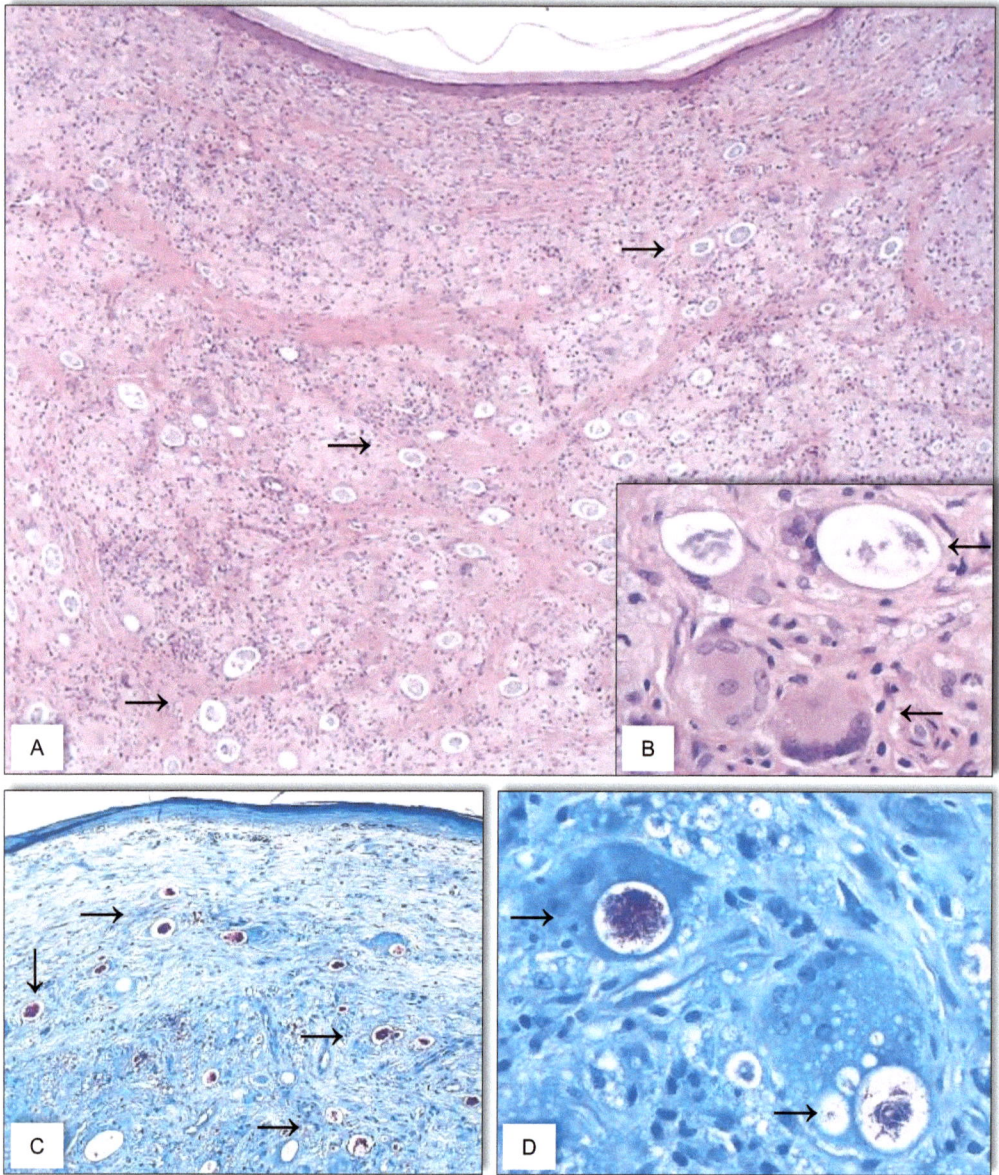

Fig. (8). Regression changes in macrophages of leprosy lesions. **(A)** An LL lesion in regression presents a large number of multinucleated giant cells containing multi-fragmented bacilli (→) (A and B). The bacilli have different staining intensities and are usually slightly stained (→) (C and D). HE (A and B) and Fite–Faraco (C and D) staining.

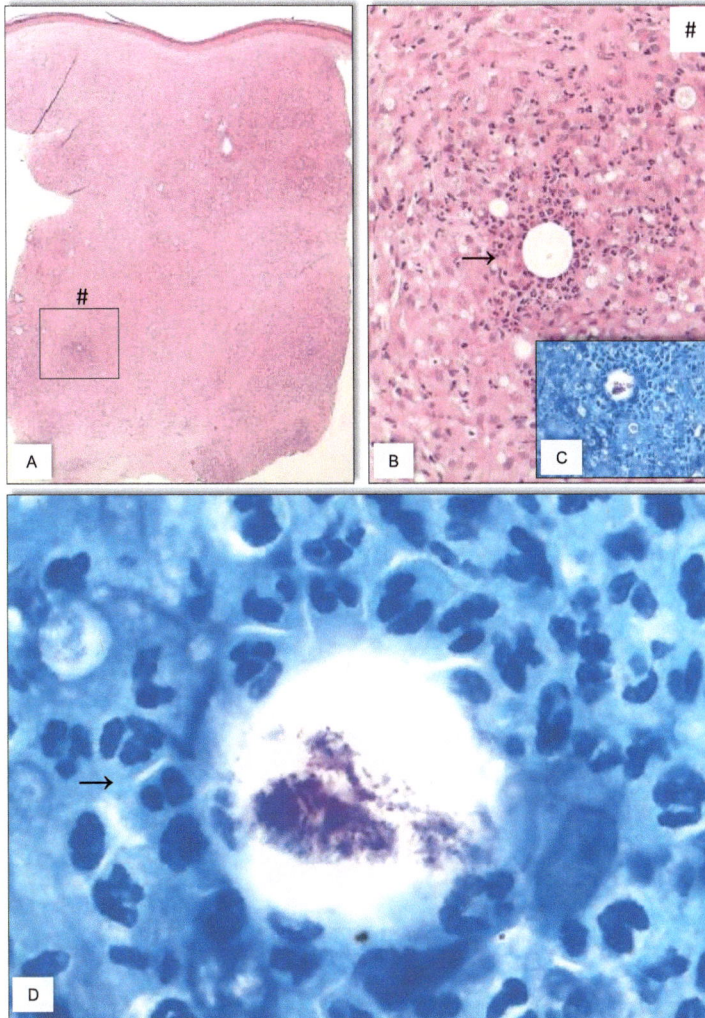

Fig. (9). Regression changes in macrophages of leprosy lesions. **(A)** A BL/LL lesion in regression presents multinucleated giant cells with a large vacuole containing multi-fragmented bacilli and surrounded by neutrophils (#) (→) (A and B). The bacilli are slightly stained (→) (C and D). HE staining (A and B) and Fite–Faraco (C and D).

The regression of leprosy lesions can cause interstitial changes. The most common alteration is the proliferation of fibroblasts accompanied by collagen bands. Two other infrequent changes consist of an important accumulation of mucin between regressive granulomas and the development of a common dermatofibroma within regressive BL or LL leprosy lesions.

A few months after treatment initiation, some lesions may appear more prominent and hardened, leading to the suspicion of development of a reaction process (T1R or T2R) or leprosy reactivation. When these lesions are biopsied, the histological sections show regressing histiocytic granulomas associated with fibroblast proliferation and formation of collagen bands or bundles, dividing the granulomas into several compartments giving the appearance of a hypertrophic or keloid scar, without any evidence of reaction or phenomenon of disease activity (Fig. **10**). Fibroblasts have prominent nuclei and inconspicuous nucleoli. The bacilloscopic examination does not show bacilli inside fibroblasts or collagen bands (Fig. **11**).

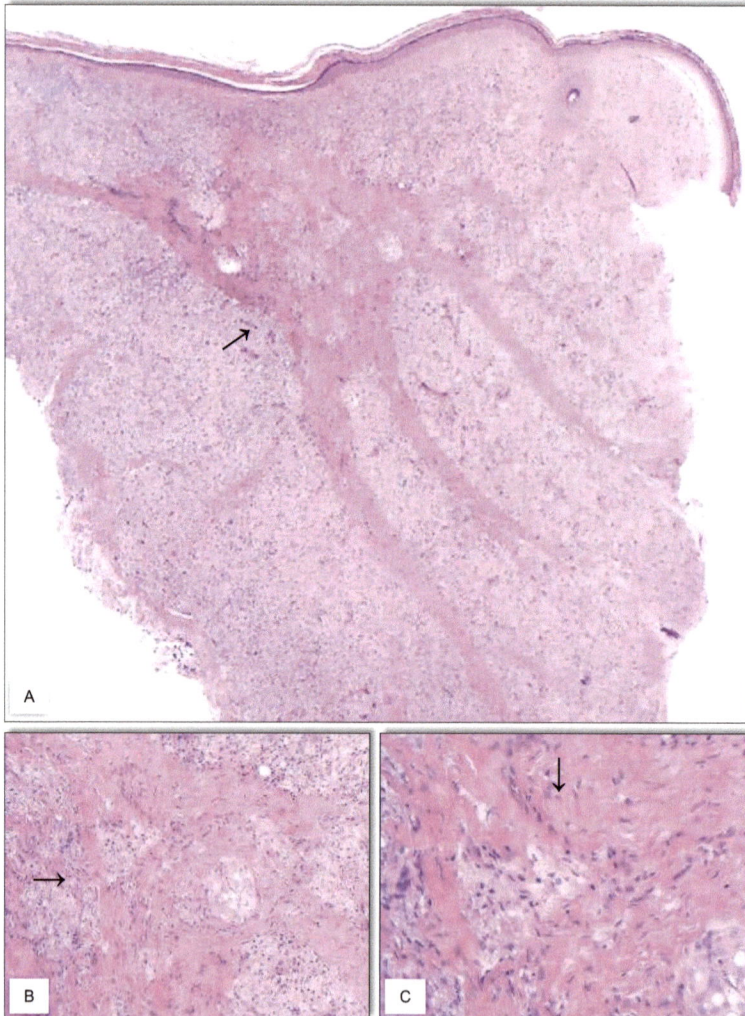

Fig. (10). LL lesion in regression with stromal reaction with hypertrophic or keloid scar appearance. **(A)** Histiocytic granulomas in regression divided by collagen bands (→). (B and C) A proliferation of fibroblasts forming collagen bands (→) divide groups of macrophages with alterations in regression. HE staining.

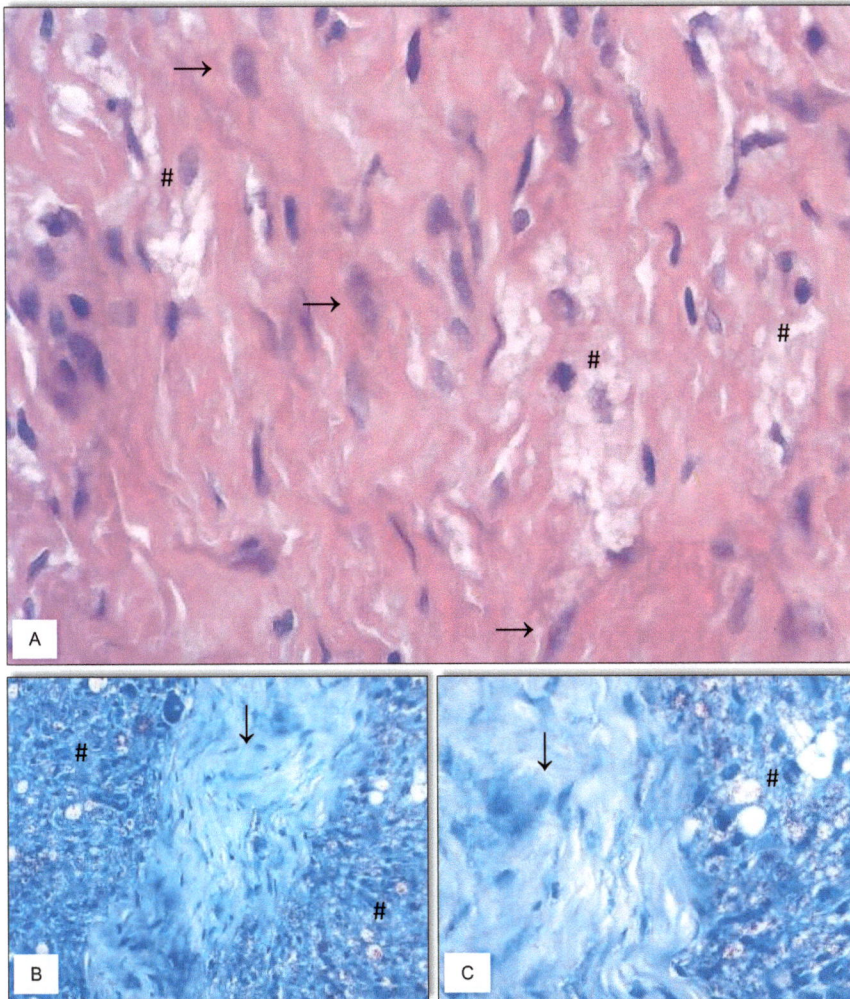

Fig. (11). Stromal reaction with hypertrophic or keloid scar appearance in a leprosy lesion in regression. **(A)** Macrophages with regression changes (#) are surrounded by collagen bands and fibroblasts with prominent nuclei and inconspicuous nucleoli. (B and C) The regressing macrophage granulomas (#) present a large number of fragmented bacilli in the macrophages and the collagen and fibroblast bands do not present bacilli (→). HE **(A)** and Fite–Faraco (B and C) staining.

Patients classified as BL and LL, especially those with a history of T2R, can develop common DF over regressive leprosy lesions [4]. Clinically, these lesions in regression with DF acquire a dark color and become raised and hardened. Histological sections demonstrate the presence of a DF at the center, generally small (≤ 0.5 cm), surrounded by the leprosy lesion in regression throughout its periphery (Fig. **12**). Bacilloscopic examination does not show DF parasitism. It is important to be attentive to the development of DF in BL and LL leprosy lesions in regression, since the regressive areas of leprosy lesions arranged on the DF periphery can be confused with areas of common DF lipidization. In histology, the vacuoles of the lipidized macrophages of the DF are regular and do not show fragmented bacilli with Fite–Faraco staining (Fig. **13**).

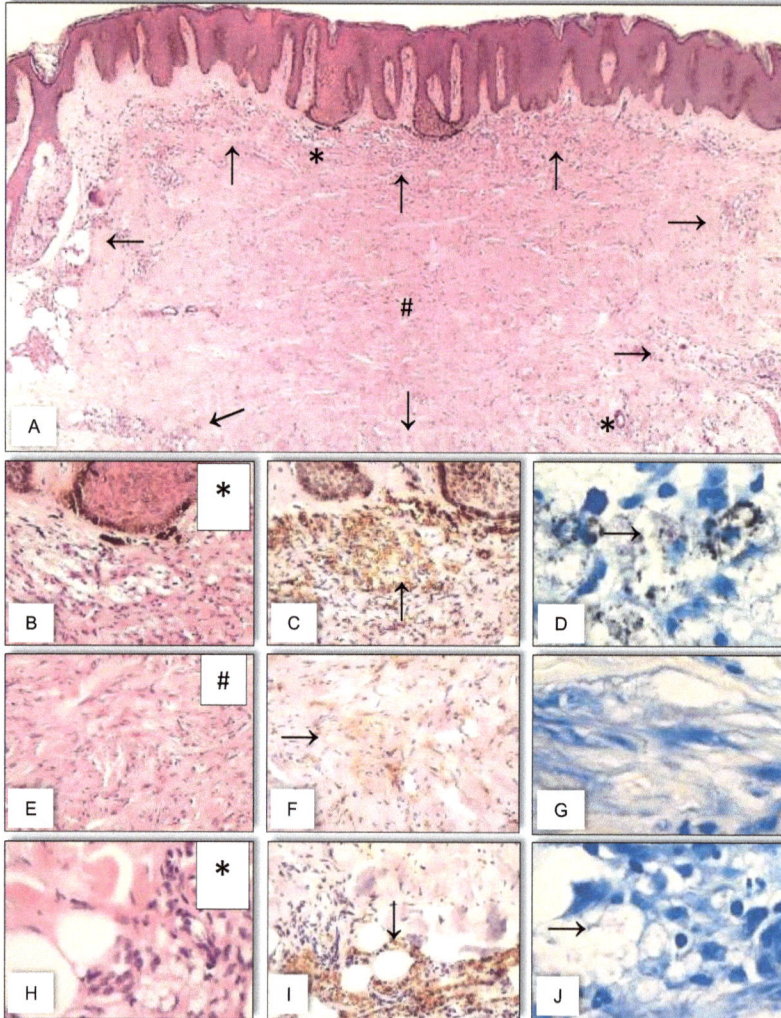

Fig. (12). Dermatofibroma originating in a leprosy lesion in regression. **(A)** Dermatofibroma common to the center (#) associated with epithelial hyperplasia of the epidermis, hyperpigmentation of the basal layer and involved by a leprosy lesion in regression (*) (→). (B, C, and D) Leprosy lesion in regression in the papillary dermis (*) **(B)**, with CD68⁺ multivacuolated macrophages (→) **(C)** showing poorly stained fragmented bacilli (→) **(D)**. (E, F, and G) Dermatofibroma consisting of spindle cells and collagen bands **(E)** positive for Factor XIIIa (→) **(F)** and absence of bacilli **(G)**. (H, I, and J) Leprosy lesion in regression in the deep and subcutaneous dermis (*) **(H)**, with CD68⁺ multivacuolated macrophages (→) **(I)** and presenting poorly stained multi-fragmented bacilli (→) **(J)**. HE staining (A, B, E, and H), IHC (C, F, and I) and Fite–Faraco (D, G, and J).

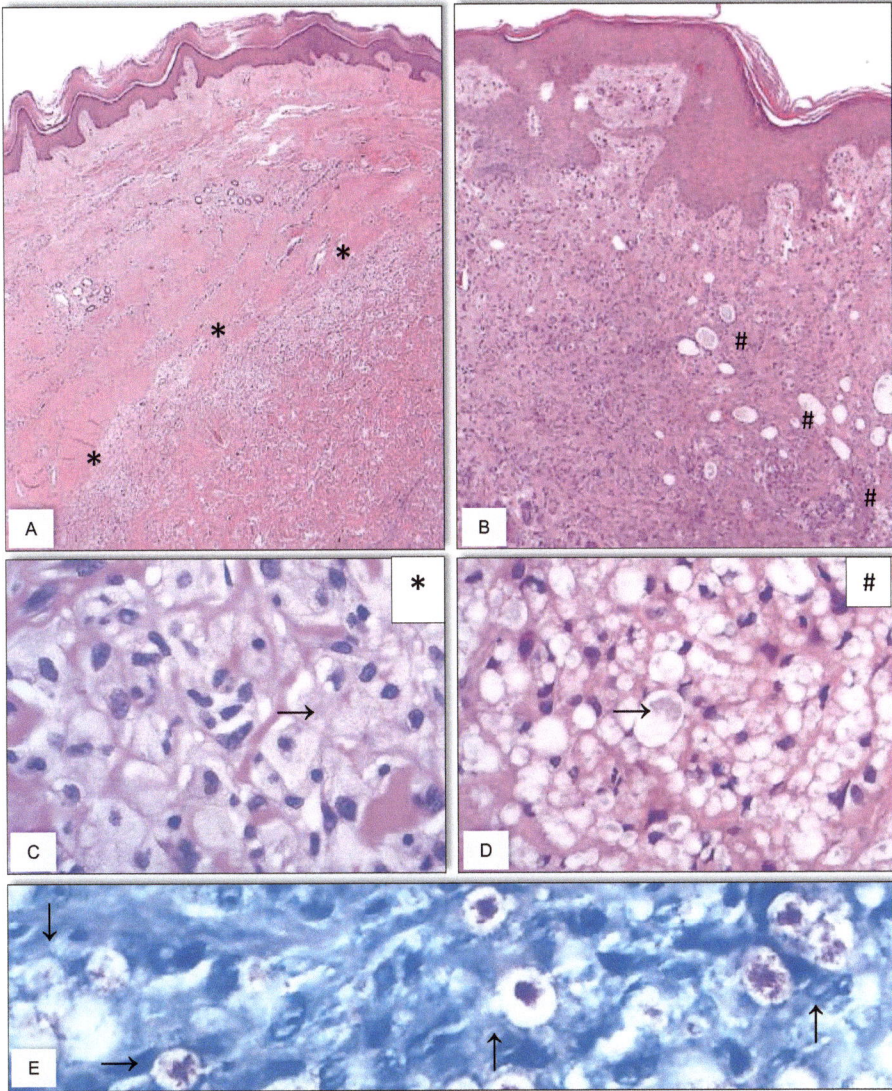

Fig. (13). Example of common dermatofibroma (DF) with lipidized macrophages (A and C) and common dermatofibroma originating in a LL lesion in regression (B, D, and E). **(C)** The lipidized macrophages (*) of the common DF have small and regular vacuoles (→). **(D)** Macrophages of the leprosy lesion in regression (#) have vacuoles of different sizes and filled with amorphous material (→) consisting of a large number of multi-fragmented bacilli poorly stained by Fite–Faraco (→) **(E)**. HE (A-D) and Fite–Faraco **(E)** staining.

In rare cases, some lesions in regression can present intense accumulation of mucin in the interstitium, divulging the collagen fibers and macrophages of the leprosy lesion in regression. Bacilloscopic examination shows fragmented bacilli inside macrophages (Fig. **14**).

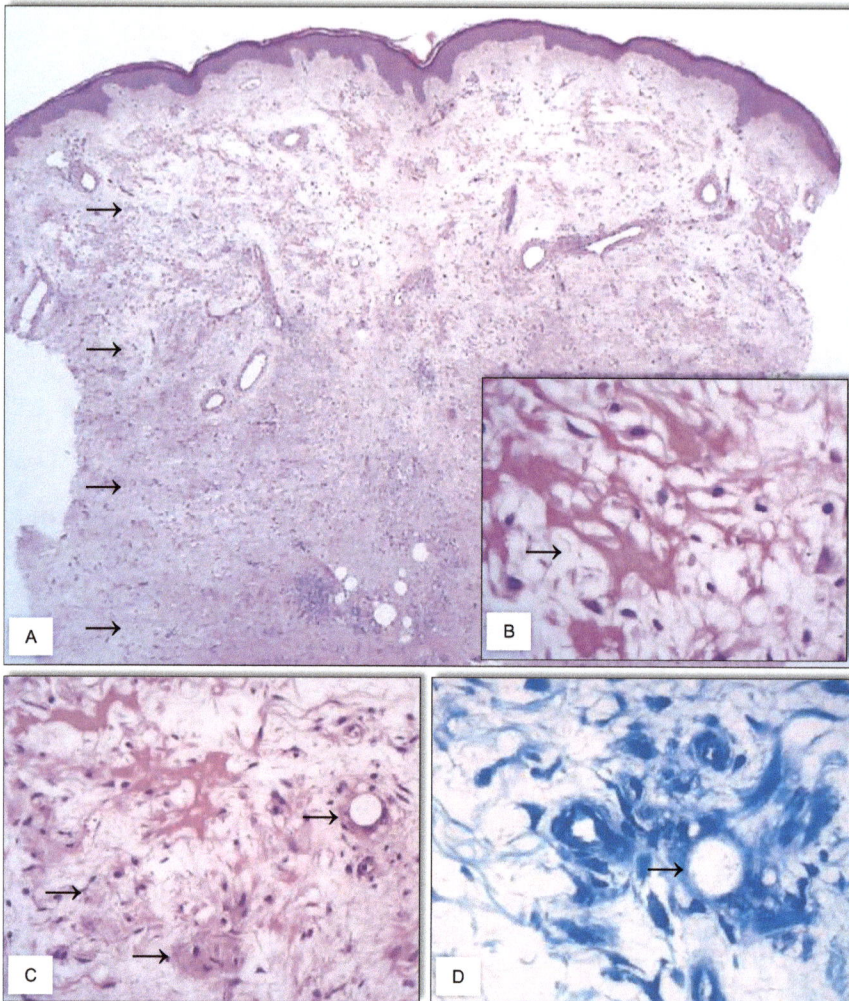

Fig. (14). Mucin deposits in the dermis of a leprosy lesion in regression. Mucin accumulation in all dermis layers **(A)** separating collagen fibers **(B)** and the macrophages from the regressing histiocytic granulomas **(C)**. Mucin involves a multinucleated giant cell with a large vacuole **(C)** showing discolored multi-fragmented bacilli (→) **(D)**. HE (A-C) and Fite–Faraco **(D)** staining.

Patients undergoing treatment for leprosy with MDT containing clofazimine progressively develop brown coloration throughout the skin that is more pronounced on leprosy lesions (Fig. **15**). The color of both skin and lesions intensifies during treatment gradually decreasing after the end of the treatment until its disappearance a few years after (Fig. **16**). In the lesions of the tuberculoid side (TT and BT) the pigmentation is intense at the edge of the few lesions present on the body (Fig. **17**). In BB and BL lesions, the pigmentation highlights various lesions in different parts of the body (Fig. **18**). In LL with extensive skin parasitism by *M. leprae*, pigmentation is diffuse (Fig. **19**). Histological sections show an intense pigmentation in macrophages of the regressing histiocytic granulomas, showing a brown coloration by HE and dark pigment granules in staining by Fite–Faraco (Fig. **20**). In some cases, interstitial changes in fibroblast proliferation with formation of collagen bands add up to changes in macrophage pigmentation in the regressing lesions (Fig. **21**). Animal studies using clofazimine show diffuse pigmentation in most tissues [5]. Due to the stigma of hyperpigmentation and the unavailability of clofazimine, it is not uncommon to replace it with ofloxacin in MDT-MB treatment regimens.

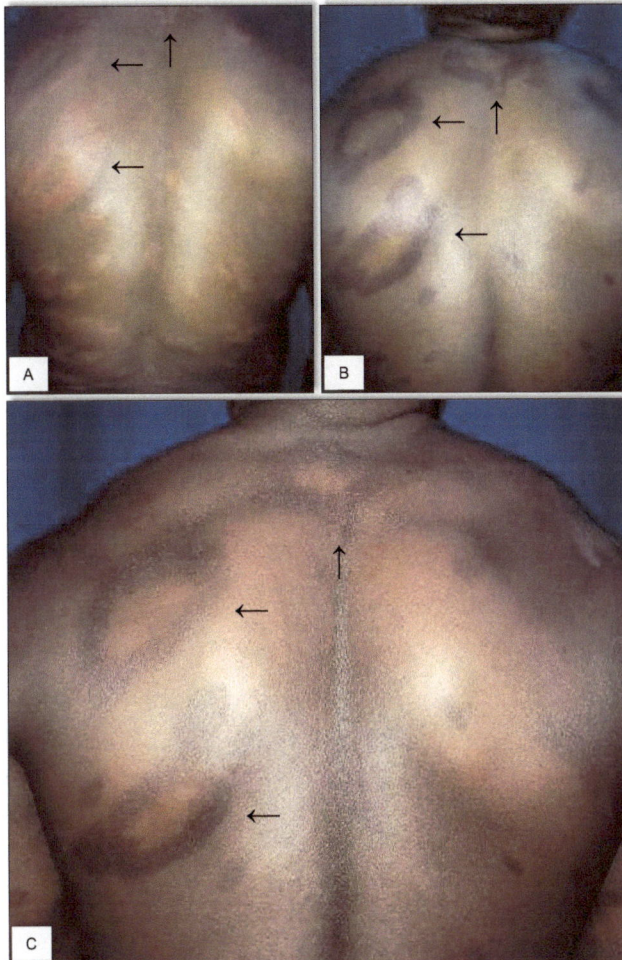

Fig. (15). Clofazimine-induced pigmentation of leprosy lesions in regression. **(A)** Leprosy lesions BB with type 1 reaction (T1R) before treatment were characterized by several erythematous annular plaques with apparently preserved central area (→). **(B)** After 12 months of MDT/MB treatment, the lesions show signs of atrophy and increased dark pigmentation (→). **(C)** One year after the end of the treatment, pigmentation is still present but less intense than in the "B" lesion (→). Courtesy of Dr. Cássio C. Ghidella.

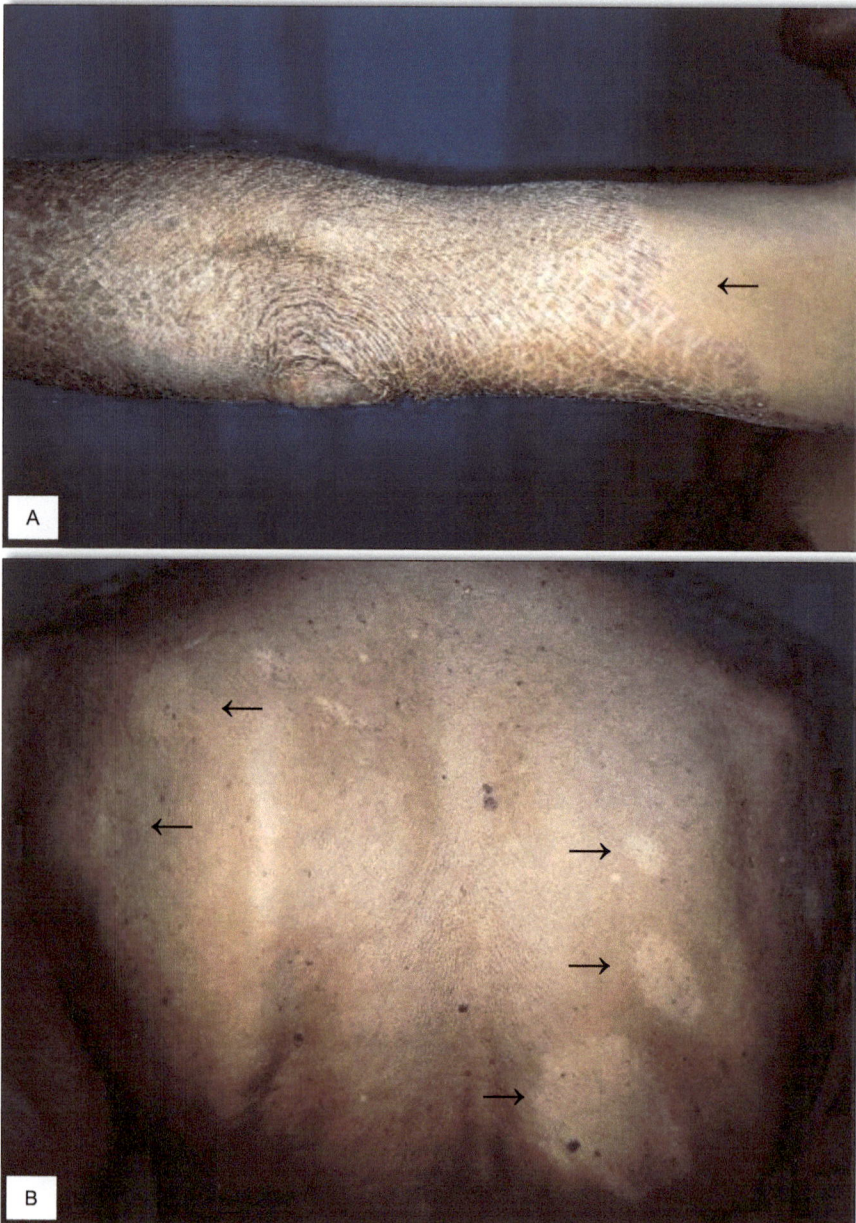

Fig. (16). Clofazimine-induced pigmentation of leprosy lesions in regression. **(A)** BB lesion in regression consisting of extensive plaque on the upper limb after 12 MDT/MB doses showing hyperpigmentation throughout the extent of the lesion (→) with associated xerosis. **(B)** BB lesion in regression three years after the end of treatment showing hypochromic and atrophic plaques on the back with disappearance of pigmentation. Courtesy of Dr. Cássio C. Ghidella.

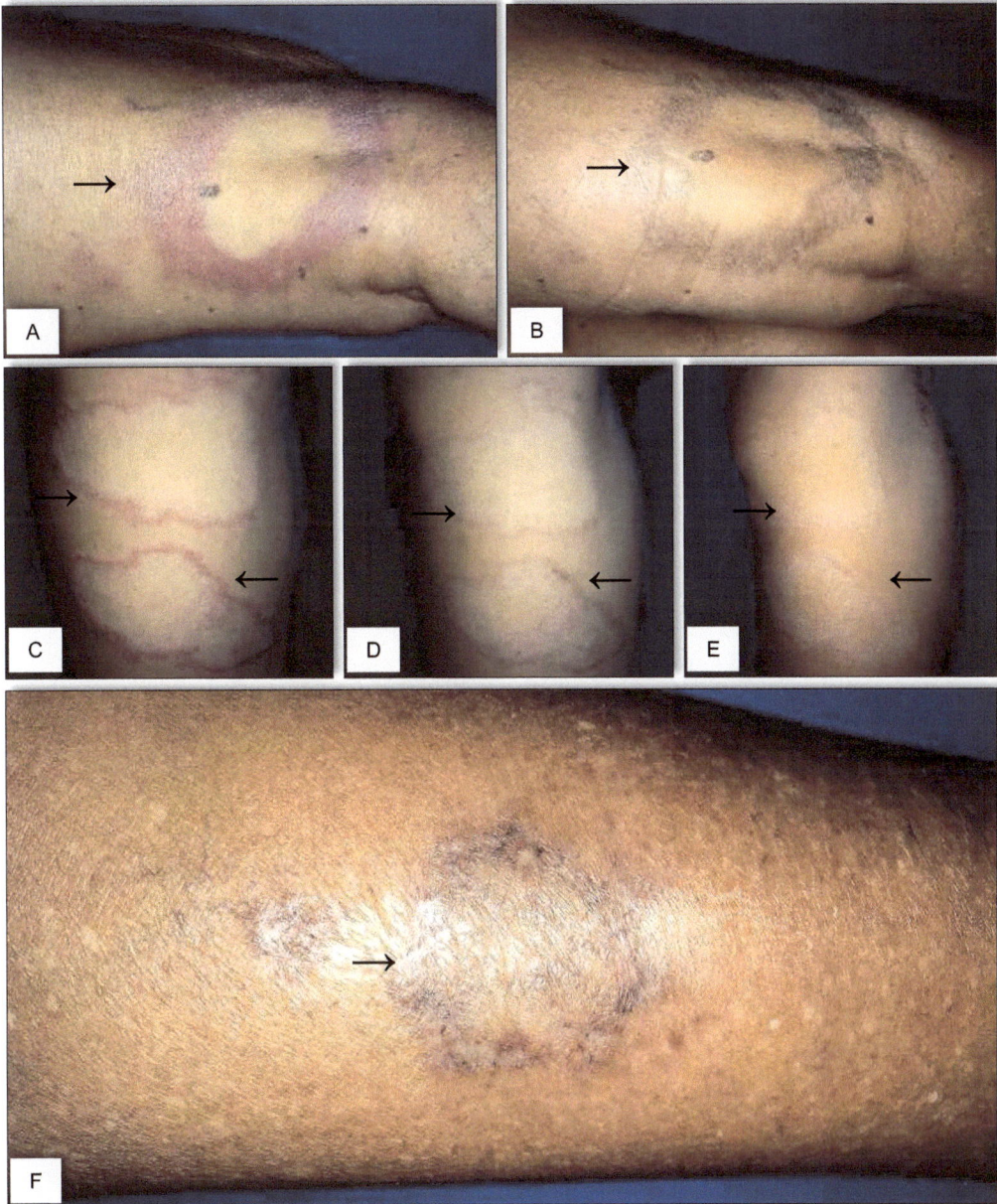

Fig. (17). Clofazimine-induced pigmentation of leprosy lesions in regression. (A and B) Active borderline lesion with T1R ($\rightarrow$) **(A)** and the same lesion ($\rightarrow$) **(B)** after 12 months of MDT/MB treatment with intense dark pigmentation drawing the entire border of the lesion. (C, D, and E) Two active TT lesions ($\rightarrow$) **(C)** formed by extensive erythematous-hypochromic plaques and the same lesion at the end of MDT/MB - 12 doses treatment ($\rightarrow$) **(D)** showing hyperpigmentation of the edges of the lesions and one year after the end of treatment ($\rightarrow$) **(E)** showing marked decrease in pigmentation. **(F)** BT lesion in regression showing atrophy, dryness and hyperpigmentation at the end of MDT/MB - 12 doses treatment ($\rightarrow$). Courtesy of Dr. Cássio C. Ghidella.

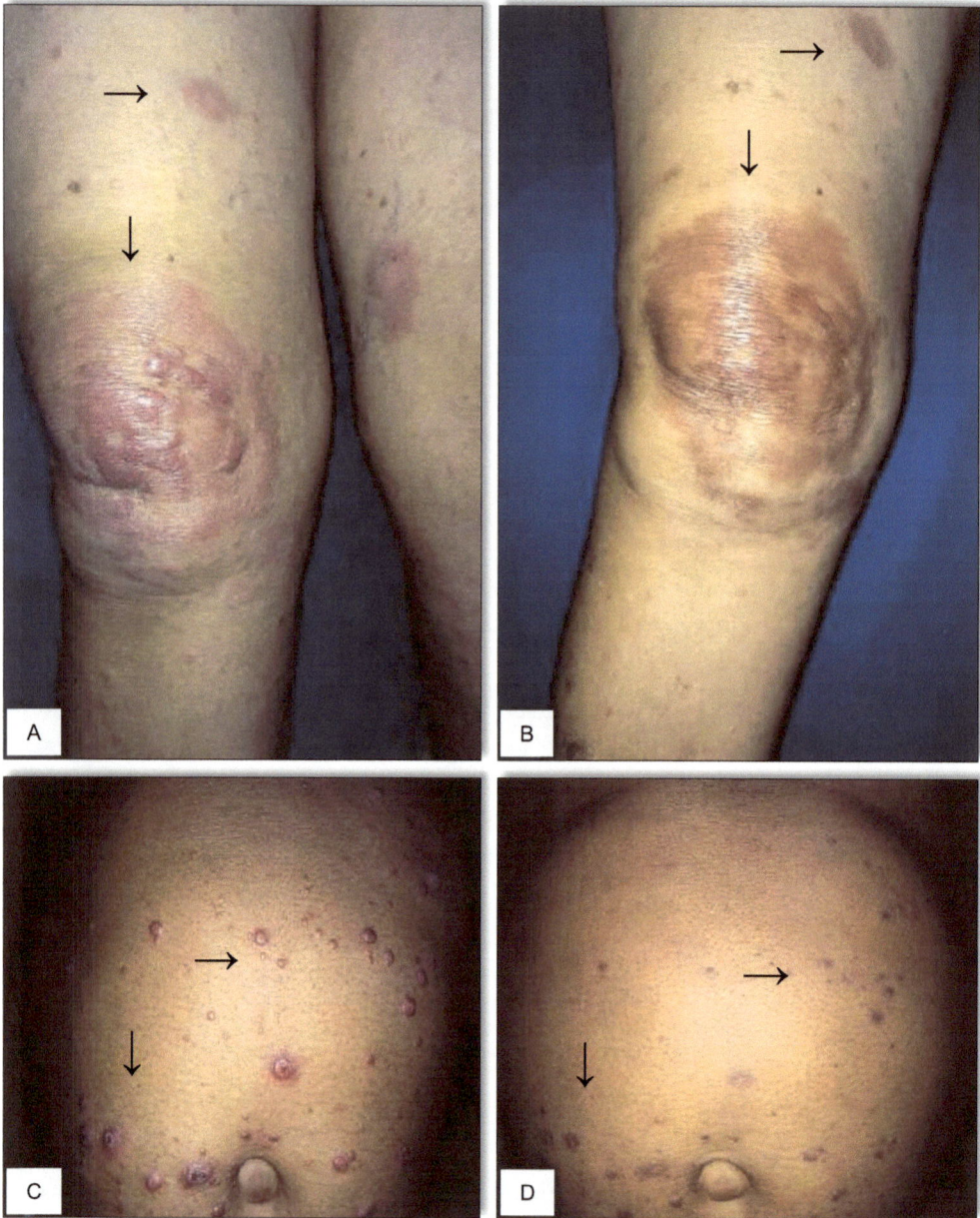

Fig. (18). Clofazimine-induced pigmentation of leprosy lesions in regression. (A and B) BL active lesions with associated T1R (→) **(A)** and the same lesion after six months of MDT/MB and corticosteroid therapy (→) **(B)** showing atrophy and hyperpigmentation of the lesions. (C and D) Active LL lesions consisting of nodules and tubercles on infiltrated skin (→) **(C)** and the same lesions three months after treatment initiation (→) **(D)** with more intense pigmentation in the most infiltrated lesions. Courtesy of Dr. Cássio C. Ghidella.

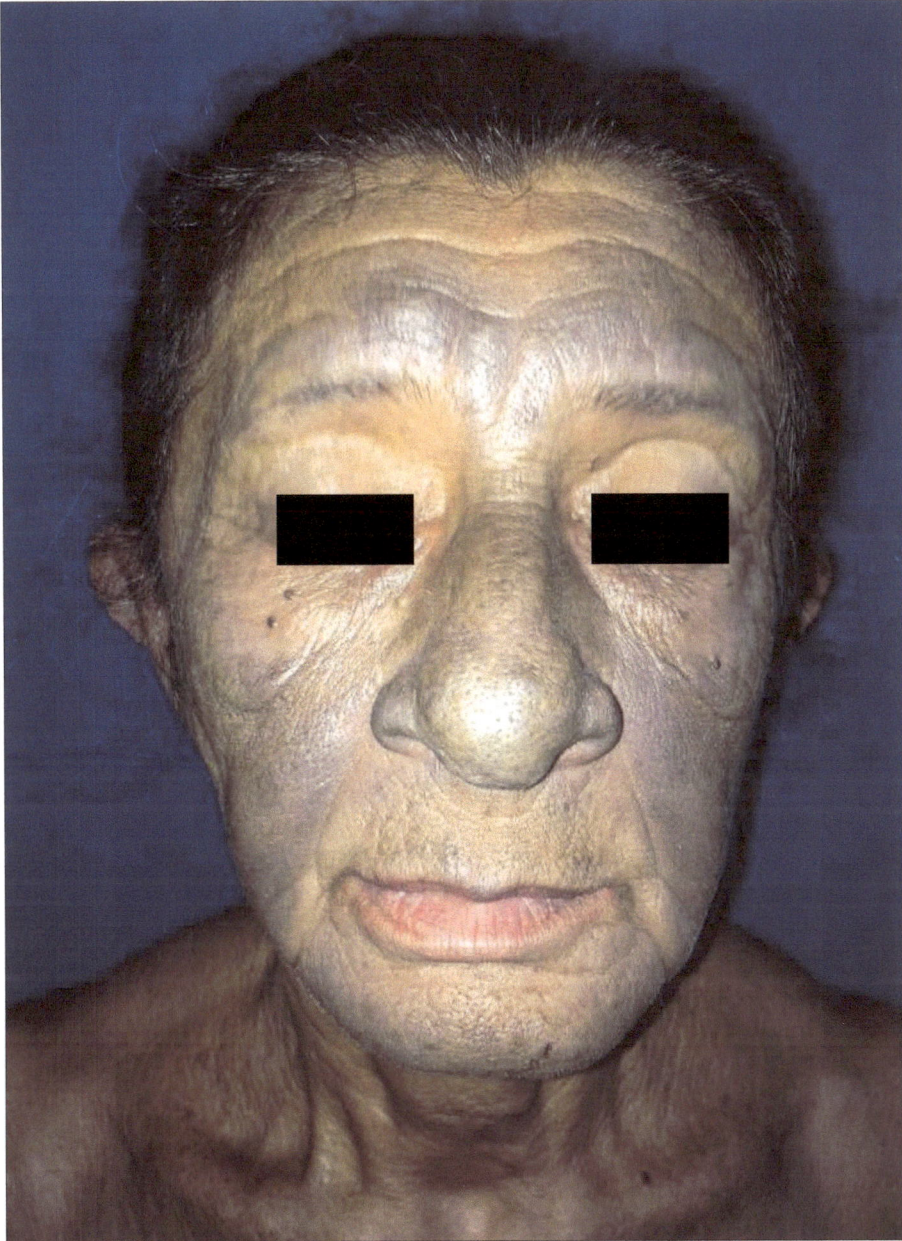

Fig. (19). Clofazimine-induced pigmentation of leprosy lesions in regression. LL patient in regression, diffuse presentation, at the end of treatment MDT/MB - 24 months showing hyperpigmentation of the entire integument. Courtesy of Dr. Cássio C. Ghidella.

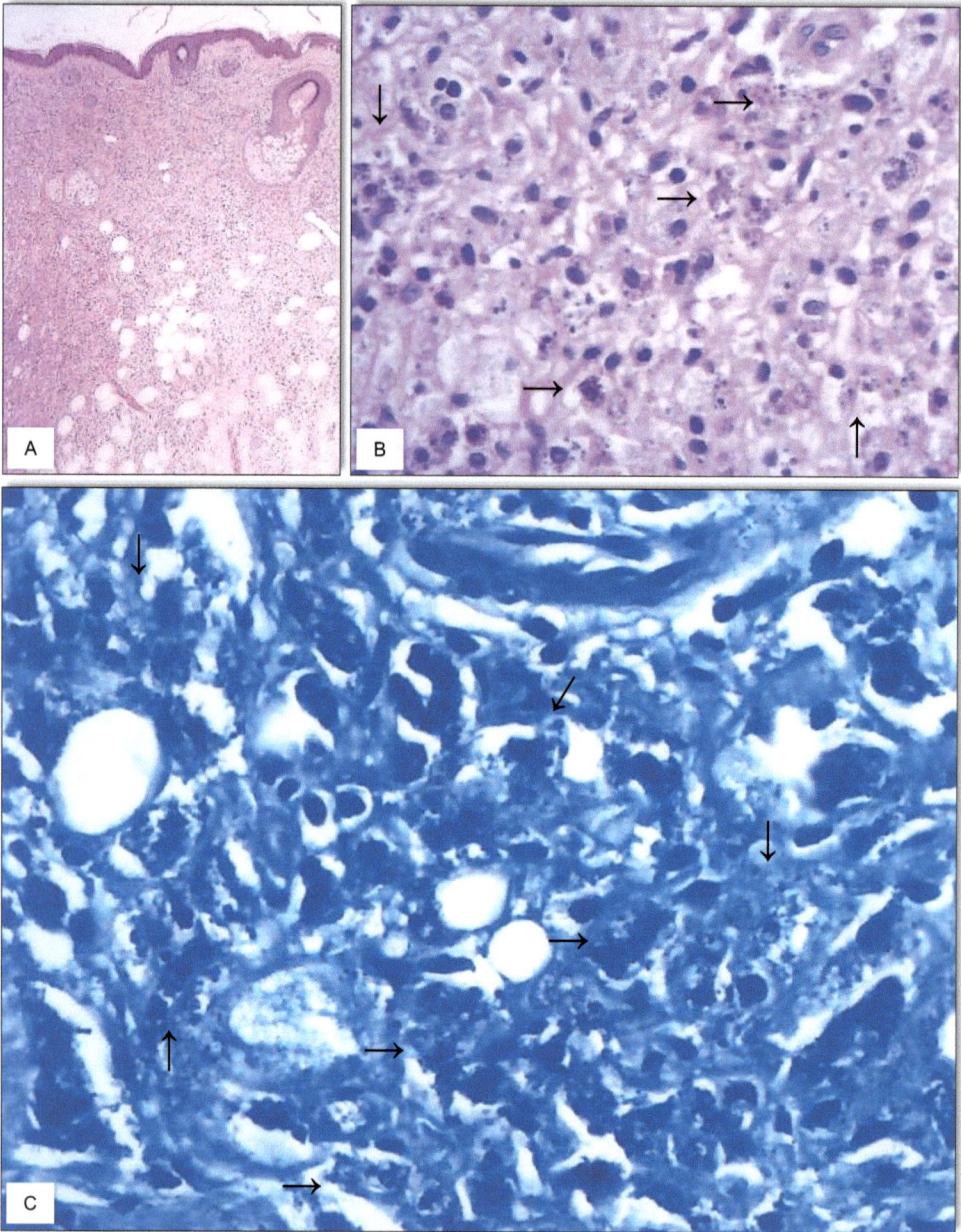

Fig. (20). Clofazimine-induced pigmentation of leprosy lesions in regression. Histological sections show intense pigmentation of macrophages by brown granules in HE staining (→) (A and B) and by dark granules in Fite–Faraco staining (→) (C).

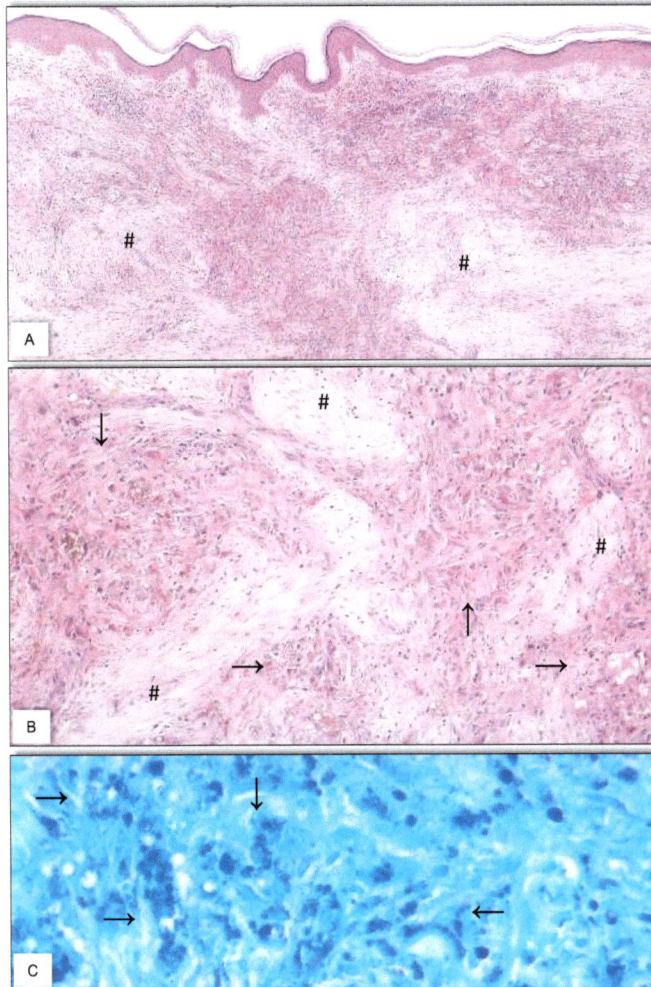

Fig. (21). Clofazimine-induced pigmentation of leprosy lesions in regression. Example of LL lesion in regression with interstitial changes in fibroblast proliferation and formation of collagen bands (#) associated with changes in pigmentation in macrophages (→). HE staining (A and B) and Fite–Faraco (**C**).

Bacilloscopic examination in regression lesions shows a constant decrease in BI and presence of fragmented bacilli with different staining intensities by Fite–Faraco in the different parasitized tissues. In our experience, bacilli fragment and disappear more quickly in endothelial cells, being rarely observed after six months of treatment initiation (MDT) and exceptionally rare after 12 months (Figs. **22** - **23**). Bacilli fragmentation is intense within macrophages, however, as they are intensely parasitized, it is common to see multi-fragmented and poorly stained bacilli in their cytoplasm for some years after treatment [6, 7]. Two years after treatment initiation, the bacilli in the macrophage's cytoplasm become weakly colored or discolored, forming something like bacillary dust (Figs. **7** and **8**). In contrast, bacilli inside neural branches and vessel walls persist longer well stained and with characteristics of solid or fragmented bacilli. It is not uncommon to identify well-stained fragmented bacilli on the vessel wall two years after treatment initiation, mainly in veins, while in adjacent tissues they are multi-fragmented and discolored (Fig. **22**).

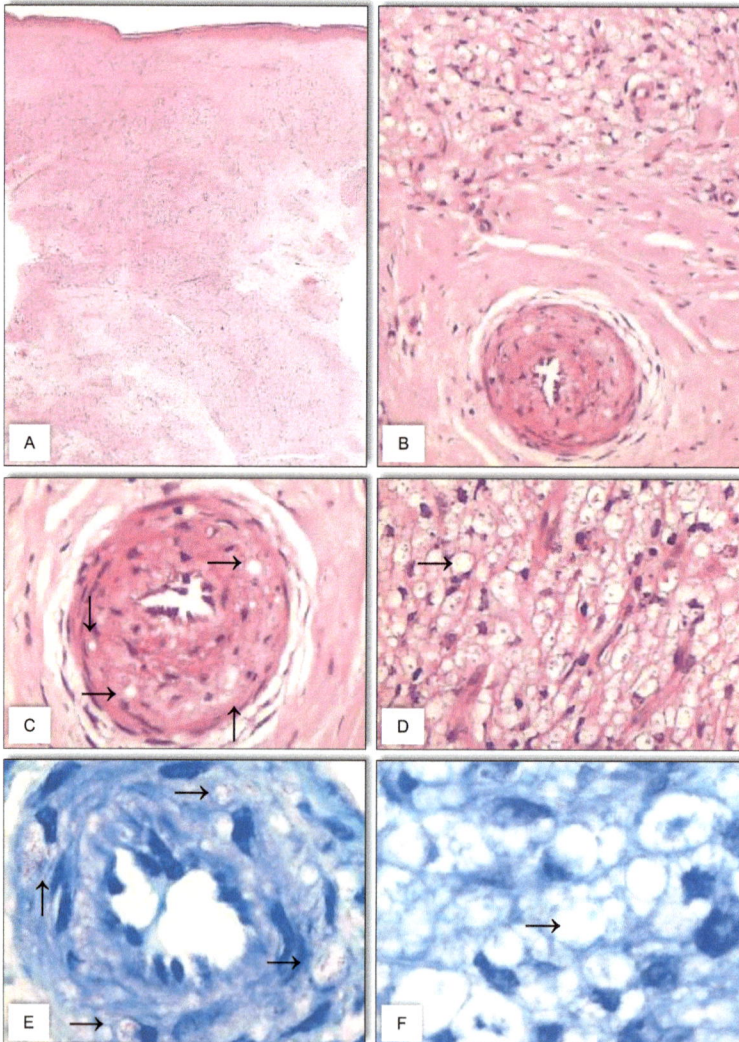

Fig. (22). Fragmentation and staining of bacilli in different parasitized tissues. (A and B) Patient LL at the end of MDT/MB - 24 doses treatment and regression changes in histiocytic granulomas and vessels. Vein with vacuoles on the wall (→) **(C)** filled with well-stained fragmented bacilli (→) **(E)**. Granulomas with vacuolated macrophages (→) **(D)** filled with multi-fragmented bacilli and discolored (→) **(F)**. HE (A-D) and Fite–Faraco (E and F) staining.

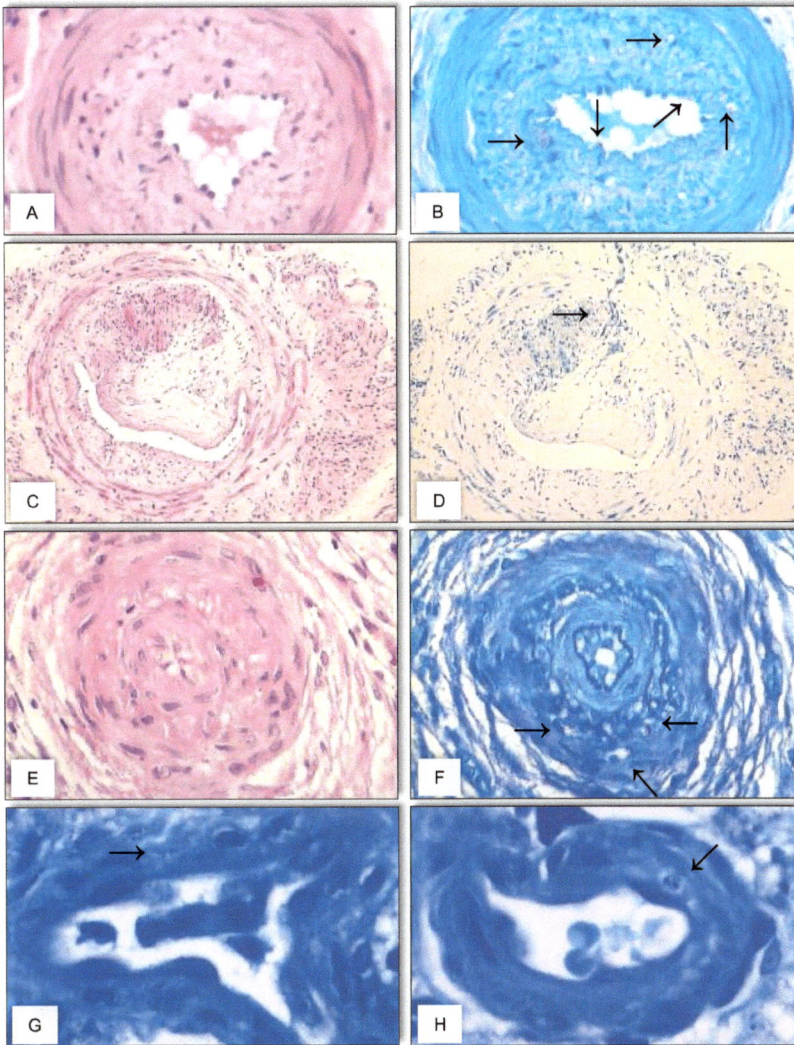

Fig. (23). Regression in parasitized vessels. (A and B) Vein with intense endothelial and subendothelial parasitism showing fragmented bacilli (→) at the beginning of treatment. (C and D) Parasitic vein at the end of MDT/MB - 24 doses treatment showing regressive changes in all layers and fragmented and slightly stained bacilli on the wall (→). (E and F) Artery at the end of treatment with fragmented bacilli on the wall (→). (G and H) Venules after treatment showing signs of parasitism of smooth muscle cells characterized by vacuoles containing discolored fragmented bacilli and clofazimine-induced pigment (→). HE staining (A, C, and E) and Fite–Faraco (B, D-F).

Part of these persistent, well-colored bacilli may be solid bacilli metabolically inactive and protected from the action of MDT drugs during treatment. At the end of the treatment, they could proliferate again, thereby reactivating the disease. This could explain how patients can suffer disease reactivation several times without bacilli with mutations for resistance to MDT/MB drugs [8, 9]. A hypothetical sequence of bacilli fragmentation and elimination in parasitized tissues would be: endothelium > macrophage > neural branch > vessel wall.

Regression changes can be identified in all parasitized cells or tissues (Figs. **23** - **26**). The histopathological and bacilloscopic characteristics observed in these tissues are the same as above and will depend mainly on the treatment protocol and the interval between its onset and biopsy performance.

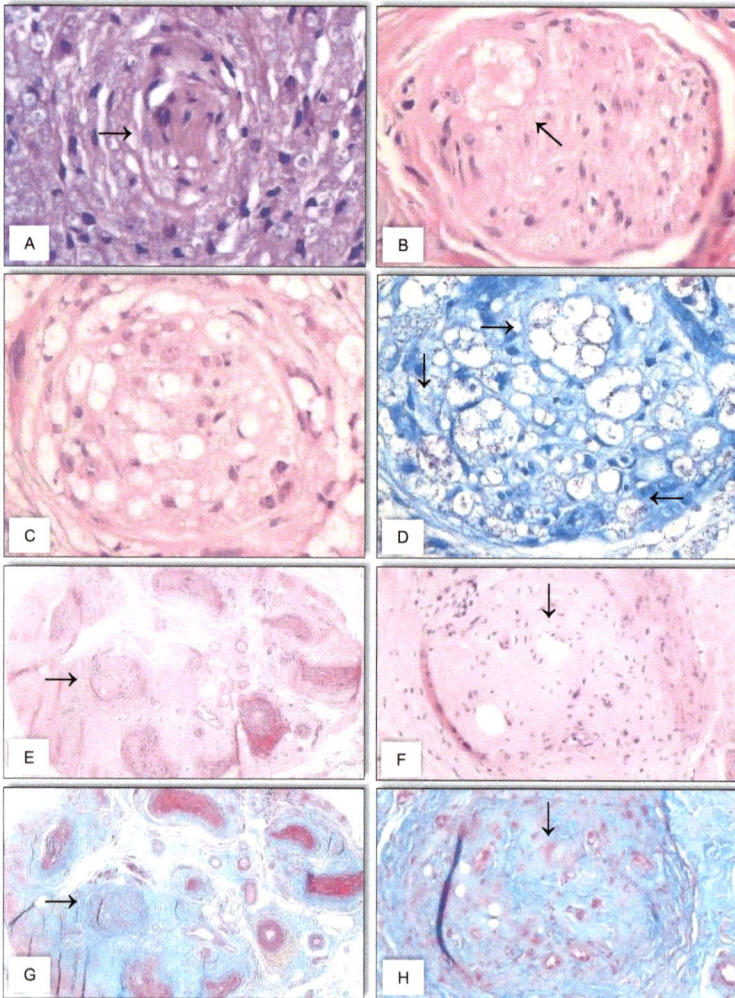

Fig. (24). Regression in parasitized nerves. **(A)** Neural branch intensely parasitized in active lesion (→). **(B)** Neural branch focally compromised with regression lesion (→). (C and D) Neural branch intensely parasitized in regression with numerous vacuoles filled with multi-fragmented bacilli (→). (E, F, G, and H) Neural branch in late phase with replacement of endoneural tissues by fibroblasts and collagen fibers (→). HE (A, B, C, E, and F), Fite–Faraco **(D)** and Masson's trichrome staining (G and H).

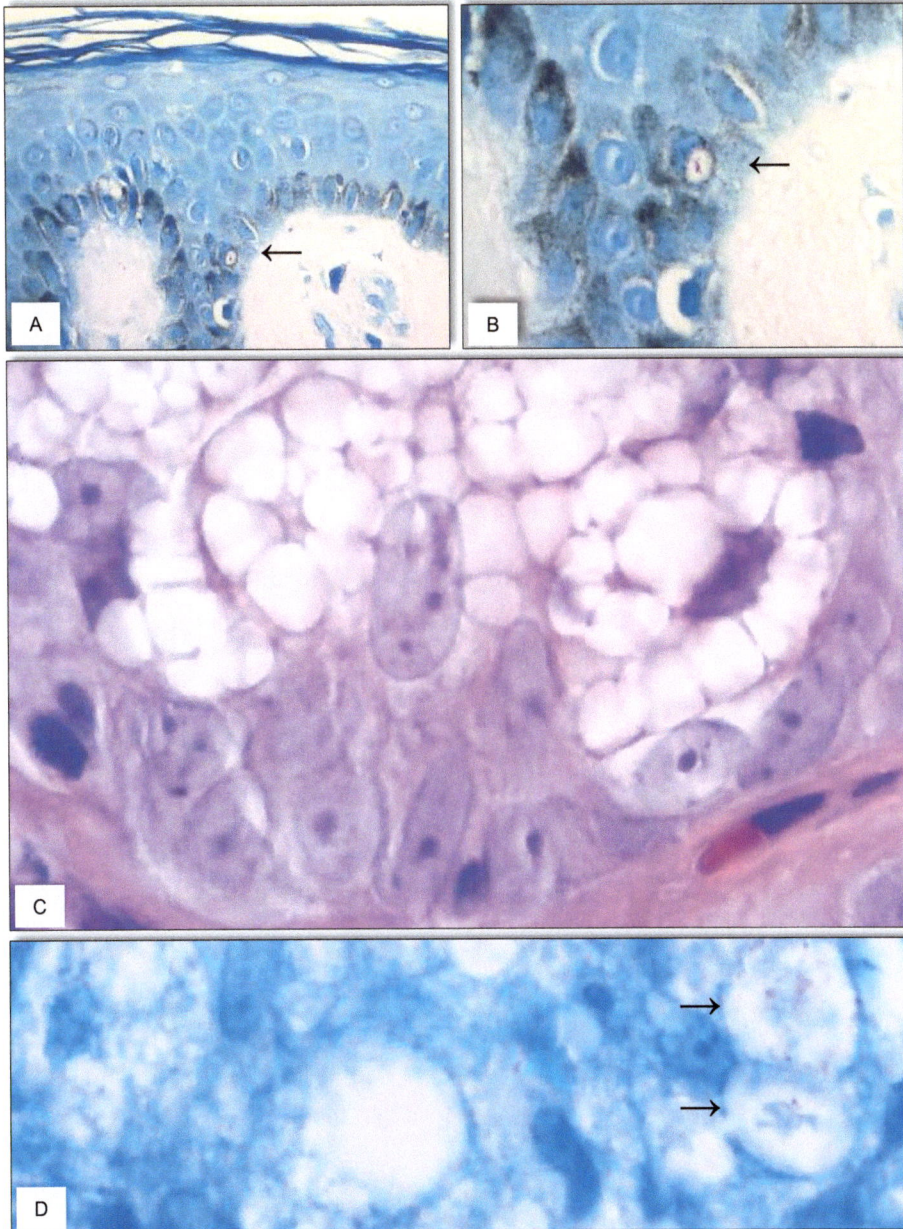

Fig. (25). Regression in squamous and sebaceous cells. (A and B) BL patient after 12 doses MDT/MB presents squamous epithelial cells with vacuole filled with fragmented and well stained bacilli in the epidermis (→). (C and D) Sebaceous cells of the hair follicle of the same patient with multi-fragmented and poorly stained bacilli in intracytoplasmic vacuoles (→). HE **(B)** and Fite–Faraco staining (A, B, and D).

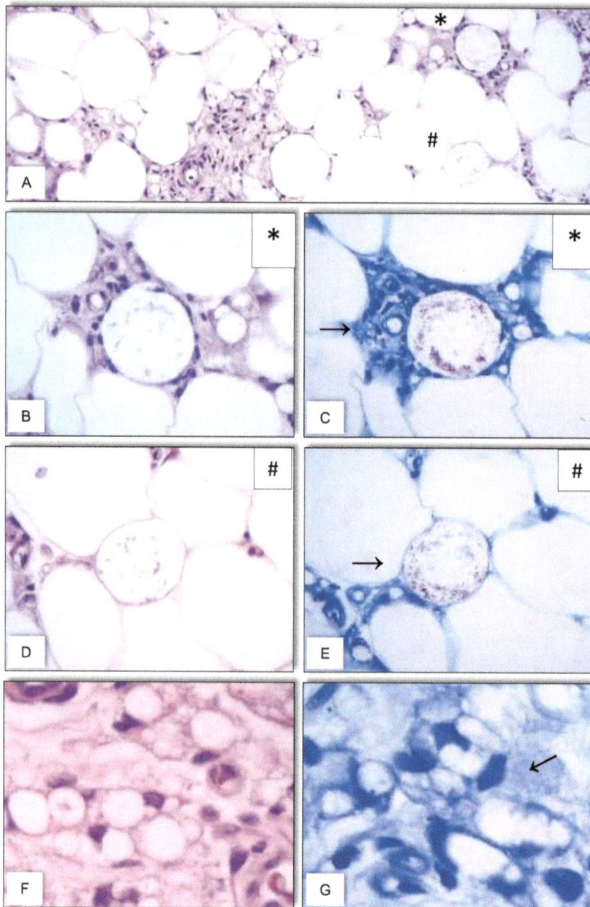

Fig. (26). Regression in adipose tissue. (A, B, C, D, and E) Patient LL after MDT/MB - 24 doses treatment showing parasitized adipose tissue with multivacuolated cells containing poorly stained multi-fragmented bacilli (→) (*) (#). All components of adipose tissue may be parasitized by *M. leprae* (macrophages, fibroblasts, vessels and adipocytes) **(A)**. (F and G) Residual LL lesion in adipose tissue with multivacuolated cells and absence of stained bacilli (→). HE (A, B, D, and F) and Fite–Faraco staining (C, E, and G).

HISTOPATHOLOGICAL AND BACILLOSCOPIC CHARACTERISTICS OF LEPROSY RELAPSE

Leprosy relapse is defined as disease resurgence by bacillary proliferation after the end of treatment. Commonly, some cutaneous or neural leprosy lesions, during or after treatment, are submitted to a biopsy to evaluate the effectiveness of the proposed treatment. In these cases, it is important to recognize which histopathological and bacilloscopic changes are diagnostic or suggestive of active leprosy lesions. The histopathological evaluation to detect leprosy activity requires a close correlation between clinical data (type of treatment, its duration and the interval between its end and the date of the biopsy procedure) and the histopathological/bacilloscopic characteristics observed in biopsies' specimens. Skin or neural lesions with signs of reactivation present active granulomatous conditions. Some findings are important to suggest an active lesion: (1) presence of vacuolated macrophages filled with thick amorphous material and permeated by lymphoplasmocytic infiltrate within regressed or residual granulomas, (2) increased BI in relation to a previous biopsy and (3) presence of solid bacilli, sometimes in the form of globi, showing bacillary proliferation (Fig. **27**). The confirmation of the presence of solid bacilli must be made very carefully and will depend on the finding of groups of morphologically solid bacilli (Fig. **27**).

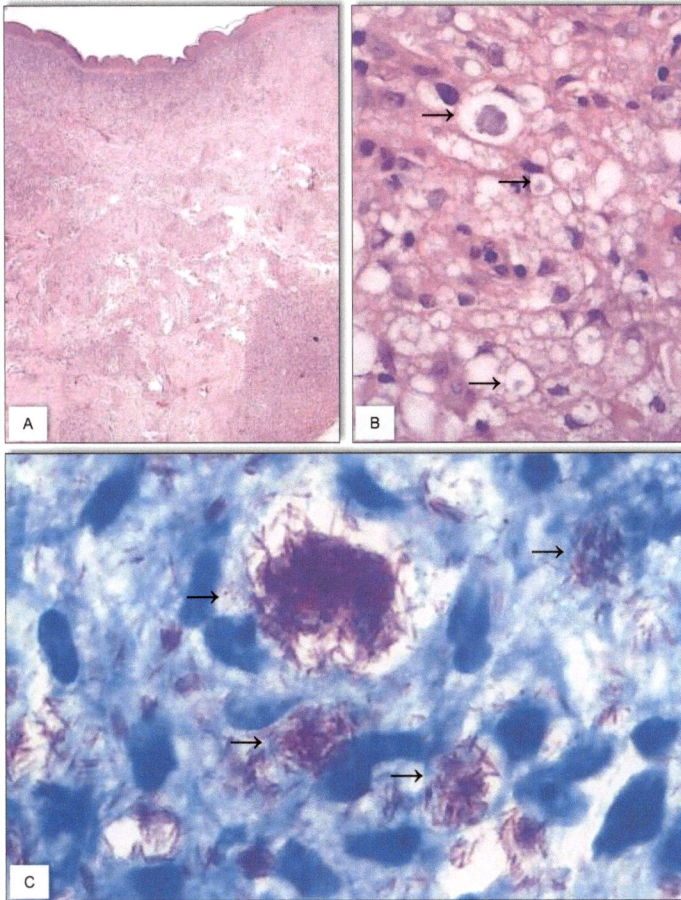

Fig. (27). Example of leprosy relapse. A 52-year-old man with a history of three previous MDT/MB - 24 dose treatments for leprosy LL in the last 37 years, the last being 12 years ago and currently with an erythematous nodule in the abdomen. Histological sections show an active LL lesion **(A)** characterized as predominantly histiocytic infiltrate with vacuolated macrophages filled with amorphous espresso material (→) **(B)**, which are morphologically solid bacilli stained by Fite–Faraco (→) **(C)**. Observe the bacilli arranged side by side, as if they were stacked, showing the bacillary proliferation and a large number of solid bacilli filling the intracytoplasmic vacuoles (globi) (→) **(C)**. HE staining (A and B) and Fite–Faraco **(C)**.

Some patients, especially those in the lepromatous side (BL/LL), even undergoing treatment MDT/MB - 24 doses in different treatment protocols may experience disease reactivation once or more (Figs. **27 - 29**). When the signs disease reactivation occur during the treatment period or shortly after its end, it is usually related to irregular or insufficient treatment or drug resistance (Fig. **30**) [10]. In late relapses, many years or decades after the end of the MDT/MB treatment, there is the possibility of proliferation of persistent bacilli or reinfection (Figs. **27 - 29**) [10]. Under adverse conditions, part of bacilli can become metabolically inactive and interrupt their multiplication process. This can prevent them from being exposed to the action of MDT drugs or causing a triggering of reaction processes. It is possible that these persistent bacilli, which can survive more protected in some tissues like neural branches or the smooth muscle of vessel walls, will proliferate again after the end of treatment and may restart the entire course of the disease.

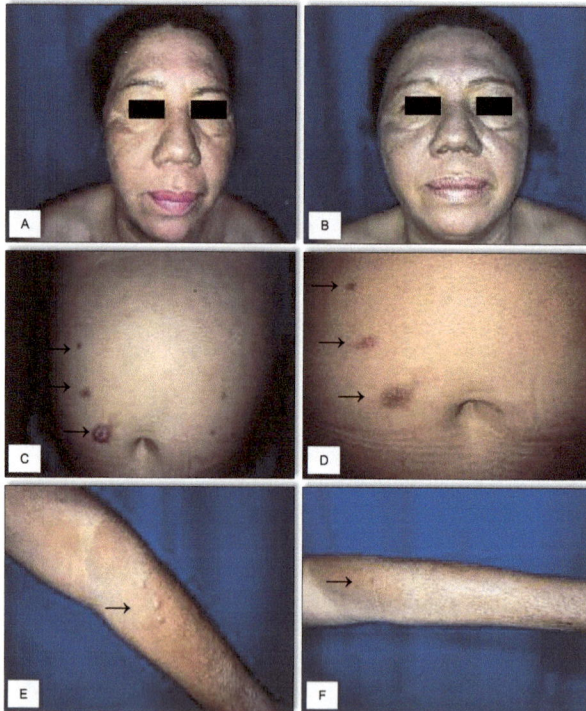

Fig. (28). Example of relapse in leprosy. 45-year-old woman with a history of previous for MDT/MB - 24 doses treatment for leprosy LL ending 14 years ago. (A, C, and E) Currently affectation with diffuse infiltration of the skin and the presence of leprosy (→), clinically compatible with recurrence and confirmed by the histopathological examination shown in Fig. **29**. (B, D, and F) After three months of MDT/MB treatment, the lesions begin to show regression characteristics, characterized by a decrease in the infiltration of the lesions and the beginning of pigmentation by the action of clofazimine. The result of the investigation of resistance by direct sequencing of resistance-related genes (*folP1*, *rpoB*, and *gyrA*) was negative. Courtesy of Dr. Cássio C. Ghidella.

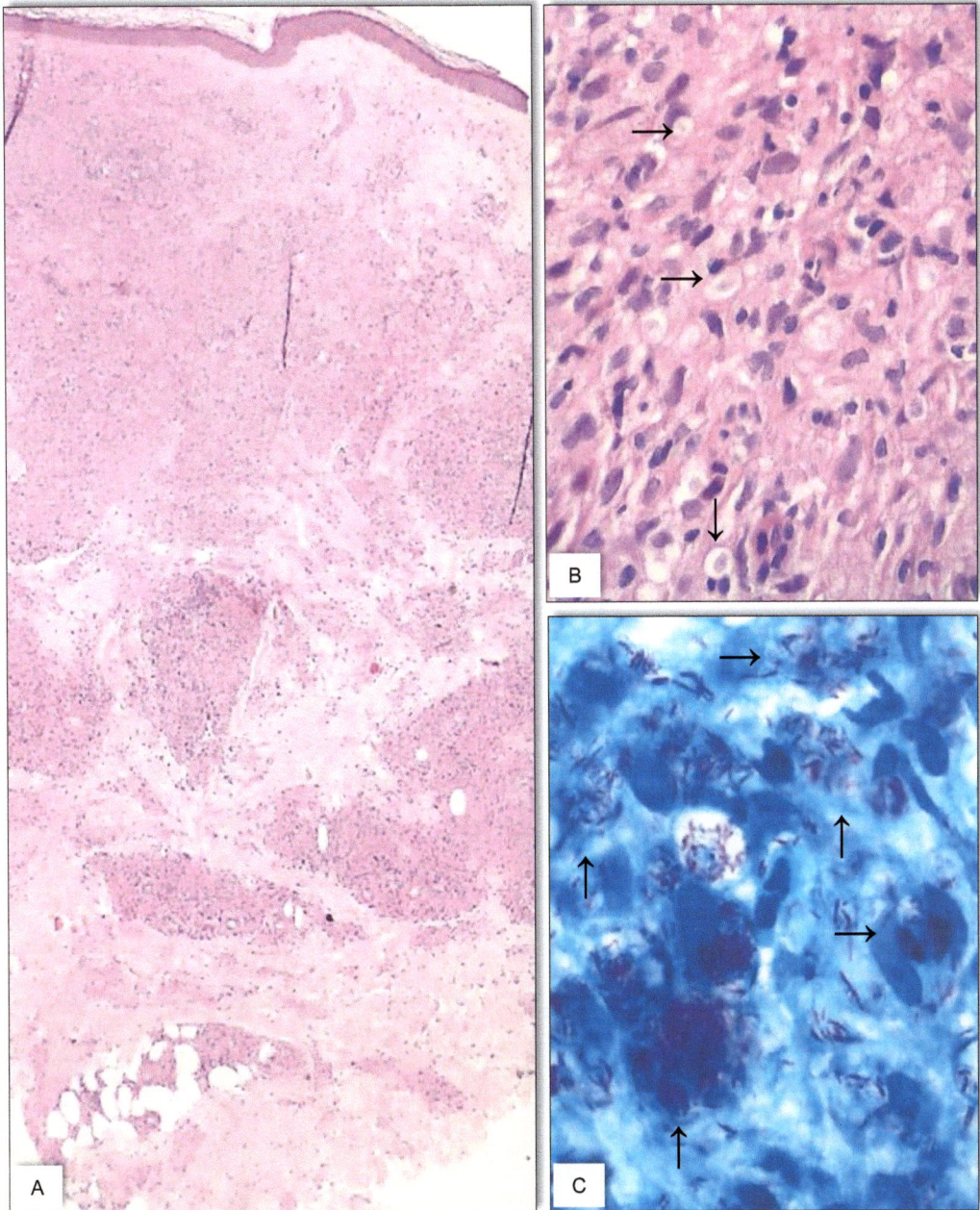

Fig. (29). Example of relapse in leprosy. Histopathological characteristics of the active abdominal injury described in Fig. **28b** . **(A)** Diffuse infiltration of the entire dermis by LL pattern histiocytic granulomas. **(B)** Part of the macrophages are fusiform, and others are vacuolated and filled with grayish amorphous material (→). **(C)** Fite–Faraco staining demonstrates that the amorphous content of vacuoles consists of numerous morphologically solid bacilli (→) (globi), characterizing an active lesion. HE staining (A and B) and Fite–Faraco **(C)**.

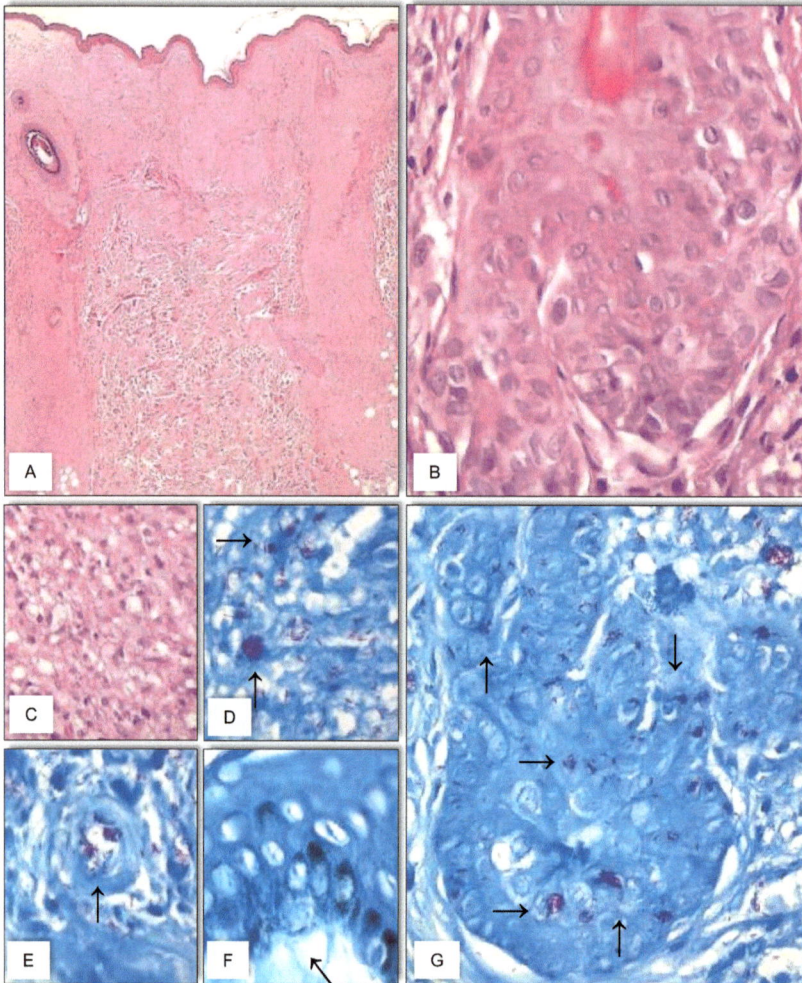

Fig. (30). Example of relapse in leprosy due to drug resistance. LL patient previously treated by MDT/MB - 24 doses and history of recurrence. He was treated 10 years ago by MDT/MB - 27 doses and currently shows signs of active lesion. Histopathological examination shows an active lesion due to diffuse infiltration of the entire skin by vacuolated macrophages (→) (A and C). The bacilloscopic examination reveals solid bacilli inside of the macrophages' vacuoles **(D)**, in the wall and endothelium of the vessels **(E)**, in a cell of the basal layer of the epidermis **(F)** and intense parasitism of the squamous epithelial cells of the hair follicle (B and G). The result of the investigation of resistance by direct sequencing of resistance-related genes (*folP1*, *rpoB*, and *gyrA*) was positive. HE staining (A-C) and Fite–Faraco (D-G).

Bacilloscopic examination of BL and LL patients may show multi-fragmented and slightly stained bacilli after the end of treatment even for several months or years, without this implying disease recurrence [7, 10]. However, modification of the histopathological characteristics of regressive granulomas and the presence of bacilli, even if fragmented, in some types of cells or tissues several years after the end of treatment is indicative of disease relapse (Figs. **31 - 33**) [10]. Also, proliferative bacilli activity should be suspected when, in a biopsy two or more years post-treatment, well-stained fragmented bacilli are detected in endothelial cells (Fig. **34**). A biopsy more than two years after the end of treatment, even in patients BL and LL, usually presents poorly stained multi-fragmented bacilli in macrophages which are discolored or absent in the endothelium.

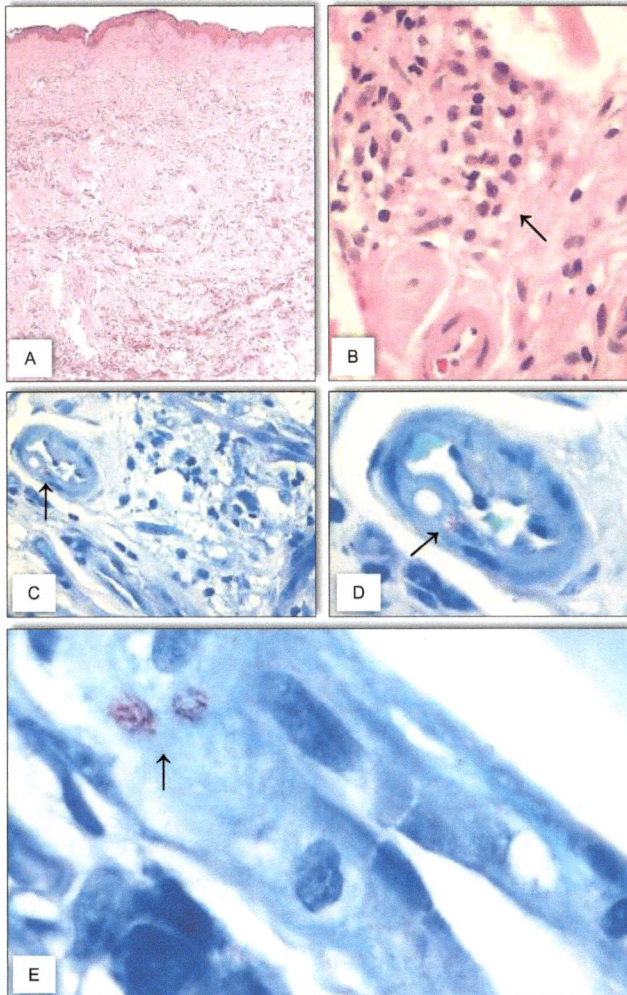

Fig. (31). Example of histopathological and bacilloscopic features suspected of relapse in leprosy. Patient treated with MDT/MB-12 doses 6 years ago for borderline leprosy (BB/BL). Currently showing clinical alterations in some lesions with histopathological examination demonstrating lesions predominantly with regression characteristics **(A)**, however, some granulomas have vacuolated macrophages permeated by lymphocytes and rare plasma cells (→) **(B)**, which are uncommon in purely residual lesions. (C, D, and E) The bacilloscopic examination shows presence of well-stained bacilli on the vessel wall, fragmented and apparently solid, suggesting disease relapse (→). HE staining (A and B) and Fite–Faraco (C-E).

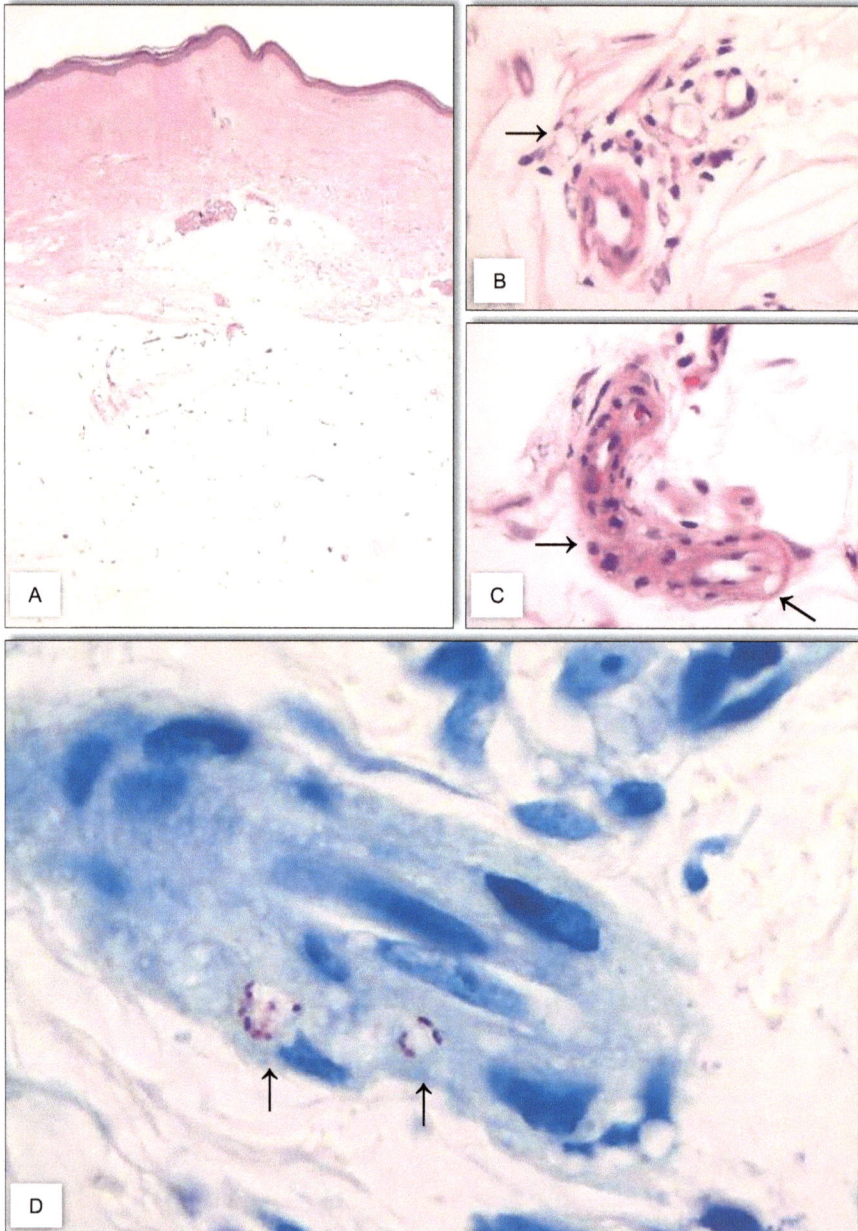

Fig. (32). Example of histopathological and bacilloscopic features that are suspected of relapse in leprosy. BL patient treated 10 years ago with MDT/MB - 24 doses. Currently with some lesions showing sensitivity changes. Histopathological examination shows a predominantly residual lesion (A and B), but some vessels have vacuoles in the vessel wall (→) **(C)**. **(D)** The bacilloscopic examination shows presence of fragmented bacilli, well stained and some apparently solid (→) inside the vacuoles, compatible with disease relapse. HE staining (A-C) and Fite–Faraco **(D)**.

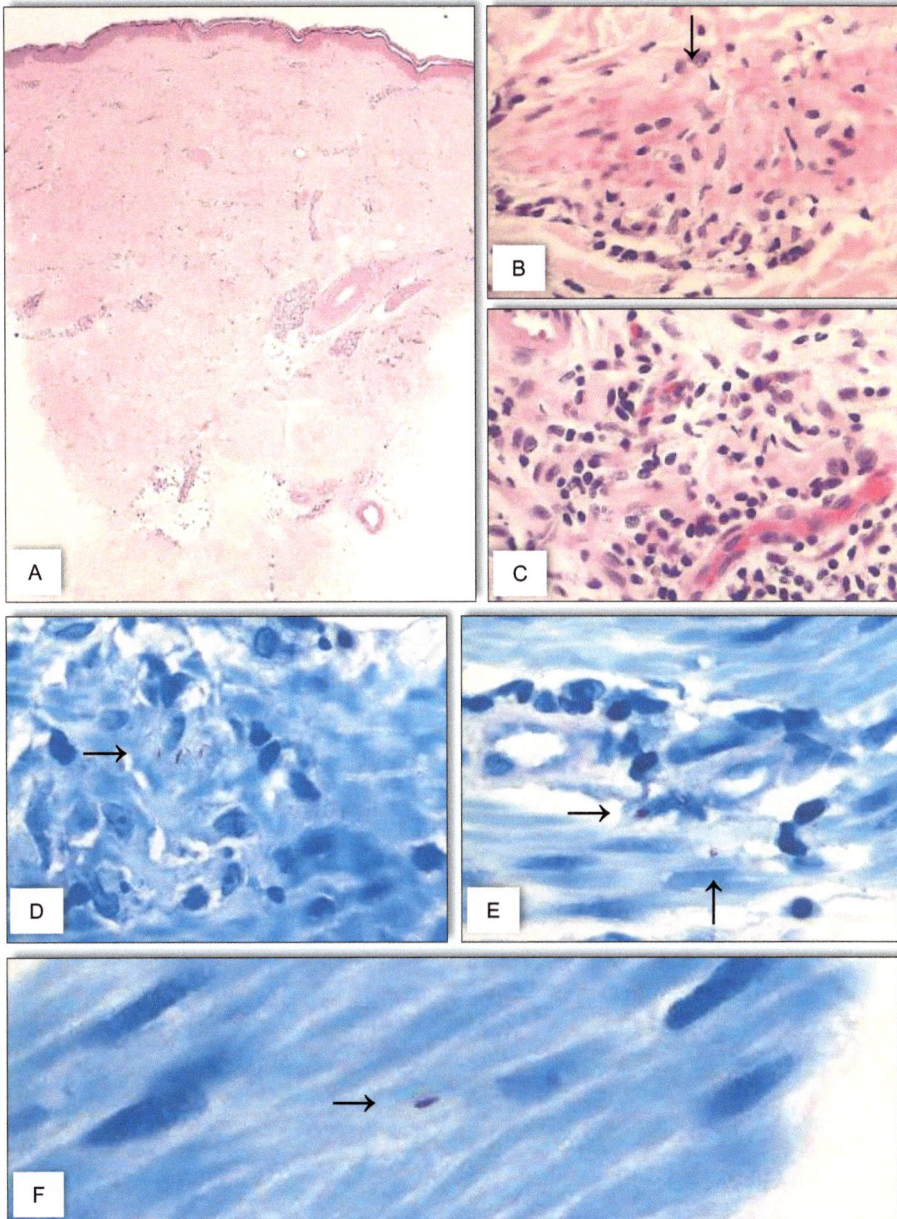

Fig. (33). Example of histopathological and bacilloscopic features of leprosy relapse. Patient treated with MDT/MB - 12 doses 8 years ago for BL leprosy. Currently presenting changes in color and sensitivity in old lesions. Histopathological exams show residual lesion **(A)**, but with several granulomas showing vacuolated macrophages permeated by lymphocytes, plasmocytes, involving neural branches, vessels and pili muscle (→) (B and C). The bacilloscopic examination shows presence of numerous fragmented bacilli, well stained and some apparently solid inside the macrophages (D and E) and in the pili muscle demonstrating recurrence (→) **(F)**. HE staining (A-C) and Fite–Faraco (D-F).

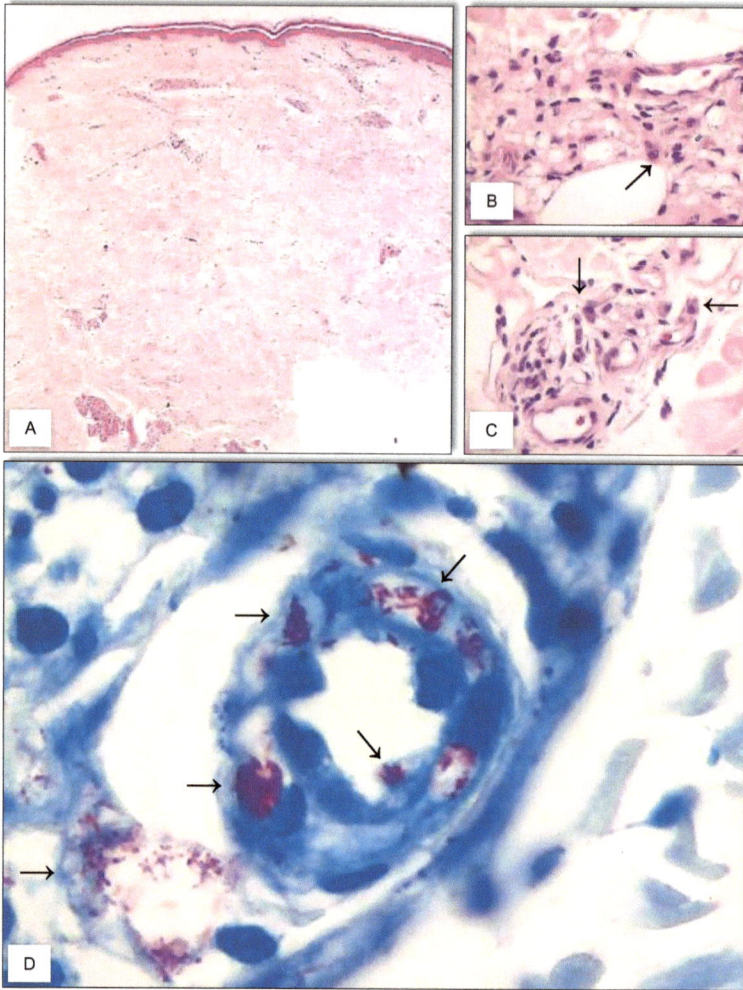

Fig. (34). Example of histopathological and bacilloscopic characteristics of leprosy relapse. Patient treated with MDT/MB - 24 doses 10 years ago for LL leprosy. Currently presenting changes in color and sensitivity in old lesions. Histopathological examination shows a residual lesion **(A)**, but with several granulomas showing vacuolated macrophages permeated by lymphocytes and plasma cells (→) (B and C). The bacilloscopic examination shows presence of fragmented and solid bacilli inside the macrophages, the vessel wall and endothelium characterizing recurrence (→) **(D)**. HE (A-C) and Fite–Faraco **(D)** staining.

Some individuals show signs of disease reactivation for the first time through a T1R. These patients develop clinical signs of T1R over old regressive leprosy lesions, usually many years after the end of treatment, and histopathological and bacilloscopic characteristics confirm T1R (Fig. **35**) [10 - 14]. A peculiar situation of leprosy reactivation is the so-called macular reverse reaction, where the individual several years after treatment begins to present an expansion of residual hypochromic leprosy lesions, or the appearance of new hypochromic lesions, suggesting recurrence [10]. In these cases, the histopathological analysis shows a non-granulomatous peri-neural infiltrate, similar to that of indeterminate leprosy (Chapter 2), or small T1R and IB "0" or 1+ pattern granulomas (Fig. **36**). Some authors believe it is a disease reactivation by bacillary proliferation of quiescent bacilli and that during this proliferation and consequent exposure of bacillary antigens the reaction process is activated [10 - 14].

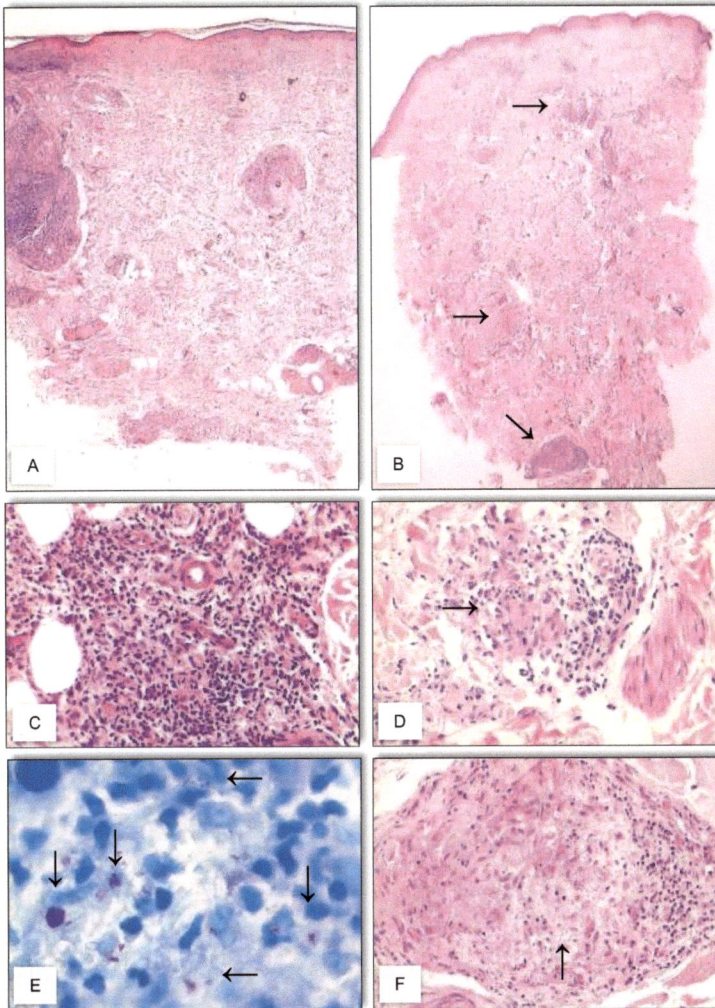

Fig. (35). Leprosy recurrence with histopathological characteristics of T1R. (A, C, and E) A 62-year-old woman presented skin lesions with histopathological characteristics (C and E) and bacilloscopic features of BB leprosy 8 years ago. She underwent treatment with MDT/MB - 12 doses. (B, D, and F) Currently shows erythematous plaques throughout the body with clinical and histopathological features of BB leprosy with associated T1R, characterized by T1R pattern granulomas. (→) and bacilloscopic index of "0." **(E)** Bacilloscopic examination of the initial lesion showed numerous solid bacilli and an IB of 4+. HE (A-D and F) and Fite–Faraco **(E)** staining.

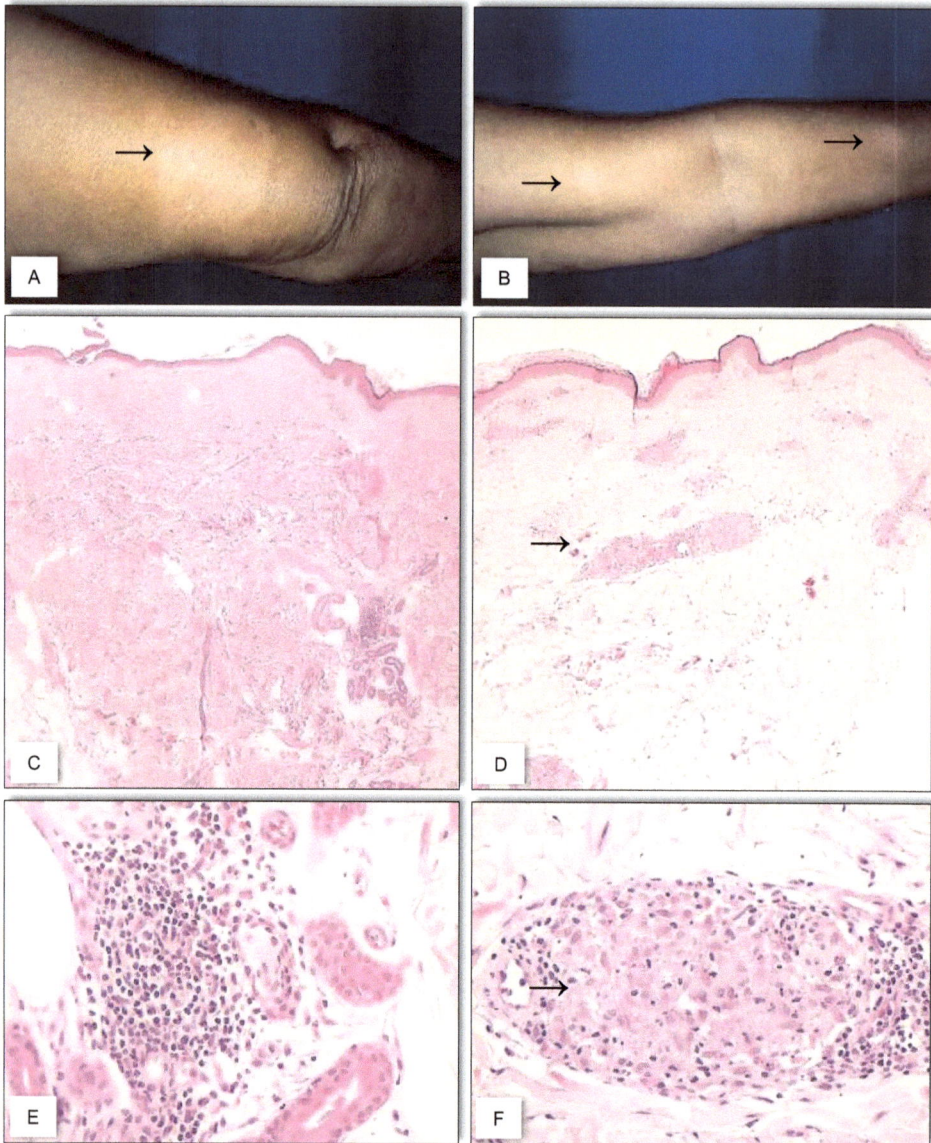

Fig. (36). Example of probable leprosy recurrence with clinic-pathological characteristics of T1R, macular type. (A, C, and E) A 66-year-old woman who seven years ago presented skin lesions with clinical **(A)** and histopathological (C and E) characteristics of BT leprosy (→). She was treated with MDT/MB - 12 doses. (B, D, and F) Currently with residual hypochromic lesions and new hypochromic lesions suggesting recurrence (→) **(B)**. Histopathological features show characteristics of T1R (→) (D and F). Courtesy of Dr. Cássio C. Ghidella (A and B). HE staining (C-F).

The first sign of recurrence may be T2R onset. Some patients in the lepromatous band, especially the LL, can reactivate the disease through bacilli proliferation without presence of clinical signs. Some of these patients can develop T2R on active lesions, especially those who used antibiotic treatment for other causes leading to fragmentation of bacilli and consequent T2R development (Fig. 37).

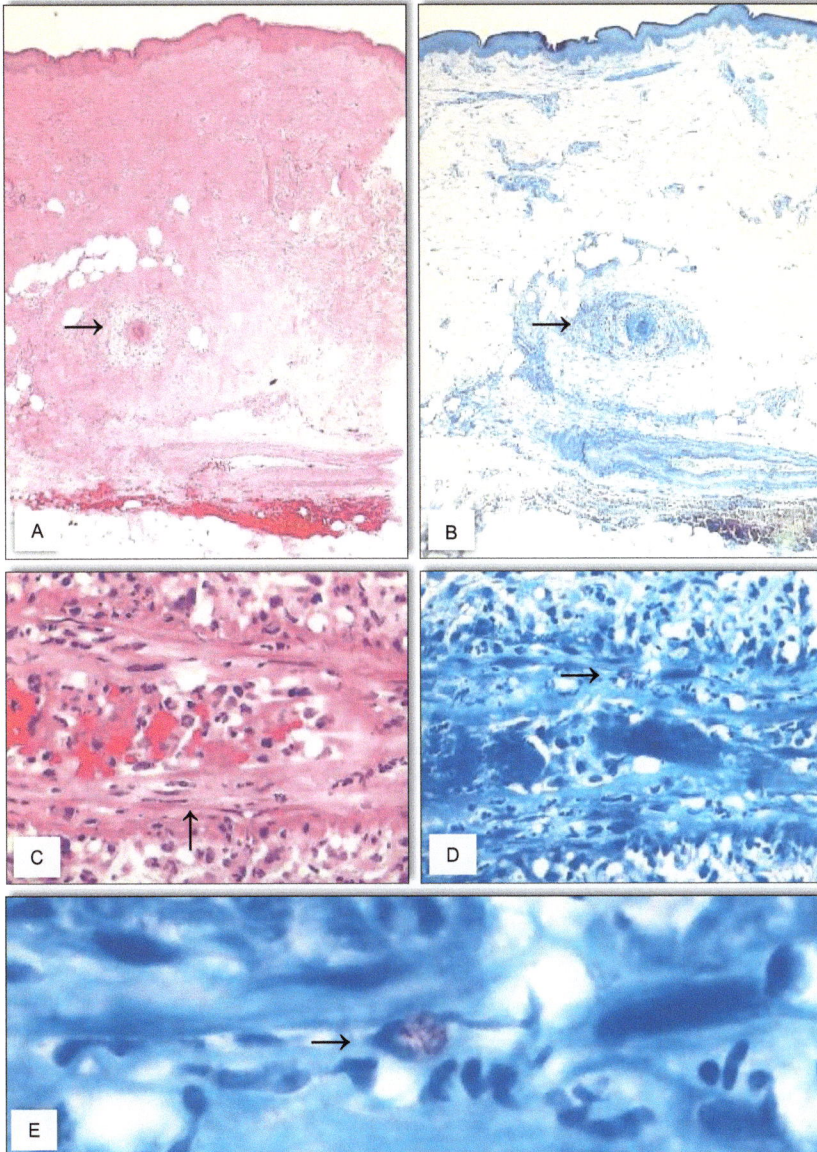

Fig. (37). Example of leprosy relapse with type 2 reaction (T2R). (A-E) Patient treated for LL leprosy 12 years ago. Currently with painful and purple lesions on the legs that started four months ago. Histological characteristics show a T2R pattern with vasculitis (→) **(C)** and fragmented bacilli well stained in macrophages surrounded by neutrophils and in the vessel wall (→) (D and E), characterizing relapse with associated T2R. HE (A and C) and Fite–Faraco (B, C, and E) staining.

Recurrence can initially occur only in deep neural branches without evidence of reactivation of skin lesions. In general, they are BL or LL patients who, long after the end of treatment, begin to show signs and symptoms of neurological disorders over a given nerve territory. Neural biopsy may show the presence of regressive changes associated with the presence of bacilli, suggesting or confirming recurrence (Fig. **38**).

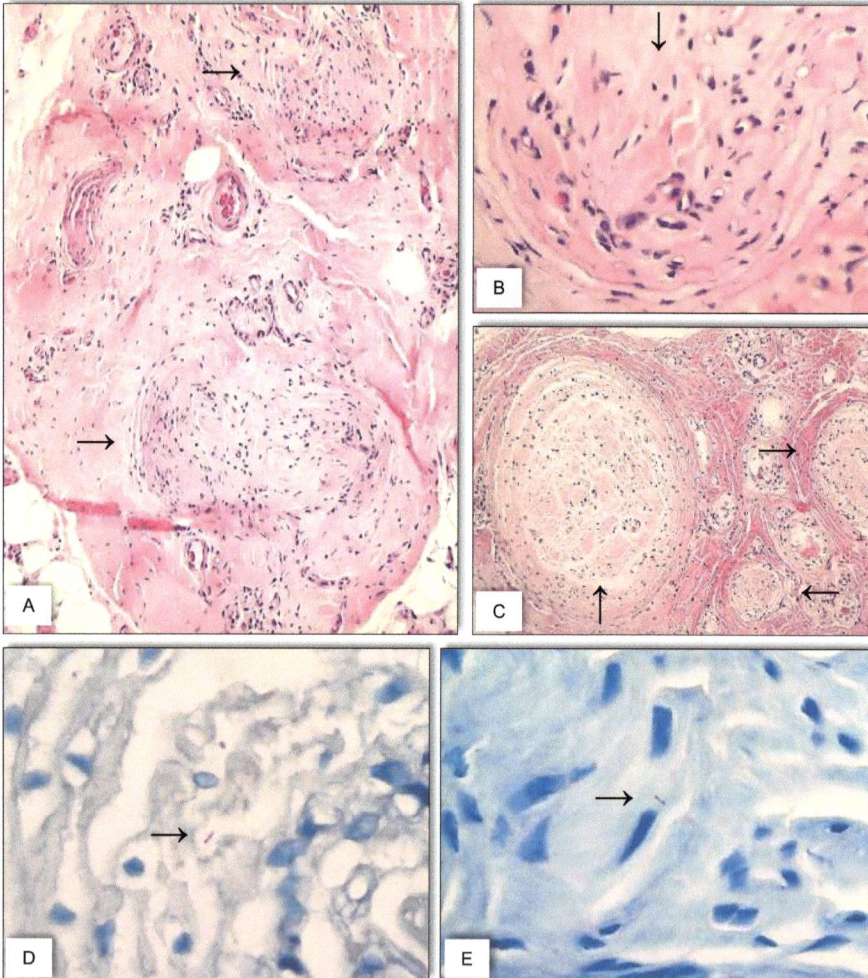

Fig. (38). Example of leprosy relapse occurring in the nerve. A 38-year-old man treated for borderline leprosy eight years ago by MDT/MB - 12 doses. A few months ago, he started to have suspected neuropathy for recurrence and absence of skin lesions. He underwent a neural biopsy procedure and the histological sections show a segment of the collagenized ulnar nerve (→) (A and B) with a discrete perineural and endoneural inflammatory infiltrate associated with important demyelination (→) **(C)**. In bacilloscopic examination, bacilli are observed inside the nerve, confirming relapse (→) (D and E). HE staining (A-C) and Fite–Faraco (D and E). Post-fixed biopsy with osmium tetroxide **(C)**.

DIFFERENTIAL CLINICAL AND HISTOPATHOLOGICAL DIAGNOSES OF REGRESSION OR RECURRENCE OF LEPROSY LESIONS

Stromal changes simulating a scar reaction in the dermis or DF originating from regressive leprosy lesions should not be confused with histoid leprosy, a special form of leprosy lesion recurrence consisting of spindle-shaped macrophages containing a large number of bacilli [15]. Histopathological characteristics and bacilloscopic examination of histoid leprosy are discussed in chapter 8.

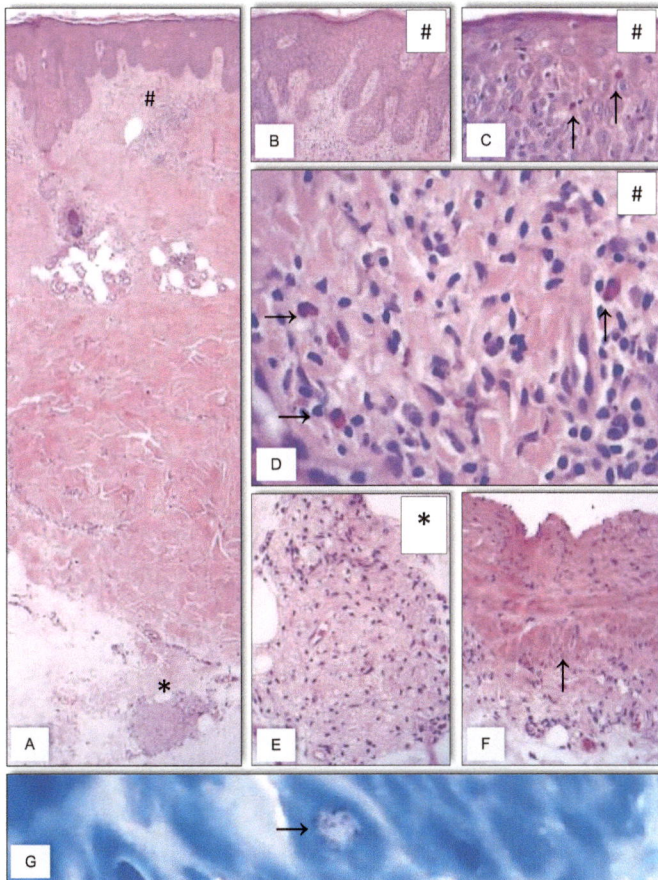

Fig. (39). Example of drug reaction on a leprosy lesion in regression. A patient treated for LL leprosy presents hyperchromic skin lesions with desquamation and continuous use of analgesics. Histopathological examination shows a mixed pattern consisting of drug reaction characteristics (#) and leprosy LL lesion in regression (*). (A, B, C, and D) Drug reaction characterized by polymorphic infiltrate with eosinophils in the papillar dermis associated with epithelial hyperplasia, hyperkeratosis, edema and exocytosis of lymphocytes and eosinophils (→). (A, D, E, and F) Leprosy lesion in regression characterized by regressive histiocytic granulomas (A and E) and regressive changes in the vessel wall **(F)** with multi-fragmented and poorly stained bacilli (→) **(G)**. HE staining (A-F) and Fite–Faraco **(G)**.

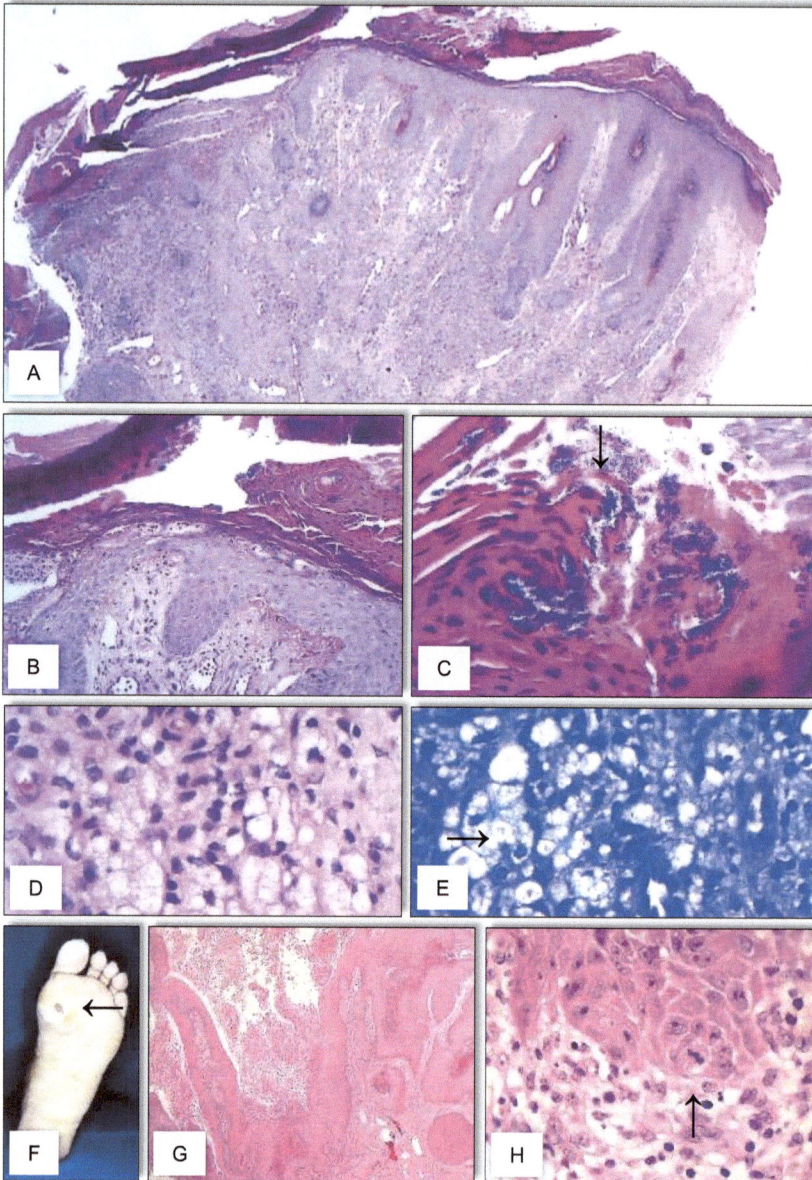

Fig. (40). Example of ulcers on the skin with leprosy lesion in regression. (A-E) Lepromatous lesion in the lepromatous band (BL/LL) in regression with ulceration due to local trauma. (B and C) Edge of the ulcer with fibrovascular hyperplasia in the dermis, epithelial hyperplasia and bacterial colonies (coccus) by secondary contamination (→). (D and E) Histiocytic granulomas in regression in the reticular dermis with multi-fragmented and discolored bacilli (→). (F) Plantar ulcer in a patient treated for leprosy (→). (G and H) Example of well-differentiated squamous cell carcinoma originating from a chronic ulcer in a patient treated for leprosy (→). HE staining (A-D, G, and H) and Fite–Faraco (E). Photo from the archives of the Lauro de Souza Lima Institute - ILSL (F).

Different types of drug reactions can affect patients with leprosy in regressive phases and simulate relapse or leprosy reactions. The reaction process can be triggered by the various drugs used in the specific leprosy treatment, by the continuous use of other drugs to treat other diseases affecting patients with leprosy or neuritis. An important type of drug reaction that affects leprosy patients is the dapsone hypersensitivity syndrome (DHS), a dose-independent idiosyncratic hypersensitivity reaction, occurring between 4 and 6 weeks after treatment initiation and presenting with the triad of fever, rash and involvement of internal organs, most often hepatitis [16]. In histopathology, DHS findings are nonspecific, and commonly present the generic characteristics of a drug reaction, characterized by polymorphic dermal inflammatory infiltrates with varying amounts of eosinophils, capillary congestion, erythrocyte leakage, aggression foci to the epidermis, spongiosis, acanthosis and epidermal edema [16]. Drug reactions in patients with leprosy are also associated with the different medications used to treat hypertension, diabetes, neuritis and other leprosy complications such as chronic ulcers (Fig. **39**). Chronic ulcers in leprosy patients are difficult to treat and after years or decades of evolution are favorable environments for the development of well-differentiated squamous cell carcinoma (Fig. **40**) [17].

CONCLUSION

In summary, it is important for the pathologist to know how to identify the histopathological and bacilloscopic changes that occur in leprosy lesions during and after treatment. This allows to determine whether the lesion is in regression or if there are signs of disease reactivation. The interpretation of the findings will depend on a close correlation among histopathological patterns, bacilloscopic characteristics, and clinical data, especially those referring to patient classification in the R&J spectrum before treatment and the interval between treatment initiation and biopsy.

REFERENCES

[1]   Maymone MBC, Venkatesh S, Laughter M, *et al.* Leprosy: treatment and management of complications. J Am Acad Dermatol 2020; S0190-9622(20): 30473-4.

[2]   Cruz RCDS, Bührer-Sékula S, Penna MLF, Penna GO, Talhari S. Leprosy: current situation, clinical and laboratory aspects, treatment history and perspective of the uniform multidrug therapy for all patients. An Bras Dermatol 2017; 92(6): 761-73.
        [http://dx.doi.org/10.1590/abd1806-4841.20176724] [PMID: 29364430]

[3]   Smith CS, Aerts A, Saunderson P, Kawuma J, Kita E, Virmond M. Multidrug therapy for leprosy: a game changer on the path to elimination. Lancet Infect Dis 2017; 17(9): e293-7.
        [http://dx.doi.org/10.1016/S1473-3099(17)30418-8] [PMID: 28693853]

[4]   Soares CT, Masuda PY, Junior DC, *et al.* A case series of dermatofibromas originating in leprosy lesions: a potentially misdiagnosed condition. Surg Exp Pathol 2019; 2: 12.
        [http://dx.doi.org/10.1186/s42047-019-0039-6]

[5]   Murashov MD, LaLone V, Rzeczycki PM, *et al.* The physicochemical basis of clofazimine-induced skin pigmentation. J Invest Dermatol 2018; 138(3): 697-703.
[http://dx.doi.org/10.1016/j.jid.2017.09.031] [PMID: 29042210]

[6]   Ridley MJ. The degradation of *Mycobacterium leprae* by a comparison of its staining properties. Int J Lepr Other Mycobact Dis 1983; 51(2): 211-8.
[PMID: 6194126]

[7]   Scollard DM. 18 September 2016, posting date. Pathogenesis and pathology of leprosy. In: Scollard DM, Gillis TP, Eds. International Textbook of Leprosy. 2016. Available from: www.internationaltextbookofleprosy.org

[8]   Cambau E, Saunderson P, Matsuoka M, *et al.* Antimicrobial resistance in leprosy: results of the first prospective open survey conducted by a WHO surveillance network for the period 2009-15. Clin Microbiol Infect 2018; 24(12): 1305-10.
[http://dx.doi.org/10.1016/j.cmi.2018.02.022] [PMID: 29496597]

[9]   Rosa PS, D'Espindula HRS, Melo ACL, *et al.* Emergence and transmission of drug-/multidru-
-resistant *Mycobacterium leprae* in a former leprosy colony in the Brazilian Amazon. Clin Infect Dis 2020; 70(10): 2054-61.
[http://dx.doi.org/10.1093/cid/ciz570] [PMID: 31260522]

[10] Fleury RN. Patologia e manifestações viscerais.Noções de Hansenologia. 2nd ed. Bauru, Brazil: Centro de Estudo Dr Reynaldo Quagliato, Instituto Lauro de Souza Lima 2000; pp. 63-71.

[11] Kaimal S, Thappa DM. Relapse in leprosy. Indian J Dermatol Venereol Leprol 2009; 75(2): 126-35.
[http://dx.doi.org/10.4103/0378-6323.48656] [PMID: 19293498]

[12] Opromolla DV. Recidiva ou reação reversa. Hansenol Int 1994; 19: 10-6.

[13] Rezende FC, Abdalla BMZ, Silveira CB, *et al.* Reação reversa macular da hanseníase: relato de caso. Hansenol Int 2014; 39: 70-4.

[14] Linder K, Zia M, Kern WV, Pfau RK, Wagner D. Relapses *vs* reactions in multibacillary leprosy: proposal of new relapse criteria. Trop Med Int Health 2008; 13(3): 295-309.
[http://dx.doi.org/10.1111/j.1365-3156.2008.02003.x] [PMID: 18397393]

[15] Canuto MJM, Yacoub CRD, Trindade MAB, Avancini J, Pagliari C, Sotto MN. Histoid leprosy: clinical and histopathological analysis of patients in follow-up in University Clinical Hospital of endemic country. Int J Dermatol 2018; 57(6): 707-12.
[http://dx.doi.org/10.1111/ijd.13926] [PMID: 29384191]

[16] Craig J, MacRae C, Melvin RG, Boggild AK. Case report: a case of type 1 leprosy reaction and dapsone hypersensitivity syndrome complicating the clinical course of multibacillary leprosy. Am J Trop Med Hyg 2019; 100(5): 1145-8.
[http://dx.doi.org/10.4269/ajtmh.18-0953] [PMID: 30915953]

[17] Bobhate SK, Madankar ST, Parate SN, Choudhary RK, Kumbhalkar DT. Malignant transformation of plantar ulcers in leprosy. Indian J Lepr 1993; 65(3): 297-303.
[PMID: 8283065]

CHAPTER 8

Lucio's Leprosy and Lucio's Phenomenon, Histoid Leprosy, Nodular Leprosy of Childhood, Primary Neural Leprosy, and Diagnosis Using Fine Needle Aspiration Cytology

Abstract: In this chapter, some special forms of the clinical and histopathological presentation of leprosy are discussed: Lucio's leprosy and Lucio's phenomenon, histoid leprosy, nodular leprosy of childhood, and primary neural leprosy. The main clinical and histopathological characteristics of these forms and the condition under which they appear within the entire spectrum of leprosy and its reaction phenomena are presented. In addition, the main differential clinical and pathological diagnoses of each of these lesions are discussed. The use of fine-needle aspiration cytology for the diagnosis of leprosy, including its reaction phenomena, has also been addressed. The identification of the histopathological features of these special forms of leprosy is important to confirm the clinical diagnosis for guiding treatment and preventing the possible misinterpretation of clinical and histopathological findings.

Keywords: Fine needle aspiration cytology, Hansen's disease, Histoid leprosy, Leprosy, Lucio's leprosy, Lucio's phenomenon, *Mycobacterium leprae*, Nodular leprosy of childhood.

INTRODUCTION

Leprosy has some rare clinical presentations. Some researchers question if they are special forms or are variants of the common forms of the disease. Therefore, from a practical point of view, it is necessary to recognize and understand where these clinical presentations occur within the spectrum of leprosy.

In this chapter, the clinico-pathologic characteristics of the special presentations of leprosy, such as Lucio's Leprosy and Lucio's Phenomenon, Histoid Leprosy, Nodular Leprosy of Childhood, and Primary Neural Leprosy, are discussed. In addition, the cytopathologic characteristics of the main forms of leprosy and their reactions are discussed as well.

The cytopathologic diagnosis of leprosy can be determined using fine-needle aspiration cytology. This technique is highly essential for the clinical management of patients with leprosy. These characteristics are described in each corresponding section of the topics described above.

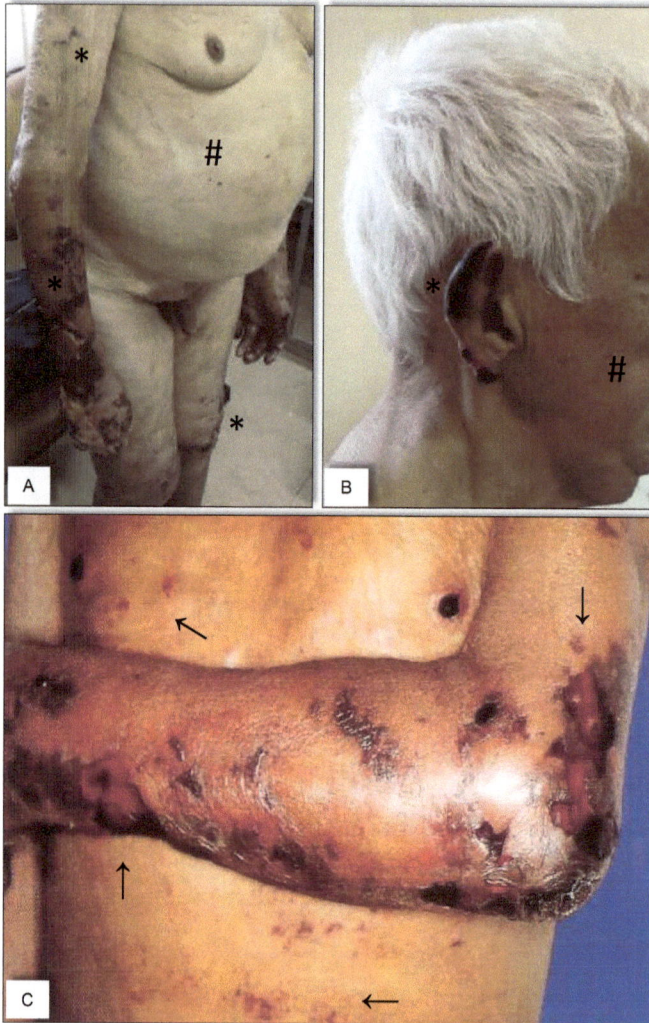

Fig. (1). Lucio's leprosy associated with Lucio's phenomenon. The patient with Lucio's leprosy presents with diffuse infiltration, without the formation of nodules, which does not modify the patient's features ("Lepra Bonita") (# A, B). The patient presented Lucio's phenomenon (*A, B) predominantly in the extremities of the lower and upper limbs and in the ear lobe characterized by ecchymotic patches that ulcerated, giving rise to superficial ulcers and irregular contours. Another example of Lucio's phenomenon with macules and flabby blisters that evolve with central necrosis and subsequent ulceration (→) **(C)**. Photos from the archives of the Lauro de Souza Lima Institute (A, B). Courtesy of Dr. Cássio C. Ghidella **(C)**.

LUCIO'S LEPROSY AND LUCIO'S PHENOMENON

Lucio's leprosy is a form of lepromatous leprosy (LL) that manifests as diffuse infiltration into the skin and absence of nodules. The skin is shiny and myxedematous in appearance; therefore, it is called "Lepra Bonita," or diffuse leprosy associated with madarosis and infiltration of the ear lobes (Fig. **1**). This lepromatous form, called Lucio's leprosy, was described in detail by Lucio and Alvarado in 1851 and was re-studied by Latapi [1 - 4]. The histopathological features of Lucio's leprosy are those of LL (Chapter 3), with diffuse infiltration into the skin by macrophages containing numerous solid bacilli (bacilloscopic index (BI) 6+) and parasitism of the vessels. All the vascular layers are infiltrated by macrophages containing bacilli associated with the parasitism of smooth muscle cells in the vessel wall, endothelium, and perivascular tissues. The endothelial proliferation and subendothelial thickening cause a reduction in vessel lumen diameter (Fig. **2**).

Lucio's phenomenon (LP), also called necrotizing erythema, is a reaction manifestation that affects patients with Lucio's leprosy and is also described as a nodular form of LL. It is characterized by multiple painful purple macules, hemorrhagic blisters, and lesions arranged in the livedoid pattern, which evolve into necrotic and ulcerated lesions, usually affecting the upper and lower limbs (Fig. **1**). In Lucio and Alvarado's description, skin lesions are accompanied by the signs of systemic impairment, such as fever, prostration, insomnia, chills, and gastrointestinal disorders that preceded death [1], and histopathological features represented a cutaneous infarction (Fig. **3**). There is coagulation necrosis that involves the epidermis, lepromatous granulomas, all dermal tissues, and subcutaneous adipose tissue. Necrotic granulomas show intense nuclear fragmentation. The small dermal vessels are dilated and intensely congested, sometimes occluded by fibrin thrombi. The red blood cells permeate the tissues adjacent to the vessels. The arterial and venous walls are infiltrated by a specific macrophage containing numerous bacilli. The lumen of the vessels is obstructed or reduced. The arteries in the deep dermis or subcutaneous cell tissue may be sub-occluded or entirely occluded by thrombi. Initial bacilloscopy examination revealed well-stained solid and fragmented bacilli. As the phenomenon is fully established, with necrosis of all the components of the skin, bacillary fragmentation is intense and sometimes not detected in the specimens stained using the Fite-Faraco method (Figs. **3** and **4**). Adjacent tissues that are not affected by LP present active lepromatous lesions, with predominantly solid bacilli and a BI of 5 or 6+ (Fig. **5**).

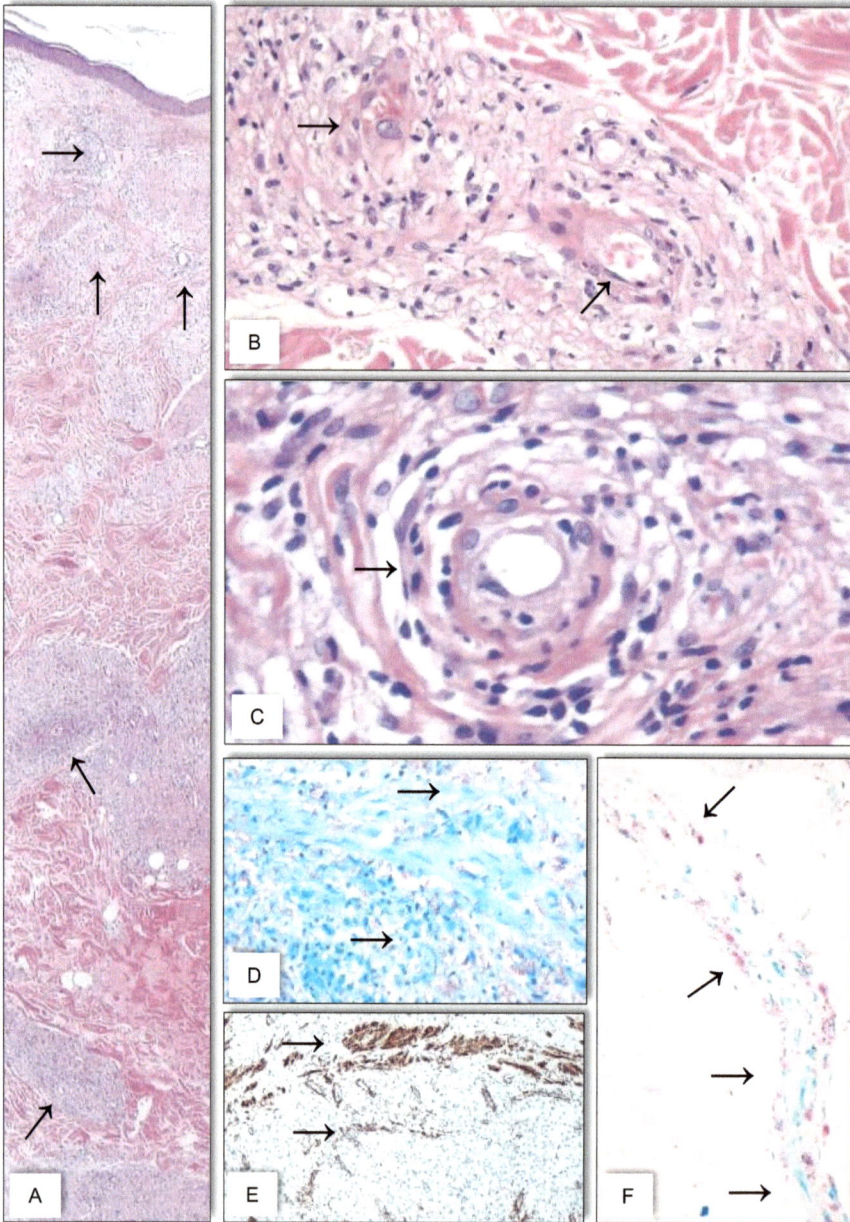

Fig. (2). Lucio's leprosy. Histopathological characteristics of diffuse tissue involvement, especially of the vessels (→) (A–C). The vessels are surrounded and permeated by multivacuolated macrophages associated with endothelial and subintimal proliferation (→) (B, C). The bacilloscopy examination shows intense parasitism (BI-6) of all the vascular layers (→) (D, F). Small-caliber vessels have intense parasitism throughout their length (→) **(F)**. Immunohistochemistry (smooth muscle actin-1A4) showing the irregular vascular wall by macrophage infiltration (→) **(E)**. Stained using hematoxylin and eosin (A–C) and the Fite-Faraco method (E, F).

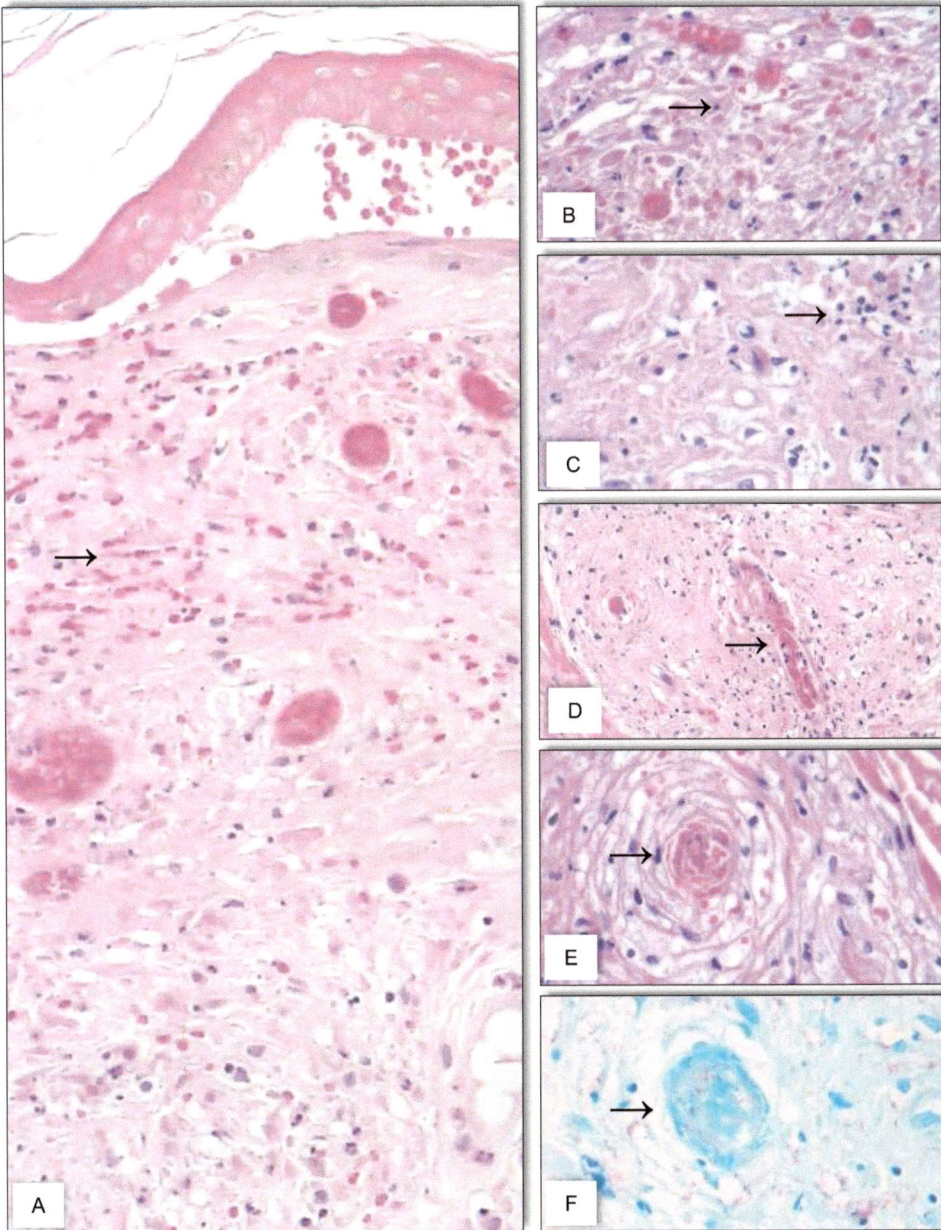

Fig. (3). Histopathological characteristics of Lucio's phenomenon. There is coagulative necrosis affecting all the skin tissues **(A)**. Necrotic granulomas show nuclear fragmentation associated with red blood cell extravasation (→) (A–C). The small vessels in the dermis are dilated and intensely congested, sometimes occluded by fibrin thrombi (→) (A–E). Note that there is no influx of lymphocytes or neutrophils or the formation of microabscesses. Bacilloscopy examination shows numerous bacilli parasitizing the adjacent vessels and tissues (BI 6). Stained using hematoxylin and eosin (A–E) and the Fite-Faraco method **(F)**.

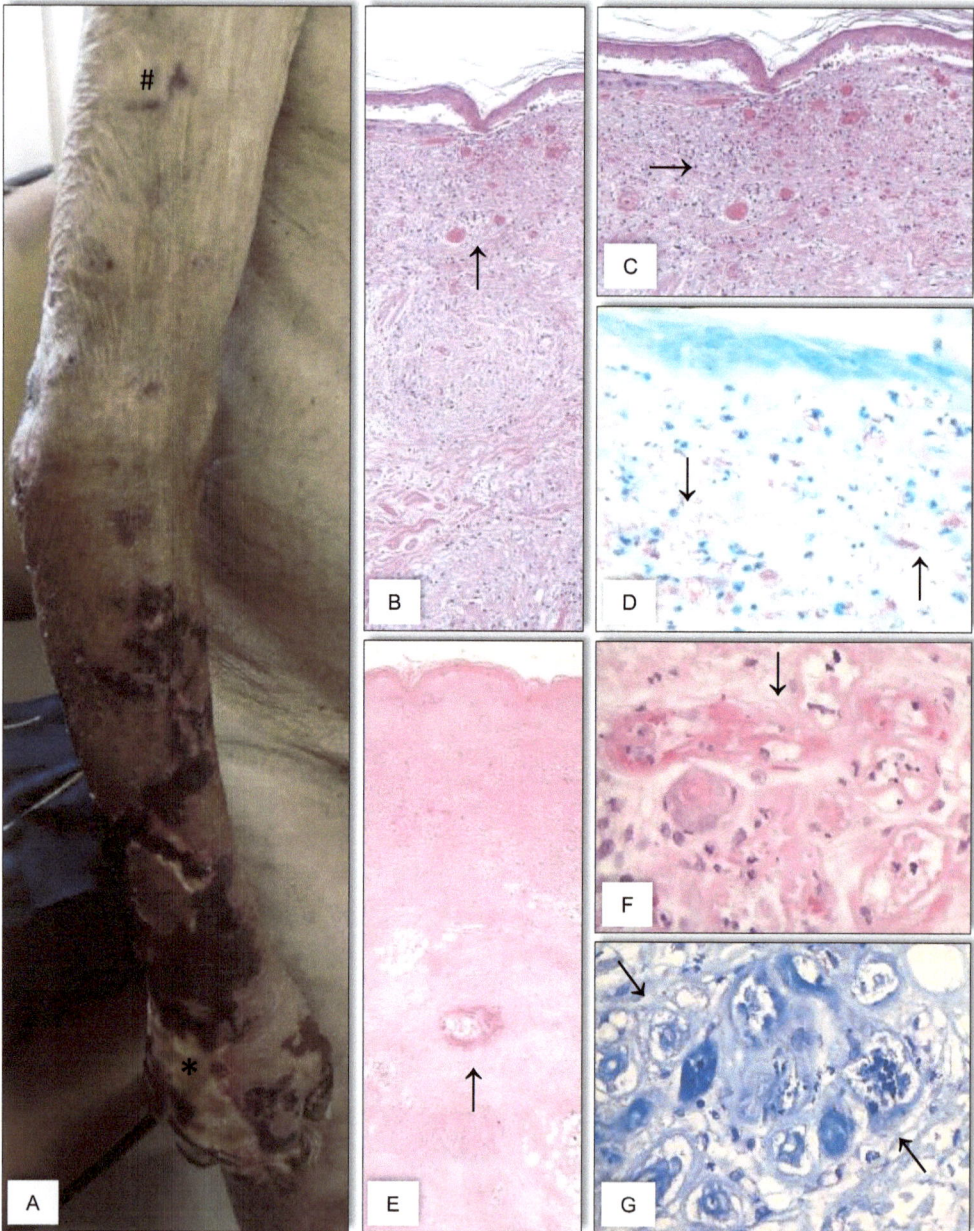

Fig. (4). Lucio's phenomenon. Histopathological characteristics of an early-stage lesion (# A, B, C, and D) and an established lesion (* A, E, F, and G). In the initial lesion (#), there is necrosis of part of the superficial tissues, congestion, overflow of red blood cells (→) (B, C), and bacilloscopy examination showing well-stained fragmented bacilli (→) **(D)**. In established or late lesions (*), there is extensive necrosis affecting all skin components, thrombosis of superficial and deep vessels (→) (E, F), and bacilloscopic examination shows discolored or slightly stained multifragmented bacilli (→) **(G)**. Stained using hematoxylin and eosin (B, C, E, and F) and the Fite-Faraco method (D, G).

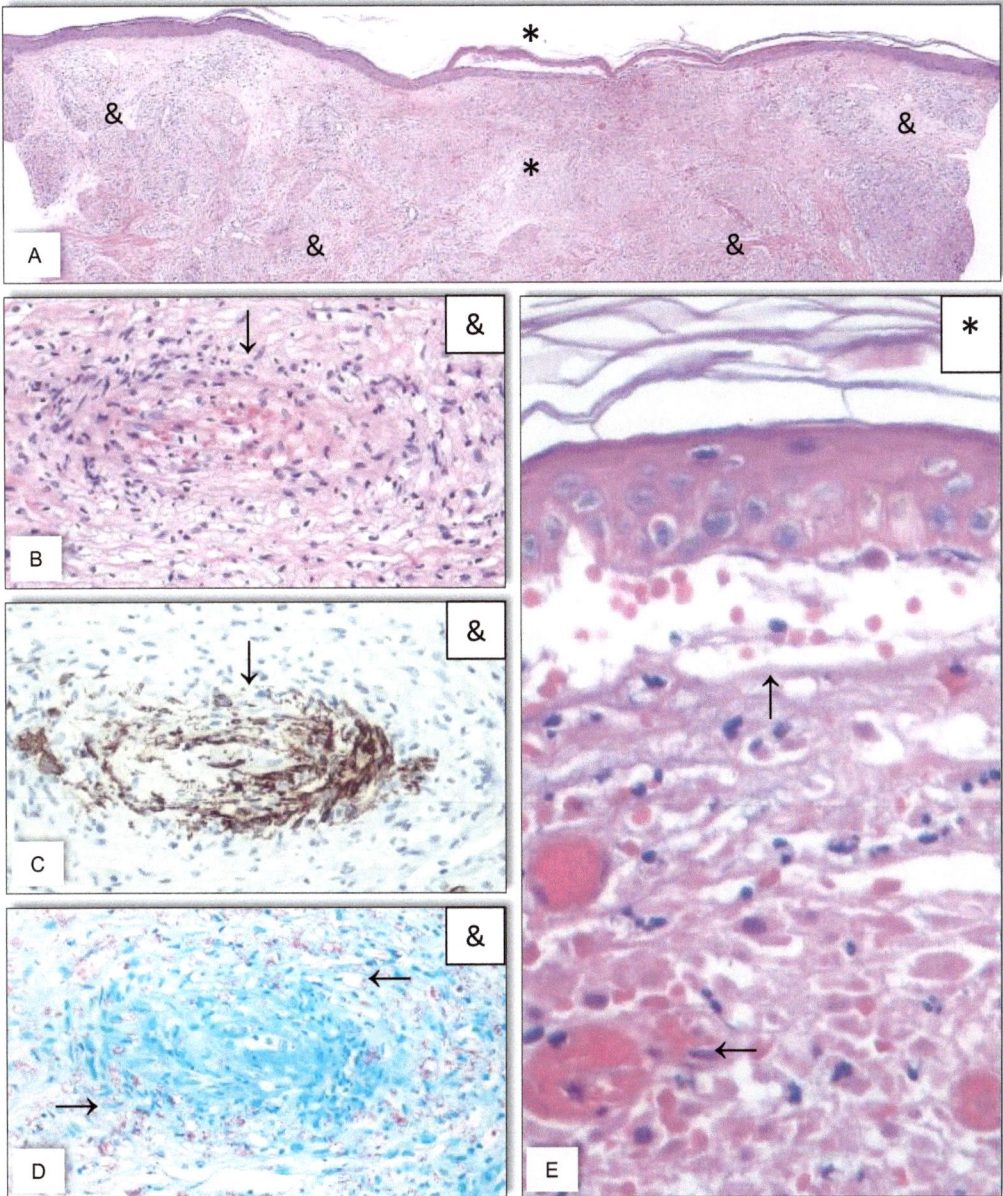

Fig. (5). Lucio's leprosy and Lucio's phenomenon (LP). Lucio´s leprosy skin lesion (→) (&, A, B, C, and D) with focal and superficial areas with LP (*A, E). The skin adjacent to the LP area has histopathological characteristics of an LL lesion with intense parasitism of the vessels characterized by intense macrophage infiltration in all the vascular layers and obstruction of the lumen (→) (A, B) and divulsion of the vessel wall by numerous macrophages parasitized by solid bacilli (→) (C, D). The area with LP shows infarction of the affected tissues, congestion, red cell leakage, and formation of a subepidermal blister (→) (A, E). Stained using hematoxylin and eosin (A, B, and E), immunohistochemistry (D; smooth muscle actin-1 A4), and the Fite-Faraco method **(D)**.

There are some hypotheses regarding the pathogenesis of LP. The most convincing, in our opinion, are those that associate cutaneous hemorrhagic infarction with the obstruction of deep cutaneous vessels (arteries or veins) by histiocytic infiltration of vascular walls associated with thrombosis [2 - 7]. Specific vascular involvement appears to be more intense in Lucio's leprosy than in common LL, thereby creating difficulty in venous return and was aggravated by thrombosis of the deepest vessels. The cause of thrombosis in LP remains unknown.

In four cases of patients with LP (necrotizing erythema) who died at the Lauro de Souza Lima Institute and underwent an autopsy, complications were observed as "causa mortis": myocardial infarction, changes in blood clotting, and opportunistic fungal infections (cutaneous moniliasis, upper airway and esophageal moniliasis, and generalized cryptococcosis). No visceral lesions were observed; the finding was similar to that observed in LP of the skin. One patient died of disseminated intravascular coagulation and another died of generalized venous thrombosis and pulmonary thromboembolism. In LP, the involvement of the terminal vascular territory and extensive tissue necrosis along with type 2 reaction (T2R) (necrotizing erythema nodosum, Chapter 6) is likely to cause severe changes in blood coagulation.

The differential clinical diagnoses of Lucio's leprosy are related to those of LL (Chapter 3) without the presence of skin nodules and alopecia associated with syphilis. Intense macrophage infiltration involving neural branches and other skin components associated with numerous bacilli (BI 6+), identified using the Fite-Faraco stain, are histopathological characteristics of leprosy. LP must be distinguished from several causes of cutaneous or systemic vasculitis, calciphylaxis, levamisole-induced cutaneous vasculitis syndrome, and T2R presenting as necrotizing erythema nodosum.

Cutaneous or systemic vasculitis does not present diffuse macrophage infiltration in the adjacent tissues, and bacilloscopy can rule out vasculitis. Calciphylaxis presents calcium deposits on the vessel wall and does not involve diffuse macrophage infiltration. Levamisole-induced vasculitis is predominantly small vessel vasculitis with thrombosis and fibrinoid necrosis surrounded by neutrophils and nuclear fragmentation (Fig. 6).

T2R in the form of necrotizing erythema nodosum leprosum (necrotizing ENL) can be clinically similar to LP. From a histopathological point of view, despite having some characteristics in common, they are two distinct entities. LP is an occlusive, non-inflammatory vasculopathy, with infarction of skin tissues and infiltration of solid bacilli, and it is a reaction phenomenon that occurs before treatment. In contrast, T2R is an inflammatory occlusive vasculopathy, with an influx of neutrophils, vasculitis, and neutrophilic micro abscesses; bacilloscopy examination reveals fragmented bacilli. T2R occurs after the initiation of treatment. The histopathological characteristics of T2R are described in detail in Chapter 6. The characteristics of LP and T2R are shown in Fig. (7). Patients with Lucio's leprosy, with or without associated LP, after receiving specific leprosy treatment may develop T2R.

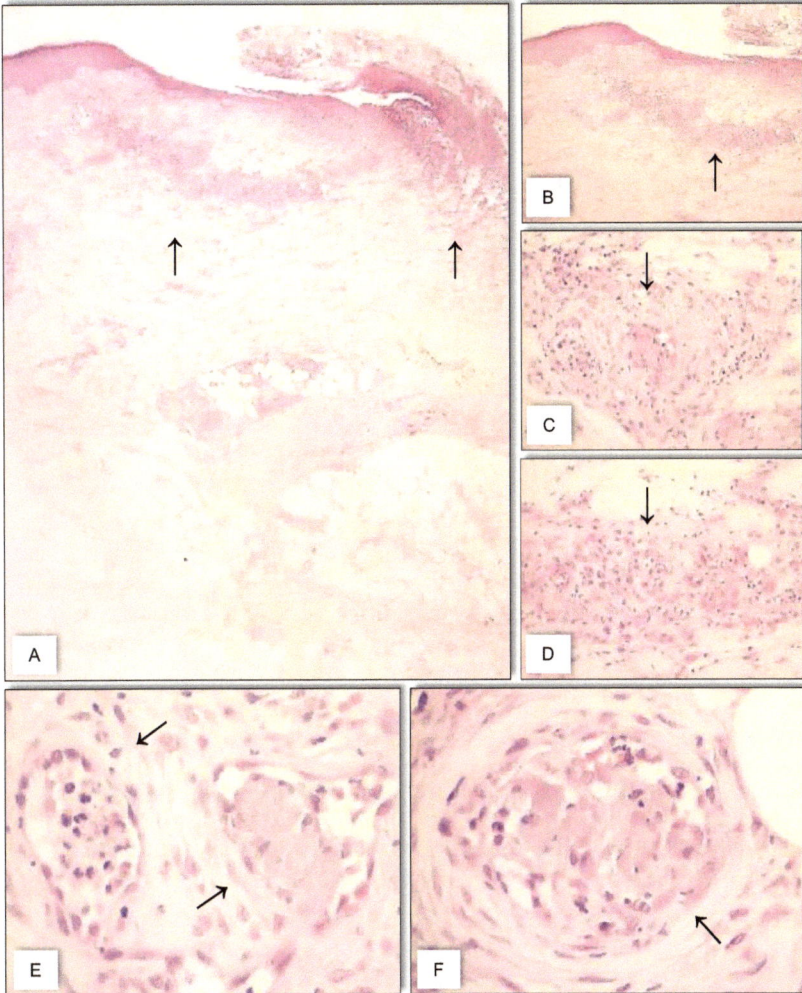

Fig. (6). Differential diagnosis of Lucio's phenomenon (LP). A frequent cocaine user started showing equimotic and necrotic lesions in the limbs and auricular pavilions. Histological sections show skin necrosis owing to vasculitis of small vessels surrounded by neutrophils and nuclear fragmentation (→) (A–D) and association with thrombosis and fibrinoid necrosis (→) (E, F). Vasculitis can be observed, which is induced by levamisole added to cocaine. Stained using hematoxylin and eosin.

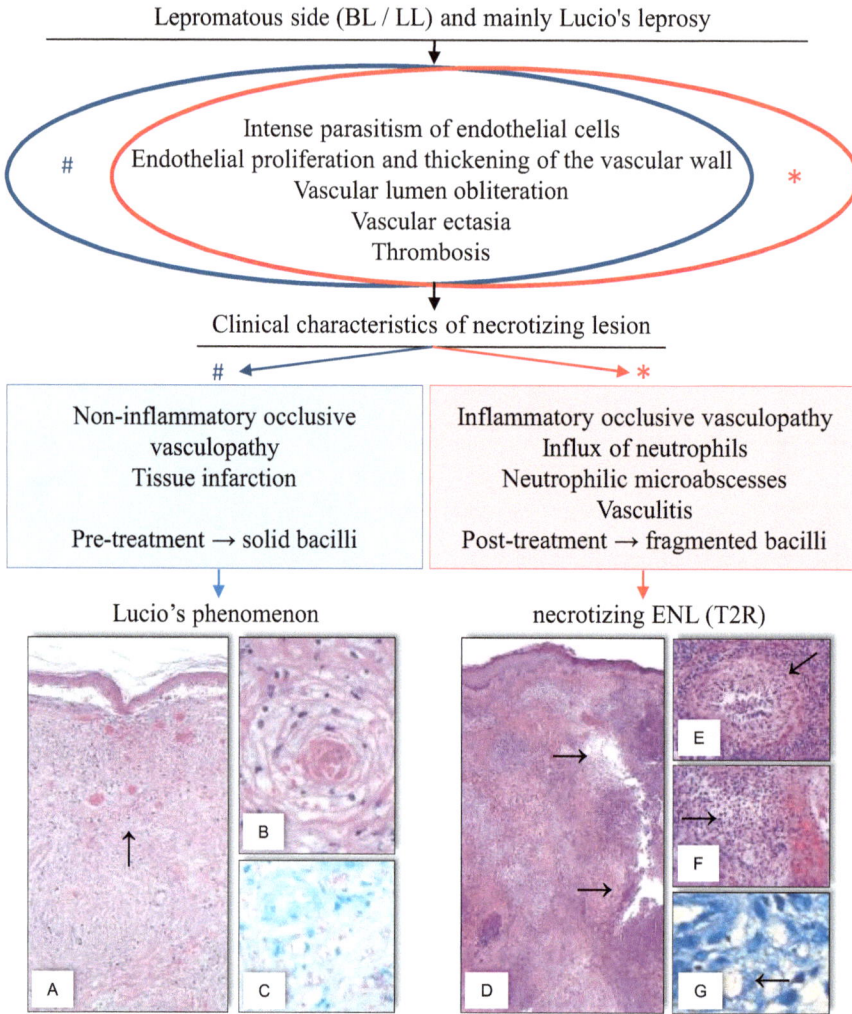

Fig. (7). Differences and similarities between Lucio's phenomenon (LP) and type 2 reaction (T2R). Lepromatous leprosy side with necrotizing skin lesions can represent both necrotizing LP and T2R. Tissue infarction, absence of neutrophilic inflammatory infiltrate, and solid bacilli are compatible with LP (→) (A–C). The presence of inflammatory vasculitis with an influx of neutrophils and multi-fragmented bacilli after treatment is characteristic of T2R (→) (D–F). Stained using hematoxylin and eosin (A, B, D, E, and F) and the Fite-Faraco method (C, G).

HISTOID LEPROSY

Histoid leprosy (HL) is a variant of LL. It was described by Wade in 1963 as a peculiar presentation characterized by well-defined cutaneous nodules of variable size and shape, which may be accompanied by tuberous or vegetative lesions with a keloid aspect (Fig. **8**) [8]. The appearance of nodules would be associated with irregular or inappropriate treatment or monotherapeutic treatment by dapsone, resulting in the development of mutant bacilli strains resistant to the drug. The etiopathogenesis of HL has not yet been defined. It is believed to be an exacerbated form of multibacillary leprosy, with an increase in the number of parasitized cells resulting in an increased humoral immune response for preventing the spread of the disease [9 - 12]. Patients initially diagnosed with LL had recurrence with histoid lesions. In addition, *de novo* cases have been described and characterized after the development of histoid lesions without any evidence of clinical features observed in other forms of leprosy [9 - 11].

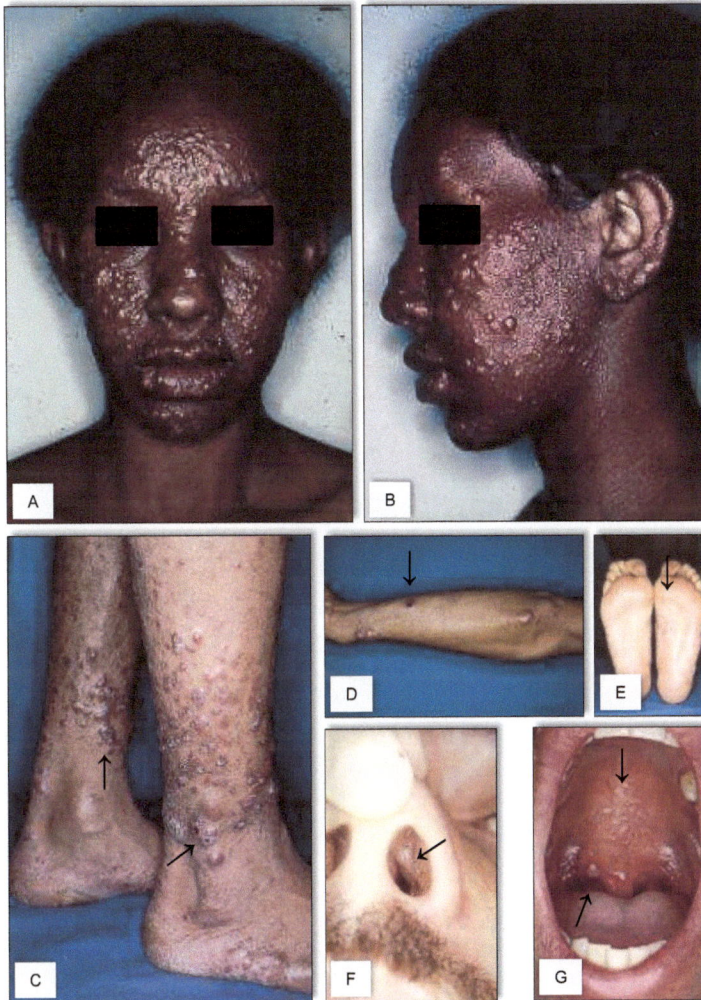

Fig. (8). Clinical characteristics of histoid leprosy. Well-defined cutaneous nodules and tuberous or vegetative lesions of varying sizes and number, sometimes with central ulceration that appear after treatment (→) (A–E). Similar lesions can appear on the mucous membranes (→) (F, G). Photos from the archives of the Lauro de Souza Lima Institute (ILSL).

Histopathological examination is characterized by spindle-shaped macrophages in a storiform arrangement resembling a dermatofibroma, and macrophages contain numerous solid bacilli (Fig. **9**). The immunohistochemical profile of spindle macrophages is positive for vimentin and CD68 and negative for factor XIIIa [11].

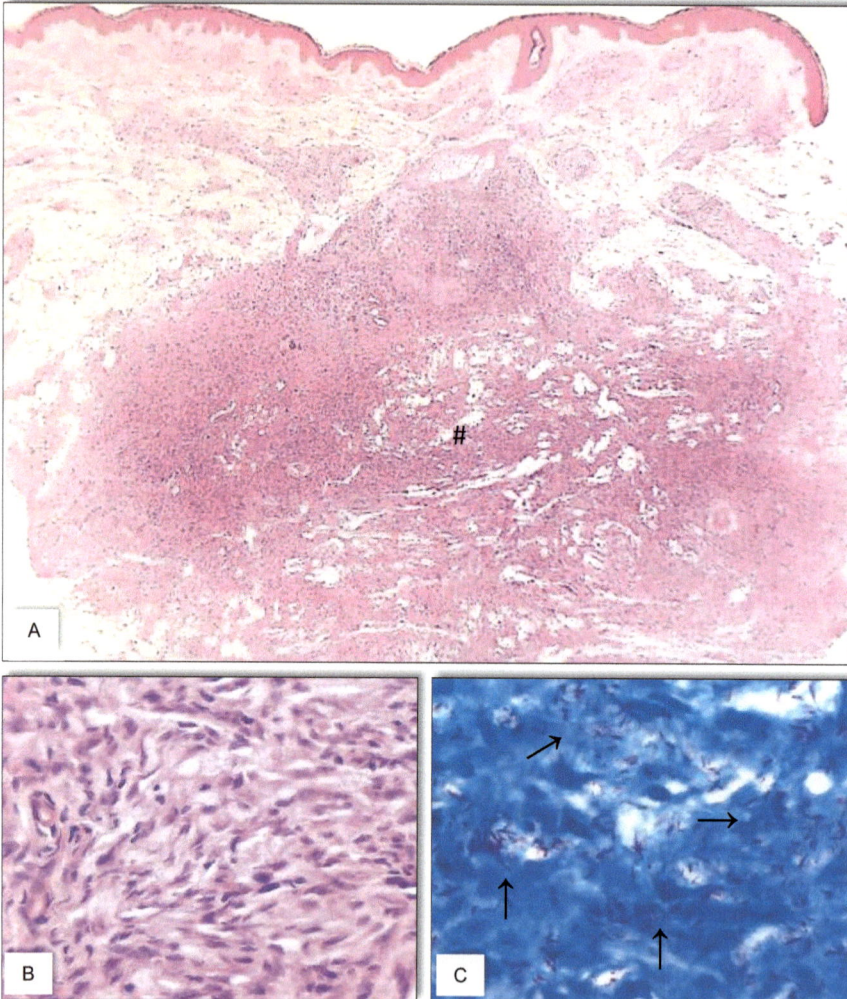

Fig. (9). Histopathological characteristics of histoid leprosy. A lepromatous leprosy pattern with numerous spindle-shaped macrophages forming a dermal nodule (#) **(A)**. Fusiform macrophages are organized in bundles in different directions, presenting a storiform aspect **(B)**. Bacilloscopy examination shows numerous solid bacilli in the cytoplasm of macrophages (→) **(C)**. Stained using hematoxylin and eosin (A, B) and the Fite-Faraco method **(C)**.

Patients with leprosy in the active and progressing lepromatous side (borderline lepromatous-BL/lepromatous leprosy-LL), with no history of previous treatment for leprosy or the use of antibiotics to treat other diseases, may present clinical and histopathological characteristics similar to HL (Fig. **10**). These lesions, which are common lepromas of the LL form, present a mixture of spindle-shaped macrophages and macrophages with broad and vacuolated cytoplasm, both containing numerous solid bacilli (Fig. **11**). The reported cases include LL patients presenting with several HL-like cutaneous nodules [13].

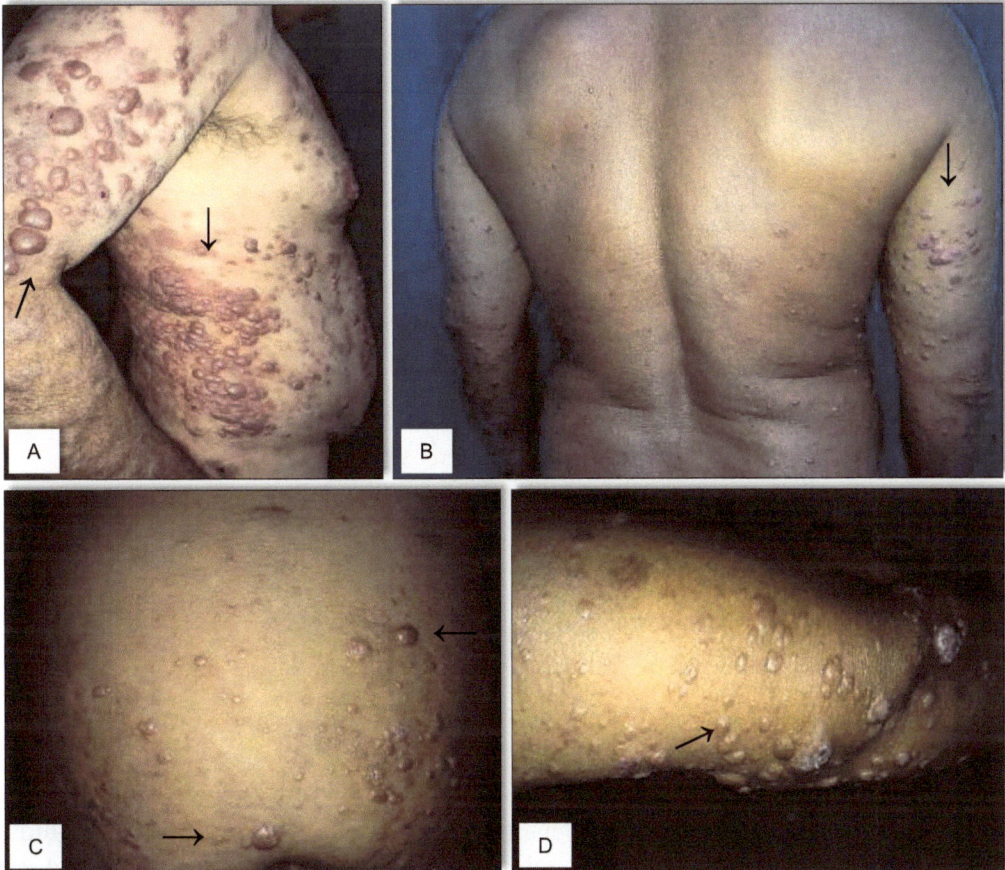

Fig. (10). Lepromatous leprosy (LL) simulating histoid leprosy (HL) (LL histoid-like). Four different patients with leprosy active LL with plaques, papules, nodules, and tubercles (→) (A–D). Some lesions are ulcerated and have a keloid aspect simulating HL. All the cases involve "virgin" treatment; the entire integument shows signs of infiltration by leprosy LL, and none presented mutations associated with drug resistance. Courtesy of Dr. Cássio C. Ghidella.

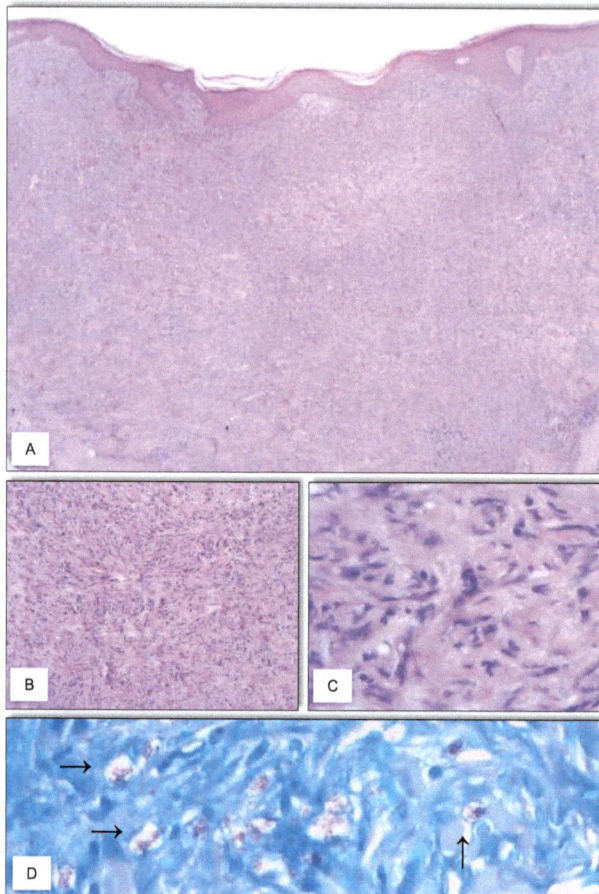

Fig. (11). Histopathological features of histoid-like lepromatous leprosy (LL). Leprosy active LL with lepromas showing diffuse infiltration of the entire dermis by spindle-shaped macrophages, which is similar to the histopathological and bacilloscopic characteristics of histoid leprosy (→) (A–D). Stained using hematoxylin and eosin (A–C) and the Fite-Faraco method **(D)**.

Clinically, HL can simulate xanthomas, neurofibromas, dermatofibroma, keloids, and skin metastases. The histopathological characteristics of spindle-shaped macrophages and, in particular, bacilloscopic examination showing numerous bacilli inside the macrophages and other skin tissues, preclude all these hypotheses. The histopathological and bacilloscopic characteristics that differentiate HL from dermatofibroma originating from leprosy lesions in the regressive lepromatous side (BL/LL) are characterized by the proliferation of spindle cells in the dermis (positive factor XIIIa and negative CD68), hyperplasia and hyperpigmentation of the epidermis, and the bacilloscopic examination (Fite-Faraco method) showing fragmented bacilli inside the macrophages of the regressed leprosy lesion in the tissues adjacent to the dermatofibroma and the fusiform cells in the center of the dermatofibroma without bacilli (Fig. **12**) [14]. Histopathological and bacilloscopic findings from dermatofibroma originating from regressive leprosy lesions and from scar/keloid stromal alterations are described in Chapter 7.

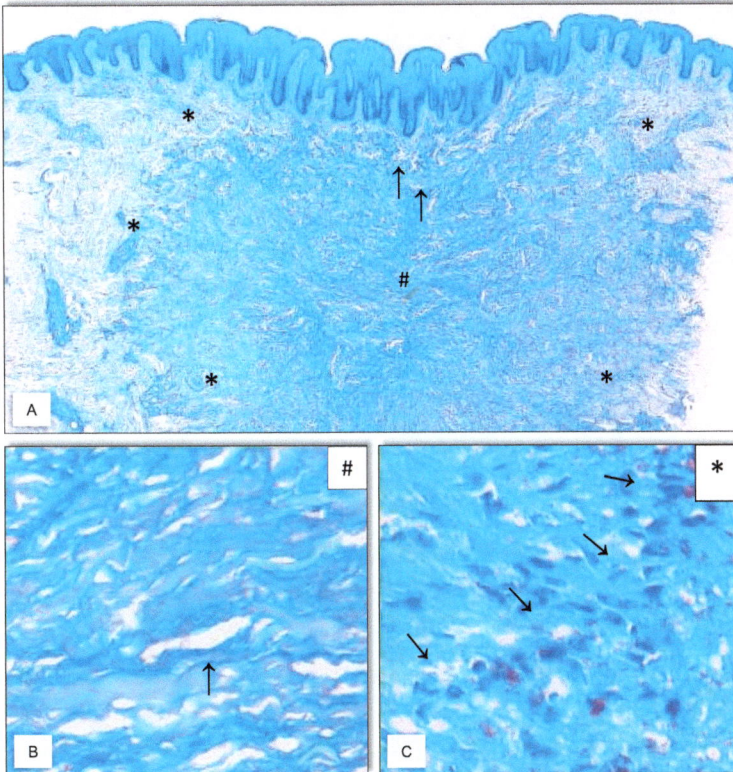

Fig. (12). Common dermatofibroma (DF) originating in leprosy injury. A lepromatous leprosy (LL) patient presented with dark papular lesion six months after treatment initiation. Histopathological features show DF common in the dermis (# A and B) and surrounded by a LL lesion in regression (*A, C). Note the epithelial hyperplasia and hyperpigmentation of the epidermis induced by DF (**A**). The spindle cells of the DF show negative bacilloscopy results (→) (**B**), and the leprosy lesion in regression in the DF periphery shows numerous fragmented and well-stained bacilli (Fite-Faraco staining) in the macrophages (→) (**C**).

NODULAR LEPROSY OF CHILDHOOD

Nodular leprosy of childhood (NLC), also known as childhood tuberculoid leprosy, was first described by Souza Campos in Brazil in 1937 [15, 16]. Considered as a benign variant of the tuberculoid spectrum, this clinical form predominantly affects children aged 1–4 years, and it is characterized by a tuberous or nodular lesion, which is dome-shaped, erythematous, and abrupt in appearance (Fig. **13**). It usually presents as a single lesion, predominantly on the face, but multiple lesions appear in various parts of the body (Fig. **13**). Clinically, NLC occurs in children living with leprosy patients in the active lepromatous side, and the appearance of the lesions would be related to possible transcutaneous inoculation of the bacilli owing to their contact with the patient. After a period of the abrupt development of a tuberous or nodular lesion, like a reactional tuberculoid lesion, the lesion regresses spontaneously until it becomes a small atrophic area, which looks similar to a scarred vaccine area (Fig. **13**). The original study conducted by Souza Campos reported the natural involution of these lesions during the period when there was no specific treatment for leprosy [15]. Unlike tuberculoid leprosy-TT/borderline tuberculoid-BT lesions, which have a marked decrease in sensitivities or are anesthetic, NLC lesions do not present significant sensitivity disorders. The smear test performed on these lesions was negative, and the Mitsuda test was positive [16]. The Mitsuda reaction is a form of granulomatous inflammatory reaction in response to intradermal inoculation of heat-killed *Mycobacterium leprae*. It is an *in vivo* test for measuring the ability to generate an immune granuloma after being sensitized by various mycobacterial infections [17].

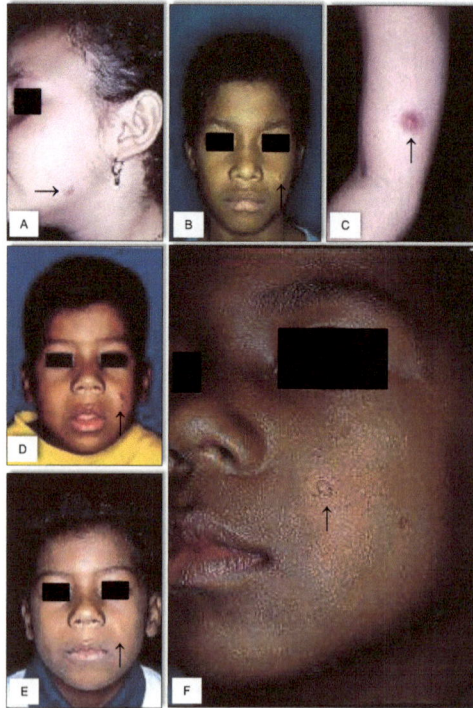

Fig. (13). Clinical features of nodular leprosy of childhood. Tuberous-nodular lesion, which is dome-shaped, erythematous, and with precise limits and abrupt appearance, is similar to reactional tuberculoid lesions (→) (A–C). After the initial phase (→) **(D)**, the lesion regresses spontaneously until it becomes a small atrophic area similar to scarred vaccine areas (→) (E, F). Photos from the archives of the Lauro de Souza Lima Institute (ILSL).

The histopathological features of NLC are nodular granulomas consisting predominantly of epithelioid macrophages in the papillary or reticular dermis, sometimes involving pilosebaceous follicles or glands (Fig. **14**). There is no involvement of neural branches by neurocentric tuberculoid granulomas following the neural pathway and with a lymphocytic mantle in the periphery as observed in TT and BT forms (Chapters 3 and 4) (Fig. **15**). It is possible to observe some neural impairment owing to the contiguity of the granulomas with the neural branches. These characteristics corroborate those reported in the initial studies published by Souza Campos, wherein significant sensitivity disorders were not identified in these lesions. From a histopathological point of view, the granulomas observed in NLC are similar to those observed in the type 1 reaction (T1R) or Mitsuda reaction (Figs. **16** and **17**). Bacilloscopy results obtained using the Fite-Faraco method were negative.

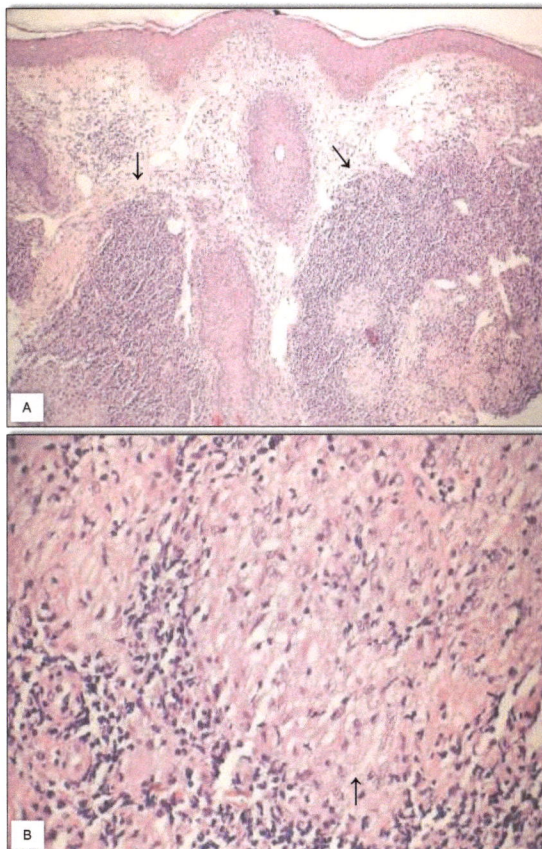

Fig. (14). Histopathological characteristics of nodular leprosy of childhood. Granulomas consisting of epithelioid macrophages and lymphocytes in the papillary or reticular dermis involving pilosebaceous follicles and glands (→) (A, B). Stained using hematoxylin and eosin.

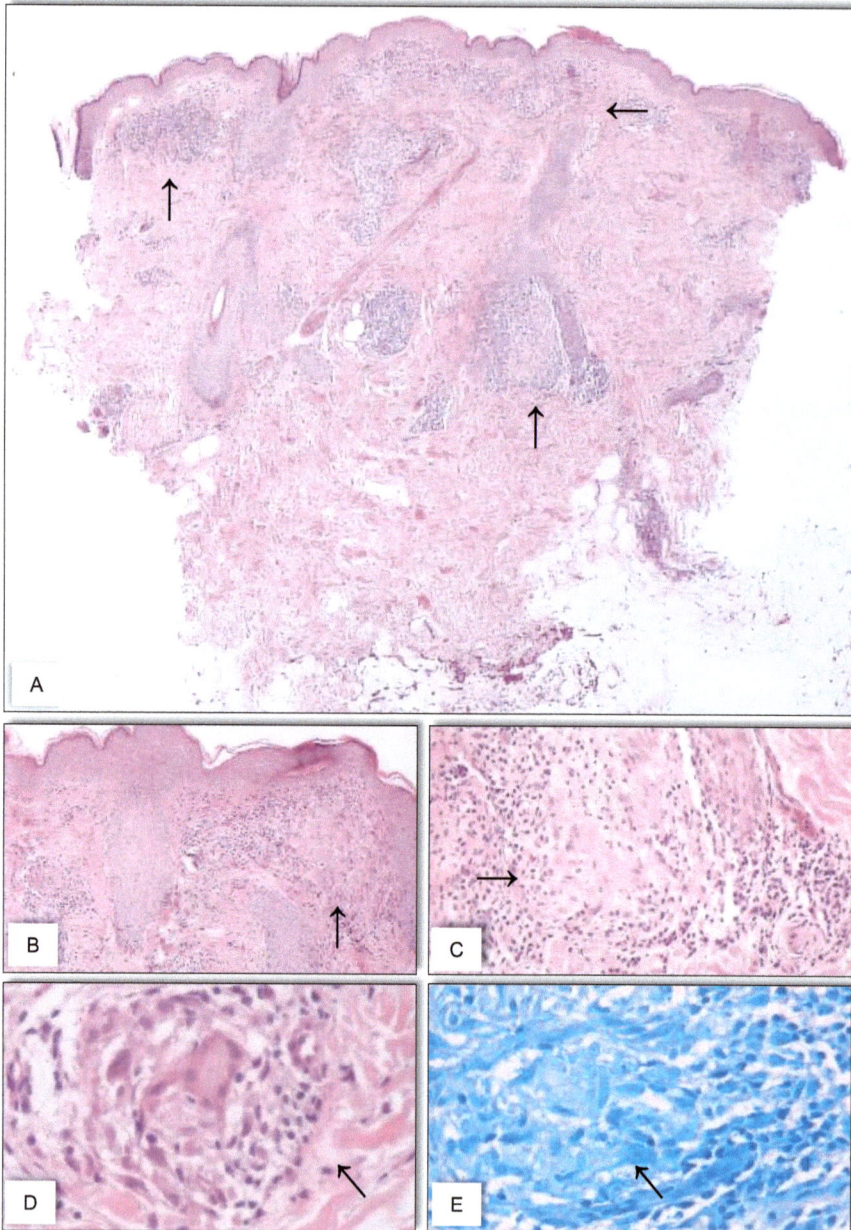

Fig. (15). Histopathological characteristics of nodular leprosy of childhood. The granulomas formed by epithelioid macrophages and lymphocytes are in the papillary or reticular dermis, sometimes involving the appendages (→) (A–C). Granulomas do not follow the path of neural branches as in TT and BT **(A)**. Granulomas resemble those of type 1 reaction (C, D). The bacilloscopic index is negative **(E)**. Stained using hematoxylin and eosin (A–D) and the Fite-Faraco method **(E)**.

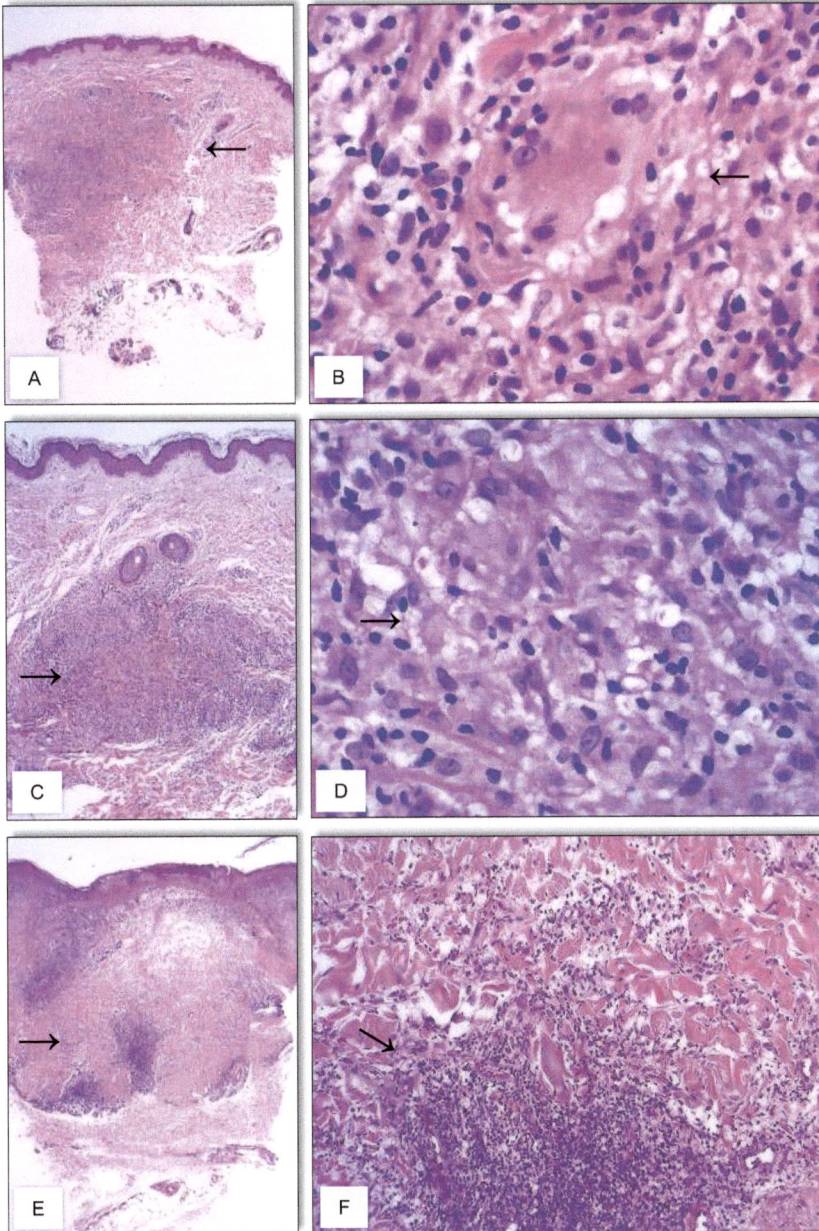

Fig. (16). Histopathological characteristics of the Mitsuda reaction. Three examples showing tuberculoid granuloma in the dermis (inoculation site), with a center constituted by epithelioid macrophages and permeated by lymphocytes (→) (A–F). Note that granulomas do not follow the path of neural branches (→) (A–C). Stained using hematoxylin and eosin (A–F).

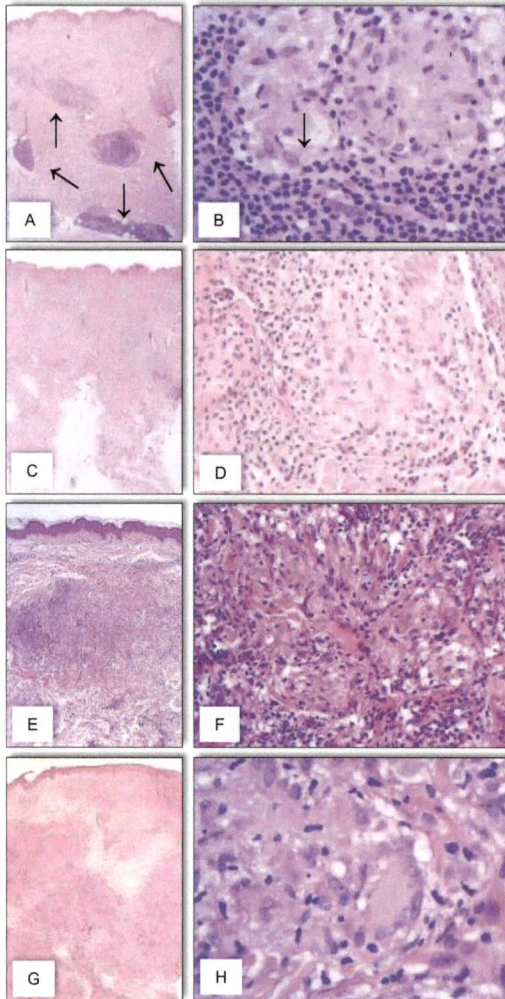

Fig. (17). Histopathological characteristics of granulomas in TT/BT forms, histoid leprosy, the Mitsuda reaction, and type 1 reaction. Note that the granulomas of the TT/BT formed in the T side follow the path of the neural branches from the depth to the superficial dermis and epithelioid macrophages are in the center and dense mantle of lymphocytes in the periphery (→) (A, B). These characteristics are not present in histoid leprosy (C, D), the Mitsuda reaction (E, F), or type 1 reaction lesions (G, H). Stained using hematoxylin and eosin (A–H).

PRIMARY NEURAL LEPROSY

Primary neural leprosy (PNL) occurs in patients with single or multiple mononeuropathies and polyneuropathy (confluent mononeuropathies) as the first manifestation of leprosy without any other identified etiology or the presence of leprosy skin lesions [18]. Although the prevalence of PNL is low, it can be overestimated when the investigation of the skin lesion is incomplete. The experience of the Lauro de Souza Lima Institute's team is that PNL is rare and affects less than 1% of cases. A careful clinical examination performed by an experienced professional can detect skin lesions or areas of sensitivity disorders in most patients referred for NLP investigation.

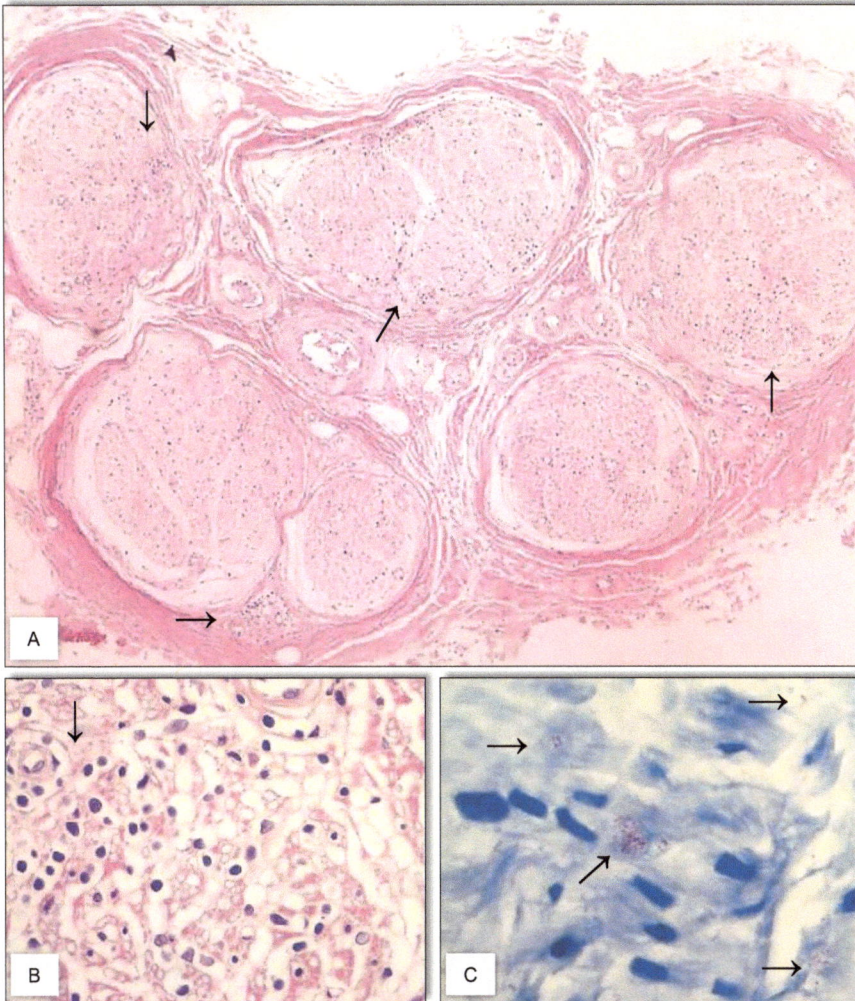

Fig. (18). Primary neural leprosy. Neural fragment with discrete endoneurial inflammatory infiltration (→) (A, B) and demyelination **(B)**. The bacilloscopy examination shows bacilli in Schwann cells (→) **(C)**. Stained using hematoxylin and eosin (A, B) and the Fite-Faraco method **(C)**. Neural fragment **(B)** post-fixed with osmium tetroxide.

The diagnosis of PNL is challenging because there are no skin lesions, and the smear test is negative [18, 19]. It is important to note that patients with suspected PNL may have a histopathological diagnosis of leprosy in skin biopsies performed in regions with some degree of sensitivity disorder or in regions with sensitivity preserved near the territory of the affected nerve [18]. In this context, skin biopsies can show histopathological characteristics of leprosy in up to 80% of cases. Skin biopsy is recommended as the first option before neural biopsy because it is a simpler and less aggressive procedure.

The histopathological characteristics of PNL are the same as those of the common forms of leprosy, including the presence of reaction phenomena (T1R and T2R). The changes range from the presence of endoneurial multivacuolated macrophages and Schwann cells parasitized by *M. leprae* detected using specific stains (*e.g.*, the Fite-Faraco stain) showing granulomatous infiltration with a tuberculoid pattern or infiltration of the neural branches by a discrete lymphohistiocytic infiltrate with negative bacilloscopy results and signs of demyelination (Fig. **18**) [18].

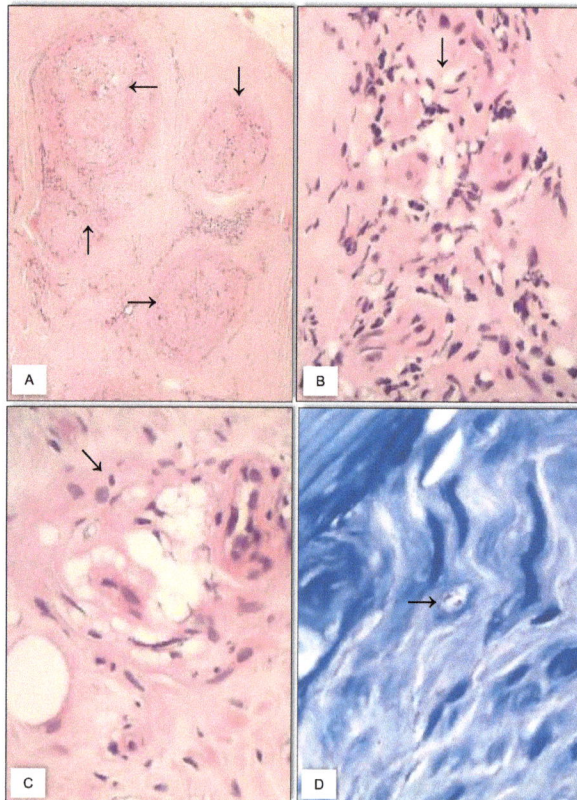

Fig. (19). Leprosy relapse with predominant neural involvement. A patient was treated for leprosy BL 16 years ago. He started presenting sensitivity disorders in the sural nerve, without clinical evidence of skin lesion. Neural biopsy shows the nerve with collagenized areas and discrete endoneurial infiltration by lymphocytes and multivacuolated macrophages (→) (A–C). Bacilloscopy examination shows fragmented and rare bacilli apparently solid in the endoneurial tissues, which confirms the recurrence (→) **(D)**. Stained using hematoxylin and eosin (A–C) and the Fite-Faraco method **(D)**.

Because leprosy can primarily affect the neural system, there is also the possibility that leprosy relapse is initially predominantly neural in origin. There are cases of patients who have been treated for leprosy, and usually, many years after completing the treatment, the patients start presenting sensitivity disorders in a certain nerve without evidence of skin lesions (Fig. **19**).

The differential diagnosis should target the causes for mononeuropathy and multiple neuropathies, including inflammatory disorders (collagen and non-systemic vasculitis); metabolic disorders (diabetes, amyloidosis, hypothyroidism, or pituitary dysfunction); infectious disease (syphilis or AIDS), traumatic injury and postural instability (acute neural compressions); chronic, congenital, or hereditary disorders (syringomyelia/syringobulbia, congenital insensitivity to pain, or hereditary neuropathy with pressure susceptibility); and tumors (schwannoma, neurofibroma, or other neural tumors) [18]. Neural biopsy should be performed for all cases excluding those of leprosy and defining the diagnosis (Fig. **20**). Molecular techniques can be used for the detection of *M. leprae* antigens, thus contributing to the diagnosis of NLP [19].

FINE NEEDLE ASPIRATION CYTOLOGY FOR LEPROSY DIAGNOSIS

Fine needle aspiration cytology (FNAC) is widely used for the diagnosis of neoplastic and non-neoplastic lesions. It is a simple, fast, and low-cost procedure compared to surgical procedures for diagnostic purposes. The use of FNAC for the diagnosis of leprosy has some limitations. Cytopathological examination of the lesions of indeterminate leprosy (I) with scarce inflammatory infiltrate is difficult. In paucibacillary lesions, the diagnosis depends on the observation of perineurial or endoneurial involvement by the inflammatory reaction, and FNAC does not provide these morphological details. Therefore, for diagnostic purposes, there is a limitation in the use of FNAC in paucibacillary forms (I, TT, and BT) where the bacilloscopy result is negative, or the bacilli are observed only in the neural branches, making it difficult to make a differential diagnosis with other cutaneous granulomatous diseases with similar patterns.

The cytopathological evaluation of leprosy lesions for diagnostic purposes has been proposed by some authors [20, 21]. The diagnostic accuracy achieved by FNAC in surgical pathology has encouraged some researchers to use this method in the diagnosis and classification of leprosy. From the standpoint of leprosy classification, studies comparing histopathological results (biopsy) with those obtained by fine needle aspiration (FNA) have shown that it is possible to obtain a good correlation between both the methods. Differentiating between the leprosy forms located at the ends of the spectrum is quite challenging, especially, for TT *versus* BT and BL *versus* LL but has a good agreement between these groups

(TT/BT *vs.* BL/LL) [21, 22]. There is also a good agreement between histopathology and FNAC for differentiating T1R and T2R [23]. FNAC can also be used for diagnosing leprosy in the lymph nodes and deep nerves [24, 25]. The specimen obtained using FNAC can be used for making a cellblock, allowing the aspirated material to be processed in the same way as that for a biopsy fragment, thus allowing several histological sections that can be used for different types of special stains for the evaluation or diagnosis using immunohistochemistry or molecular techniques [26, 27]. FNA is useful in obtaining material for inoculation in animals, with results similar to those obtained using biopsy or excision [28].

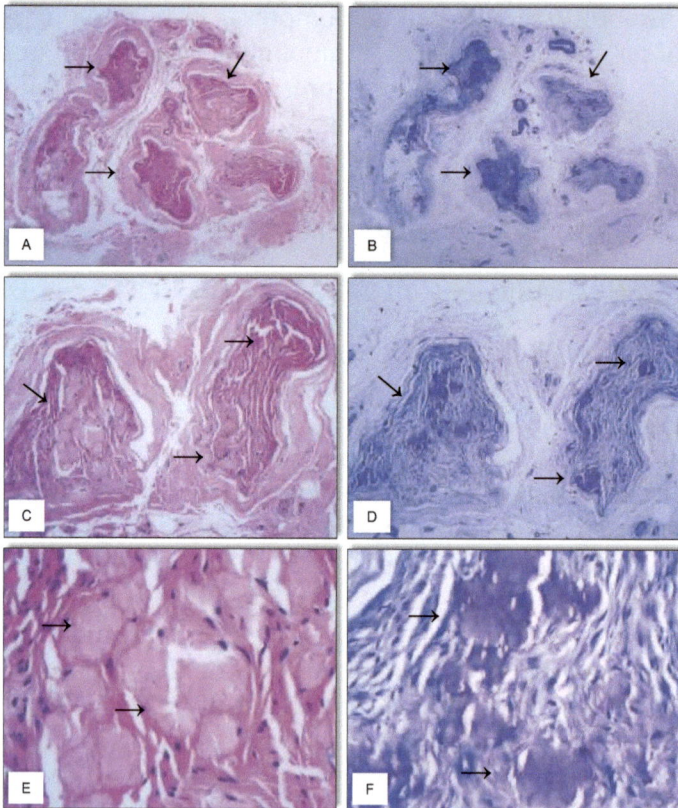

Fig. (20). Differential diagnosis of primary neural leprosy. Neural biopsy was performed for assessing clinical suspicion of primary amyloidosis. Histological sections show nerve without inflammation and endoneurial deposits of amyloid substance compatible with primary amyloidosis (→) (A–F). Stained using hematoxylin and eosin (A, C, and E) and crystal violet (B, D, and F).

In the context that the use of FNAC has some limitations and that the histopathological examination using biopsies is the "gold standard" for the diagnosis of leprosy, FNAC can be used for the diagnosis of the forms of leprosy, its reaction, and differentiation from other infectious or neoplastic lesions that may affect the skin, deep nerves, or lymph nodes. Generally, in the leprosy forms occurring on the tuberculoid side (TT/BT) and T1R, the smears and histological sections of the cellblock material present epithelioid macrophages, lymphocytes, and sketches of granulomas. Lesions occurring on the lepromatous side (BL/LL) show few lymphocytes, plasma cells, and numerous multivacuolated macrophages containing numerous bacilli when stained using the Fite-Faraco method. T2R lesions show multivacuolated macrophages with multifragmented bacilli and neutrophils, the latter being present in large numbers only in T2R (Figs. **21 – 25**).

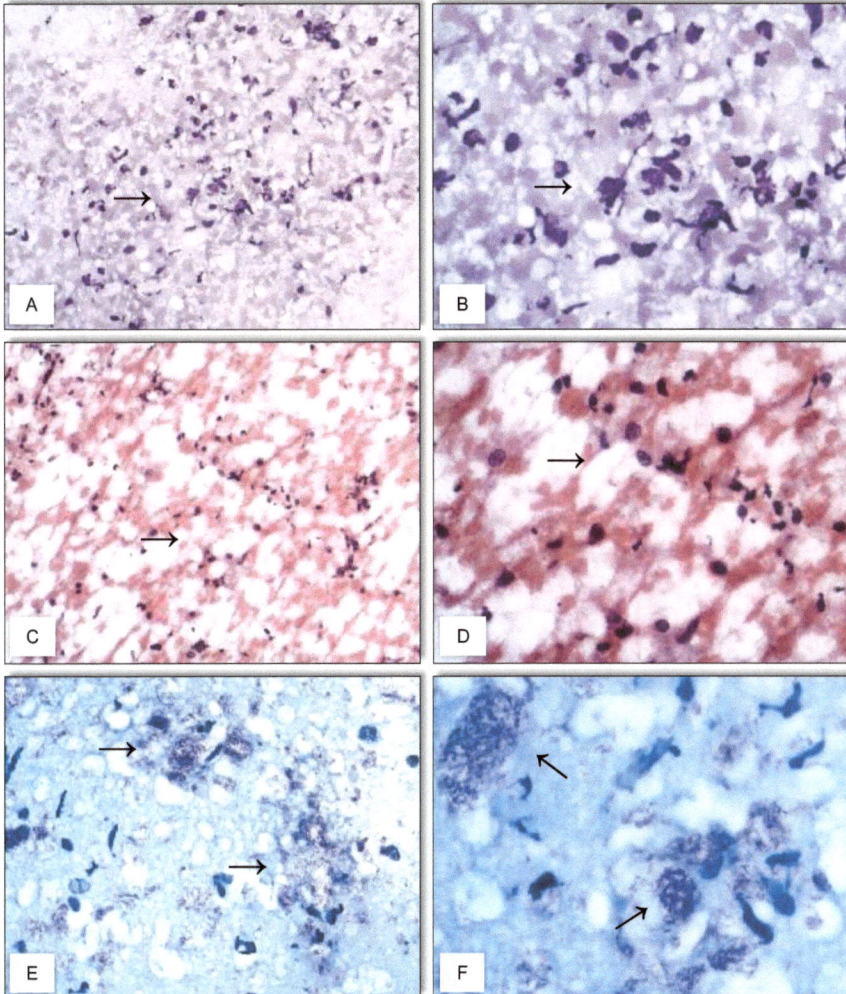

Fig. (21). Fine needle aspiration cytology for the diagnosis of leprosy occurring on the lepromatous side (BL/LL). Smears stained using May-Gründwald-Giemsa (MGG) (A, B) and hematoxylin and eosin (C, D) show multivacuolated macrophages and rare lymphocytes (→). The vacuoles are filled with numerous bacilli when stained using the Fite-Faraco method (→) (E, F).

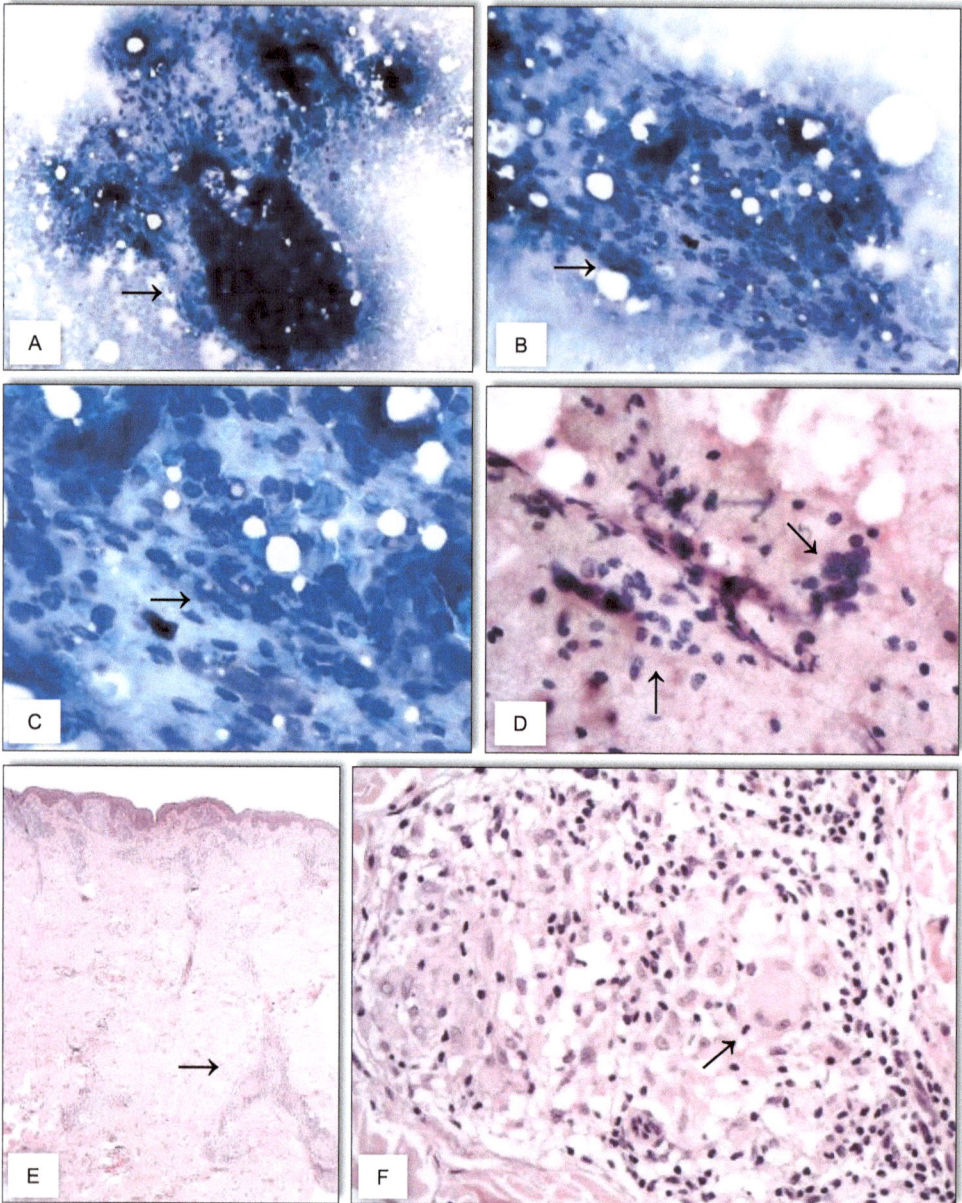

Fig. (22). Fine needle aspiration cytology for the diagnosis of borderline leprosy with associated type 1 reaction (T1R). A patient had borderline leprosy with clinical signs of T1R. Smears have epithelioid macrophages permeated by lymphocytes and the outline of granulomas with epithelioid macrophages (→) (A–C) and the presence of multinucleated giant cells (→) **(D)** are compatible with T1R. Histological sections of the skin lesion corresponding to fine needle aspiration cytology show borderline leprosy with associated T1R characterized by granulomas with epithelioid macrophages permeated by lymphocytes and presence of multinucleated giant cells (→) (E, F). Stained using May-Gründwald-Giemsa (A–C) and hematoxylin and eosin (D–F).

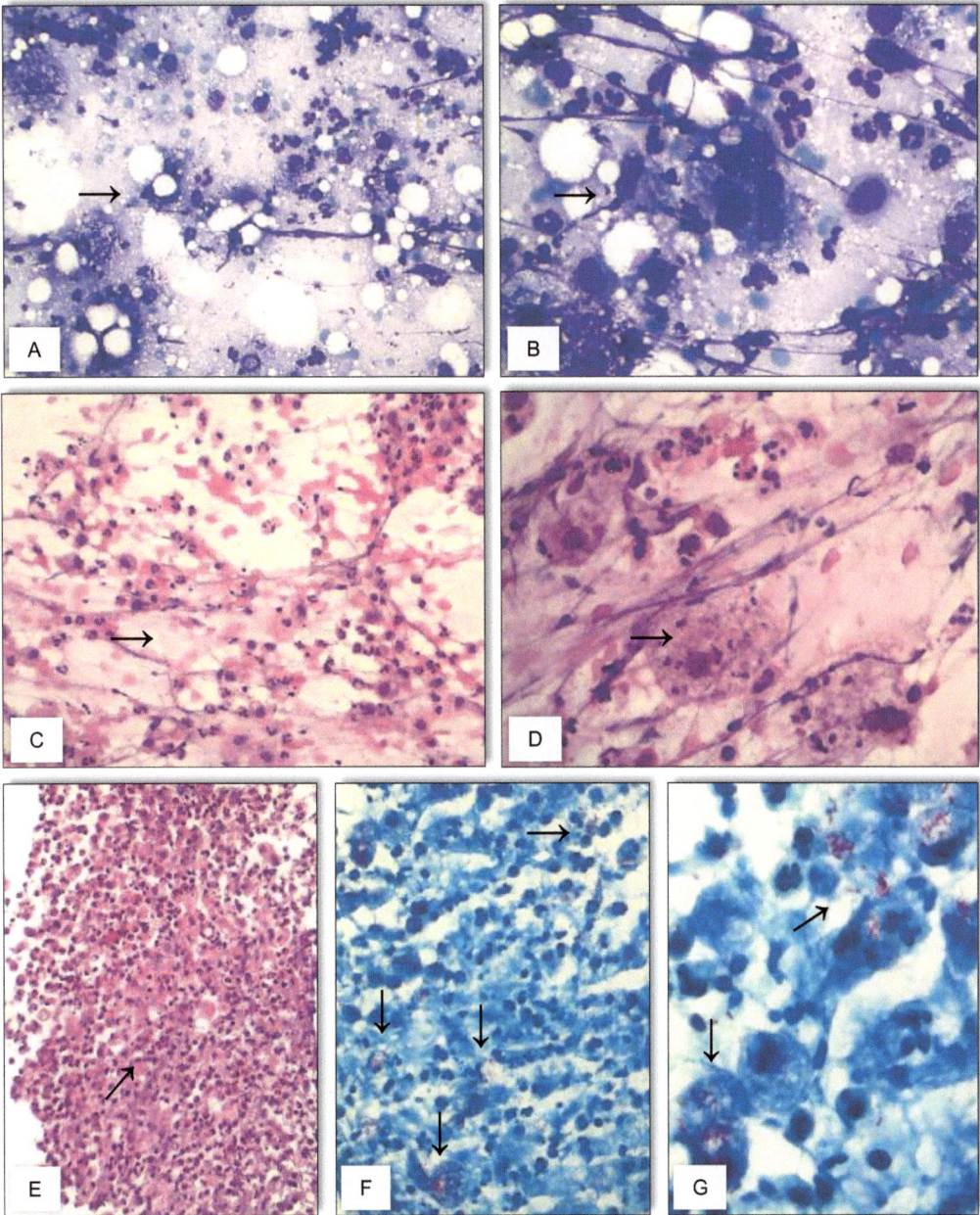

Fig. (23). Fine needle aspiration cytology for the diagnosis of type 2 reaction (T2R) in the skin lesion. The skin nodule with T2R characteristic was submitted to fine needle aspiration. The smears show multivacuolated macrophages containing cell debris associated with neutrophils (→) (A–D). Cell block histological sections (E-G) show a suppurative process with neutrophils and numerous bacilli inside macrophages characterizing T2R. Stained using May-Gründwald-Giemsa (A, B), hematoxylin and eosin (C–E), and the Fite-Faraco method (F, G).

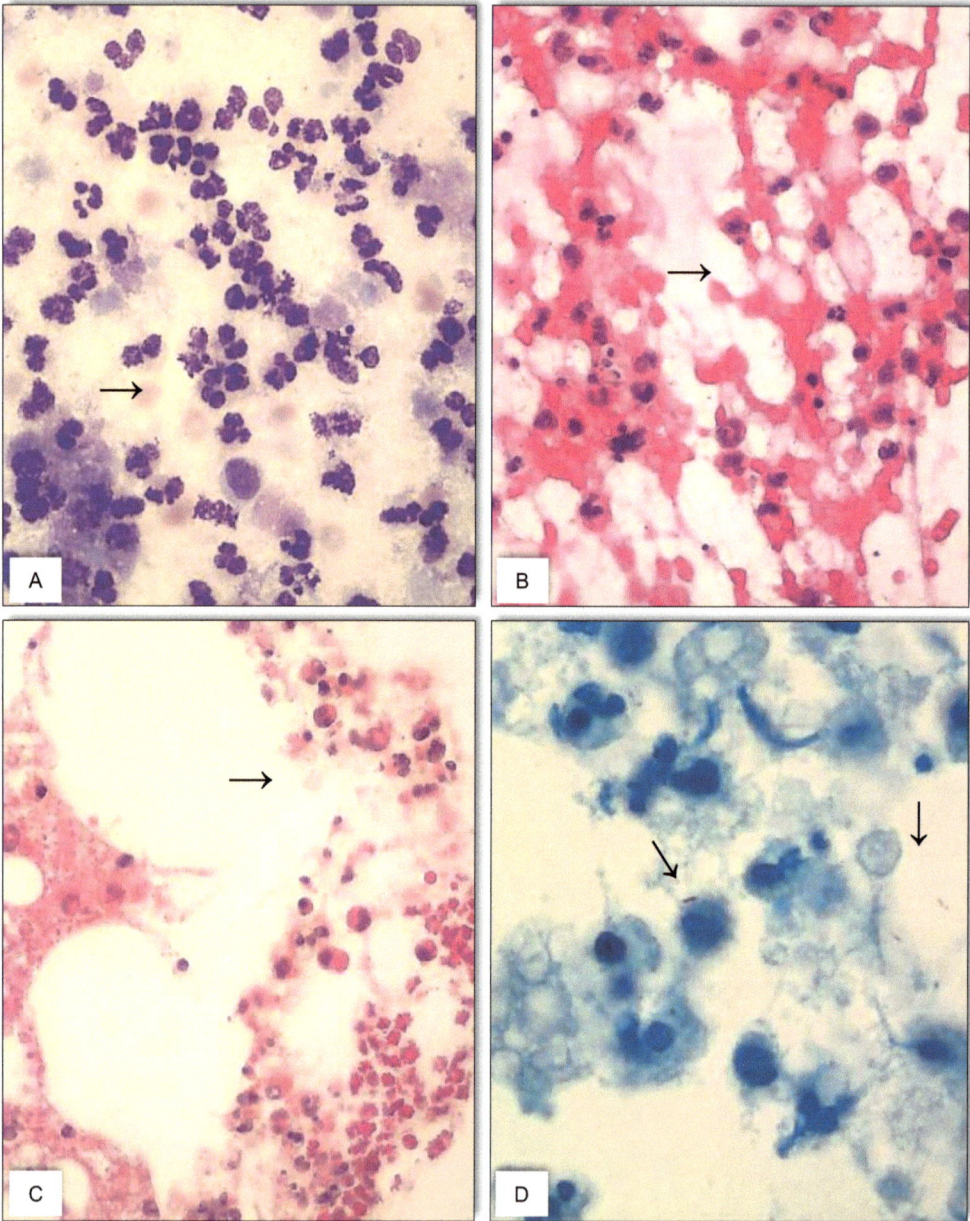

Fig. (24). Fine needle aspiration cytology for the diagnosis of type 2 reaction in the neural lesion. A borderline leprosy patient undergoing treatment had neuritis and abrupt thickening of the popliteal nerve. He underwent fine needle aspiration cytology guided by ultrasound for the neural lesion. The smears show multivacuolated macrophages containing cell debris associated with neutrophils (→) (A, B). Histological sections of the cell block (C, D) show cell debris, neutrophils, and multivacuolated macrophages containing fragmented bacilli (→) **(D)**, which are compatible with type 2 reaction. Stained using May-Gründwal--Giemsa **(A)**, hematoxylin and eosin (B, C), and the Fite-Faraco method **(D)**.

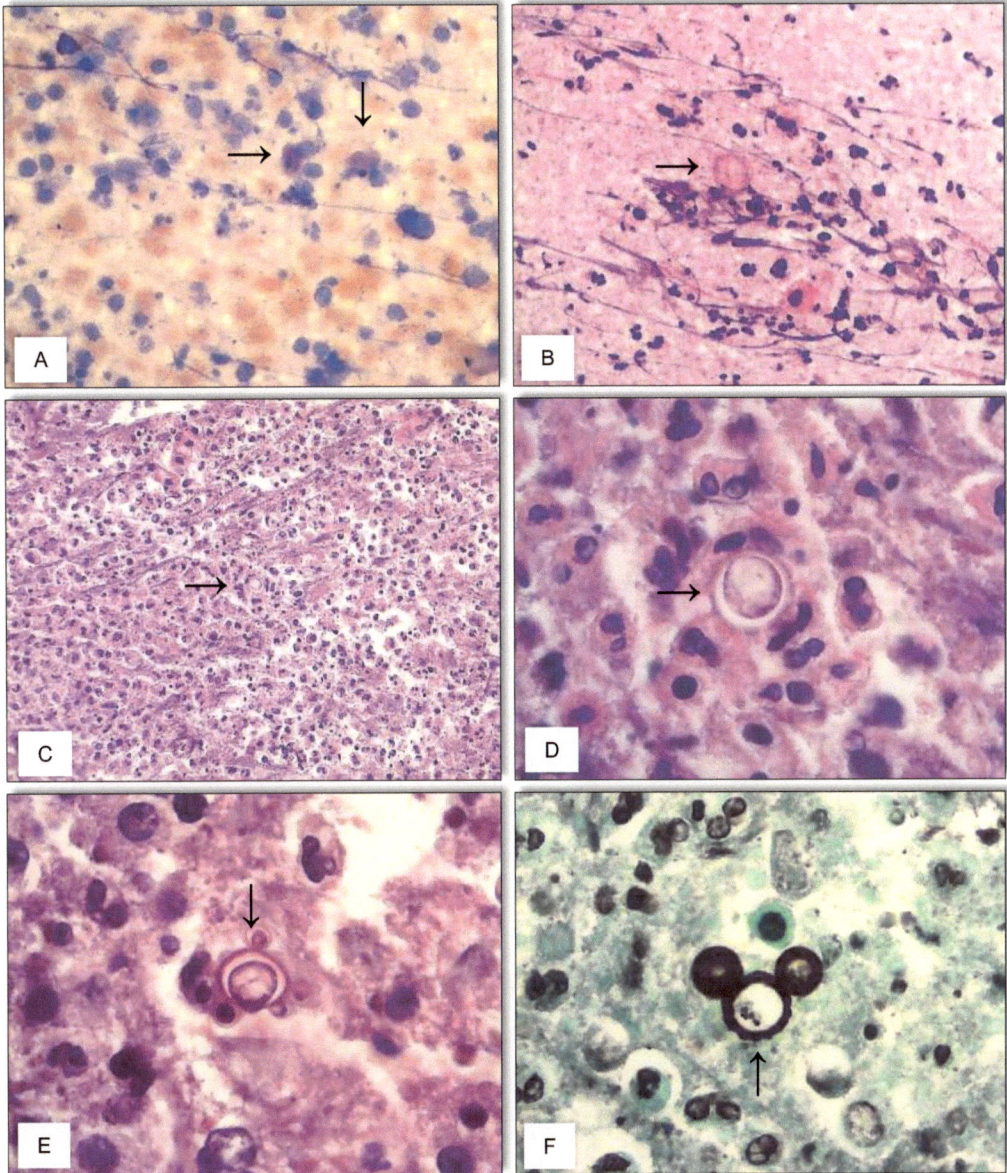

Fig. (25). Fine needle aspiration cytology for the differential diagnosis of leprosy. A patient with a history of borderline leprosy treated 15 years ago started to present generalized lymph node enlargement, splenomegaly, and hepatomegaly. Fine needle aspiration cytology was performed on the cervical lymph node. The smears (A, B) appear rounded and are suppurative. The histological sections of the cell block material (C–F) show the predominance of neutrophils and macrophages containing rounded fungi, which are compatible with paracoccidioidomycosis (→). May-Gründwald-Giemsa staining **(A)**, hematoxylin and eosin staining (B–D), periodic acid-Schiff with diastase **(E)** staining a fungus, giving it a "pilot's wheel" appearance, and silver methenamine **(F)** staining a fungus, giving it a "mickey mouse" appearance, both are typical of *Paracoccidioidis brasiliensis*.

CONCLUSION

Special presentations of leprosy, such as Lucio's leprosy and Lucio's phenomenon, histoid leprosy, nodular leprosy of childhood, and primary neural leprosy are significant within the context of the disease and thus need to be recognized. In general, their clinical and histopathologic characteristics allow them to be detected among and distinguished from other forms of leprosy. Lucio's phenomenon has both pathophysiologic mechanisms and histopathologic characteristics distinct from those of T2R (Chapter 6). Fine needle aspiration cytology, under certain conditions, may be used in the diagnosis of leprosy and its reaction phenomena.

REFERENCES

[1]   Lucio R, Alvarado I. Opusculo sobre el mal de San Lazaro o elephantiasis de los Griegos. México: Murguía e Cia 1852.

[2]   Azulay-Abulafia L, Spinelli L. Revendo a Hanseníase de Lucio e o Fenômeno de Lucio. Med Cutan Ibero Lat Am 2005; 33: 125-33.

[3]   Vargas-Ocampo F. Diffuse leprosy of Lucio and Latapí: a histologic study. Lepr Rev 2007; 78(3): 248-60.
[http://dx.doi.org/10.47276/lr.78.3.248] [PMID: 18035776]

[4]   Jurado F, Rodriguez O, Novales J, Navarrete G, Rodriguez M. Lucio's leprosy: a clinical and therapeutic challenge. Clin Dermatol 2015; 33(1): 66-78.
[http://dx.doi.org/10.1016/j.clindermatol.2014.07.004] [PMID: 25432812]

[5]   Fleury RN, Ura S, Opromolla DVA. Fenômeno de Lucio (eritema necrotizante). Hansenol Int 1995; 20(2): 60-5.

[6]   Rea TH, Ridley DS. Lucio's phenomenon: a comparative histological study. Int J Lepr Other Mycobact Dis 1979; 47(2): 161-6.
[PMID: 572350]

[7]   Rea TH, Jerskey RS. Clinical and histologic variations among thirty patients with Lucio's phenomenon and pure and primitive diffuse lepromatosis (Latapi's lepromatosis). Int J Lepr Other Mycobact Dis 2005; 73(3): 169-88.
[PMID: 16830639]

[8]   Wade HW. The histoid variety of lepromatous leprosy. Int J Lepr 1963; 31: 129-42.
[PMID: 14086699]

[9]   Nair SP, Nanda Kumar G. A clinical and histopathological study of histoid leprosy. Int J Dermatol 2013; 52(5): 580-6.
[http://dx.doi.org/10.1111/j.1365-4632.2012.05753.x] [PMID: 23590373]

[10]   Gupta SK. Histoid leprosy: review of the literature. Int J Dermatol 2015; 54(11): 1283-8.
[http://dx.doi.org/10.1111/ijd.12799] [PMID: 26094829]

[11]   Canuto MJM, Yacoub CRD, Trindade MAB, Avancini J, Pagliari C, Sotto MN. Histoid leprosy: clinical and histopathological analysis of patients in follow-up in University Clinical Hospital of endemic country. Int J Dermatol 2018; 57(6): 707-12.
[http://dx.doi.org/10.1111/ijd.13926] [PMID: 29384191]

[12]   Shaw IN, Ebenezer G, Rao GS, Natrajan MM, Balasundaram B. Relapse as histoid leprosy after receiving multidrug therapy (MDT); a report of three cases. Int J Lepr Other Mycobact Dis 2000; 68(3): 272-6.

[PMID: 11221089]

[13]   Andrade TCPC, Itimura G, Vieira BC, Oliveira AMN, Silva GV, Soares CT, *et al.* Hanseníase histoide símile: desafio diagnóstico. Hansenol Int 2014; 39(1): 66-9.

[14]   Soares CT, Masuda PY, Junior DC, Belachew WA, Wachholz PA. A case series of dermatofibromas originating in leprosy lesions: a potentially misdiagnosed condition. Surg Exp Pathol 2019; 2: 12.
[http://dx.doi.org/10.1186/s42047-019-0039-6]

[15]   Souza CN. Aspects cliniques de la lèpre tuberculoïde chez l'enfant. Rev Bras Leprol 1937; 5: 33-113.

[16]   Fakhouri R, Sotto MN, Manini MI, Margarido LC. Nodular leprosy of childhood and tuberculoid leprosy: a comparative, morphologic, immunopathologic and quantitative study of skin tissue reaction. Int J Lepr Other Mycobact Dis 2003; 71(3): 218-26.
[http://dx.doi.org/10.1489/1544-581X(2003)71<218:NLOCAT>2.0.CO;2] [PMID: 14608817]

[17]   Alecrim ES, Chaves AT, Pôrto LAB, Grossi MAF, Lyon S, Rocha MODC. Reading of the Mitsuda test: comparison between diameter and total area by means of a computerized method. Rev Inst Med Trop São Paulo 2019; 61e5
[http://dx.doi.org/10.1590/s1678-9946201961005] [PMID: 30785559]

[18]   Garbino JA, Marques W Jr, Barreto JA, *et al.* Primary neural leprosy: systematic review. Arq Neuropsiquiatr 2013; 71(6): 397-404.
[http://dx.doi.org/10.1590/0004-282X20130046] [PMID: 23828524]

[19]   Santos DFD, Mendonça MR, Antunes DE, *et al.* Revisiting primary neural leprosy: Clinical, serological, molecular, and neurophysiological aspects. PLoS Negl Trop Dis 2017; 11(11)e0006086
[http://dx.doi.org/10.1371/journal.pntd.0006086] [PMID: 29176796]

[20]   Singh N, Bhatia A, Gupta K, Ramam M. Cytomorphology of leprosy across the Ridley-Jopling spectrum. Acta Cytol 1996; 40(4): 719-23.
[http://dx.doi.org/10.1159/000333945] [PMID: 8693892]

[21]   Rao IS, Singh MK, Gupta SD, Pandhi RK, Kapila K. Utility of fine-needle aspiration cytology in the classification of leprosy. Diagn Cytopathol 2001; 24(5): 317-21.
[http://dx.doi.org/10.1002/dc.1068] [PMID: 11335960]

[22]   Singh N, Manucha V, Bhattacharya SN, Arora VK, Bhatia A. Pitfalls in the cytological classification of borderline leprosy in the Ridley-Jopling scale. Diagn Cytopathol 2004; 30(6): 386-8.
[http://dx.doi.org/10.1002/dc.20012] [PMID: 15176024]

[23]   Malik A, Bhatia A, Singh N, Bhattacharya SN, Arora VK. Fine needle aspiration cytology of reactions in leprosy. Acta Cytol 1999; 43(5): 771-6.
[http://dx.doi.org/10.1159/000331290] [PMID: 10518129]

[24]   Cavett JR III, McAfee R, Ramzy I. Hansen's disease (leprosy). Diagnosis by aspiration biopsy of lymph nodes. Acta Cytol 1986; 30(2): 189-93.
[PMID: 2421510]

[25]   Singh N, Malik A, Arora VK, Bhatia A. Fine needle aspiration cytology of leprous neuritis. Acta Cytol 2003; 47(3): 368-72.
[http://dx.doi.org/10.1159/000326535] [PMID: 12789916]

[26]   Bueno Angela SP, Viero RM, Soares CT. Fine needle aspirate cell blocks are reliable for detection of hormone receptors and HER-2 by immunohistochemistry in breast carcinoma. Cytopathology 2013; 24(1): 26-32.
[http://dx.doi.org/10.1111/j.1365-2303.2011.00934.x] [PMID: 22220518]

[27]   De A, Hasanoor Reja AH, Aggarwal I, *et al.* Use of fine needle aspirate from peripheral nerves of pure-neural leprosy for cytology and polymerase chain reaction to confirm the diagnosis: a follow-up study of 4 years. Indian J Dermatol 2017; 62(6): 635-43.
[http://dx.doi.org/10.4103/ijd.IJD_115_17] [PMID: 29263539]

[28]   Rosa PS, Belone AdeF, Lauris JR, Soares CT. Fine-needle aspiration may replace skin biopsy for the collection of material for experimental infection of mice with *Mycobacterium leprae* and *Lacazia loboi*. Int J Infect Dis 2010; 14 (Suppl. 3): e49-53.
[http://dx.doi.org/10.1016/j.ijid.2009.11.003] [PMID: 20149978]

ABBREVIATIONS

BB   Borderline Borderline leprosy or mid-borderline leprosy

BL   Borderline lepromatous leprosy

BT   Borderline tuberculoid leprosy

BI   Bacilloscopic index

FF   Fite–Faraco

FNAC   Fine-needle aspiration cytology

HL   Histoid leprosy

I   Indeterminate leprosy

IHC   Immunohistochemistry

LL   Lepromatous leprosy

LP   Lucio's phenomenon

ML   *Mycobacterium leprae*

NLC   Nodular leprosy of childhood

PCR   Polymerase chain reaction

PNL   Primary neural leprosy

RR   Reversal Reaction

TT   Tuberculoid leprosy

T1R   Type 1 reaction

T2R   Type 2 reaction

SUBJECT INDEX

www.ingramcontent.com/pod-product-compliance
Lightning Source LLC
Chambersburg PA
CBHW050820220326
41598CB00006B/271